Abedin • Conner

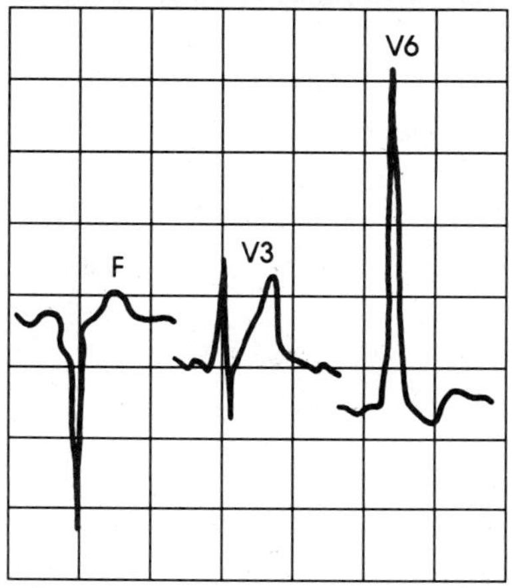

12 Lead ECG Interpretation:

The Self-Assessment Approach

Zainul Abedin, MD, FACC, FRCP(C)
Associate Clinical Professor of Medicine
Division of Cardiology
Texas Tech University Health Sciences Center
El Paso, Texas

Robert P. Conner, RN, CCRN
Coronary Care Unit
Providence Memorial Hospital
El Paso, Texas

W.B. SAUNDERS COMPANY
A Division of Harcourt Brace & Company
Philadelphia ▪ London ▪ Toronto ▪ Montreal ▪ Sydney ▪ Tokyo

W.B. SAUNDERS COMPANY
A Division of
Harcourt Brace & Company

The Curtis Center
Independence Square West
Philadelphia, Pennsylvania 19106

Library of Congress Cataloging-in-Publication Data

Abedin, Zainul.
12 lead ECG interpretation: the self-assessment approach/Zainul Abedin, Robert P. Conner.
p. cm.
Includes index.
ISBN 0-7216-2846-X
1. Electrocardiography–Examinations, questions, etc. I. Conner, Robert P. II. Title. III. Title: Twelve lead ECG interpretation.
RC683.5.E5A24 1989
616.1′207547–dc19 88-36588

Listed here is the latest translated edition of this book together with the language of the translation and the publisher.

Indonesian—*1st Edition*—Yayasan Essentia Medica, Yogyakarta, Indonesia

Editor: Michael Brown
Developmental Editor: Martha Tanner
Designer: Paul Fry
Production Manager: Pete Faber
Manuscript Editor: Ann Houska
Illustration Coordinator: Peg Shaw
Indexer: Helene Taylor
Cover Designer: Michaelle Maloney

TWELVE LEAD ECG INTERPRETATION:
The Self-Assessment Approach ISBN 0-7216-2846-X

Last digit is the print number: 9 8 7 6 5 4 3

PREFACE

Intelligent use of a book presupposes an understanding of the author's intent. This book has been designed for use in a classroom or as a primary source for rapid, independent study of the normal 12-lead electrocardiogram and its most common abnormalities. A deliberate effort has been made to avoid the exhaustive treatment expected of a reference textbook, and to concentrate instead on those conditions for which the electrocardiogram is the primary diagnostic tool. Critical care nurses, as well as physicians-in-training, will find this book useful.

Many conditions, ranging from severe head injury to hypothermia to serum electrolyte imbalance, are potential causes of electrocardiographic abnormalities. In none of these conditions, however, does the electrocardiogram represent the primary diagnostic tool. Therefore, the description of electrocardiographic findings associated with the list of physical derangements in which the electrocardiogram does not serve as the primary diagnostic tool is left to the larger textbooks. This book ignores the peripheral issues of electrocardiography, the better to concentrate on the central core.

It is assumed that the reader possesses a knowledge of basic arrhythmias. However, essential points regarding the measurement of complexes and intervals, and the derivation and orientation of leads are developed progressively in the text. The frontal plane leads are introduced early and with them the calculation of the mean QRS axis is explained using the vector approach. This is followed by an introduction of the horizontal plane leads and an explanation of the genesis of the normal electrocardiogram illustrated by selected instantaneous vectors.

After the normal electrocardiogram is described, the text progresses in turn through discussions of intraventricular conduction delays, ischemia and infarction, chamber enlargement and hypertrophy, acute pericarditis, and the basic elements of the Wolff-Parkinson-White syndrome. These abnormalities are amply illustrated in the text, and the student is given many opportunities to diagnose them independently in the self-assessment sections. In all, 330 electrocardiograms appear in the text, 312 of them in the self-assessment sections.

The authors have used several methods to enhance the value of the text as a learning tool. Each section begins with a list of learning objectives that we have called **cognitive goals**. The goals help identify what is essential in the text and are tested for in the multiple choice questions that accompany each section. In addition, an answer key, which identifies the mean QRS axis within a range of 10 degrees and pinpoints the major abnormalities of each tracing is provided at the end of each self-assessment section.

This text has the feature, unique to this type of book, of employing sequential tracings, taken hours to years apart, to illustrate the evolution of abnormalities. Particular emphasis has been placed on the hyperacute phase of infarction, intermittent bundle branch blocks, and the Wolff-Parkinson-White syndrome. The development of conduction defects in patients with anterior wall infarction is represented by a number of sequential tracings.

No attempt at exhaustive referencing has been made. Those references that are cited mark the progress of current thinking in the field and are included to give the interested reader a feeling for how new correlations and criteria emerge from the controversy that inevitably surrounds the findings of ongoing studies.

Illustrations are frequently used, and the text is closely keyed to these line drawings, which are designed to illustrate relationships that exist between anatomical parts, such as the arterial supply and the conduction system, or between electrical events and the recordings produced. In an attempt to further facilitate the synthesis of data, electrocardiographic entities, such as fascicular blocks, are correlated with the findings of histopathological studies, echocardiographical data, hemodynamic findings, or the insights gained from long-term epidemiological studies.

Finally, numerous examples of arrhythmias are given in conjunction with the 12-lead tracings. These serve, in some cases, to demonstrate the continuity of events, such as conduction loss as a consequence of infarction, or to illustrate the association of 12-lead findings with certain classes of arrhythmias. The rhythm strips serve the added purpose of testing the student's diagnostic proficiency, and can be used to advantage in a class as a basis for discussing interventions.

ZA
RC

CONTENTS

CHAPTER ONE

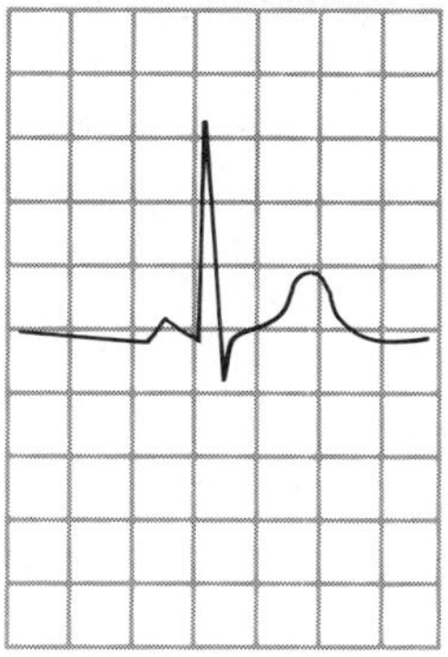

COMPLEXES AND INTERVALS

COGNITIVE GOALS

1. Identify the elapsed time and voltage equivalent for each millimeter on the ECG graph paper.
2. Identify the cardiac electrical events represented by the P wave, the QRS complex, and the T wave.
3. Define the terms **Q wave, R wave,** and **S wave** and describe how they are measured.
4. Define the term **QS complex.**
5. Describe the characteristics of the normal T wave.
6. Define the terms **PR interval, QR interval, QRS interval, ST segment,** and **QT interval.**
7. Discuss how **R:S** and **Q:R ratios** are obtained.
8. Define **slurring** and **notching.**
9. Describe the characteristics of a **delta wave.**

An electrocardiogram (ECG) is a recording of cardiac electrical activity displayed on graph paper that is scored horizontally and vertically in 1-millimeter (mm) increments. Each millimeter on the horizontal axis represents 0.04 second of elapsed time and each millimeter on the vertical axis represents 0.1 millivolt (mV) of electrical force (Fig. 1–1). Each 5-millimeter mark is scored with a heavier line and represents 0.20 second on the horizontal axis or time line and 0.5 millivolt on the vertical axis or amplitude line. Paper used for routine cardiac monitoring is marked across the top by small vertical lines placed at 3-second intervals. Heart rate per minute can be rapidly estimated by counting the number of beats in a 6-second strip and multiplying that number by 10. An ECG tracing consists of two elements: **complexes** and **intervals.** The normal complexes are the P wave, the QRS complex, the T wave, and the U wave.

The **P wave** represents atrial depolarization. It normally assumes the shape of a truncated pyramid with rounded contours, does not exceed 0.25 mV (2.5 mm) amplitude in any lead or 0.11 second in duration, and has a mean electrical axis of 0 to +70 degrees in the frontal plane. The amplitude of the P wave is measured from the top of the baseline to the top of the P wave (Fig. 1–2).

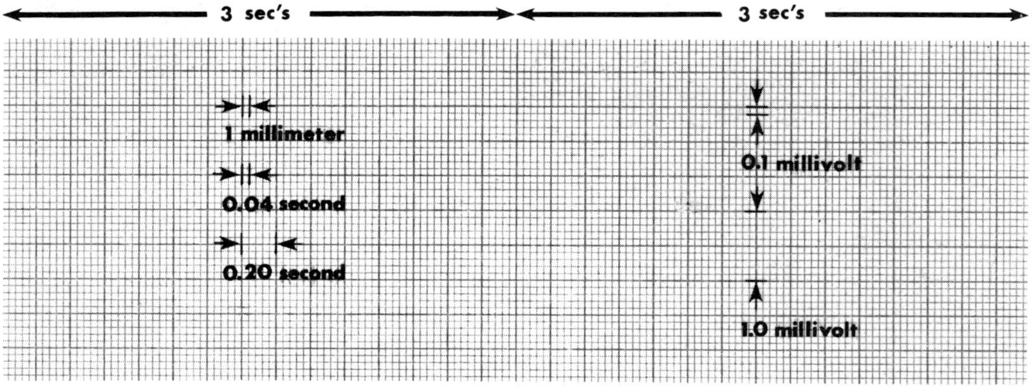

Figure 1–1. Time and voltage measurements.

The **QRS complex** represents ventricular myocardial depolarization. The QRS amplitude exhibits a wide range of normal values, but an amplitude greater than 1.1 mV (11 mm) in lead aVL, greater than 2.0 mV (20 mm) in lead aVF in the frontal plane leads, or greater than 3.0 mV (30 mm) in the horizontal plane (precordial) leads is considered abnormally high. Abnormalities of amplitude are discussed in greater detail in subsequent sections. The duration (width) of the normal QRS complex ranges from 0.05 to 0.10 second.

The positive and negative deflections of the QRS complex are named according to certain universal conventions. The first deflection of the QRS complex, if *negative*, is called the **Q wave.** The Q wave amplitude is measured from the bottom of the baseline to the deepest point of the written waveform (Fig. 1–2). Small, narrow Q waves are expected findings in leads I, III, aVL, aVF, V5, and V6. Normally Q waves do not exceed 0.03 second in duration in any lead. The Q wave may be represented by a lower case **(q)** or upper case **(Q)** letter, according to its size in relation to other QRS deflections (Fig. 1–3). Completely negative QRS complexes or QRS complexes in which no positive deflection reaches more than 1 millimeter above the baseline are called **QS complexes** (Fig. 1–3).

The first *positive* deflection of the QRS complex, whether preceded by a negative deflection (Q wave) or not, is called the **R wave.** The R wave amplitude is measured from the top of the baseline to the peak of the written waveform (see Fig. 1–2). In the case of polyphasic QRS complexes, subsequent positive deflections are labeled **R′** (read "R prime"). Examples of R′ waves are shown in panels **7** and **9** of Figure 1–3. An R wave may be represented by an upper or lower case letter according to its relative size (Fig. 1–3).

A negative deflection *following* an R wave is called an **S wave.** The S wave amplitude is measured from the bottom of the baseline to the deepest point of the written waveform (see Fig. 1–2). In the case of polyphasic QRS complexes, a subsequent negative deflection following the first S wave is called an S′ (read "S prime") wave. Like Q waves and R waves, an S wave may be represented by a lower or upper case letter, according to its size (Fig. 1–3).

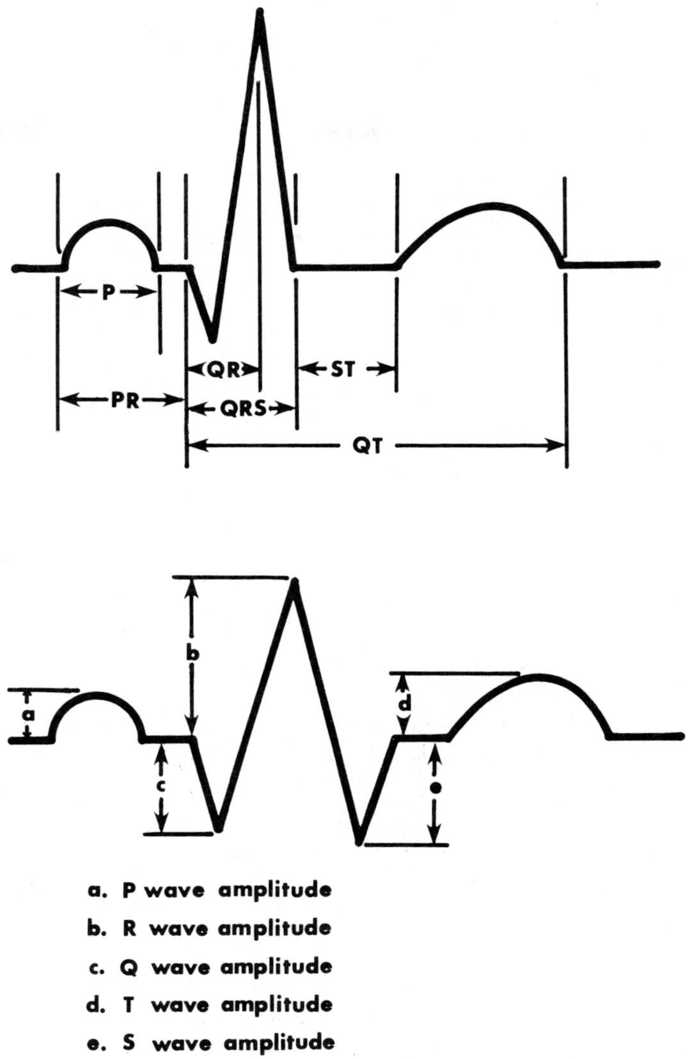

Figure 1–2. Measurements of wave amplitude and duration.

The **T wave** represents ventricular myocardial repolarization. The amplitude of the T wave is measured from the top of the baseline to the highest point of the written waveform and does not normally exceed 0.5 mV (5 mm) in any frontal plane lead or 1.0 mV (10 mm) in any horizontal plane lead. The proximal limb of the normal T wave exhibits a gentle upward slope, while the distal limb, or descending component, exhibits a steeper slope as it returns to the baseline. Normal T waves are illustrated in panels **1a, 2a,** and **3a** of Figure 1–4. Normal T waves are not sharply pointed, nor are they symmetrical. The polarity of T waves varies according to lead, being normally positive (upright) in leads I, II, and V3–V6 in adults, negative (inverted) in aVR, and variable in III, aVL, aVF, V1, and V2.

The **U wave** is a low-voltage deflection of uncertain origin sometimes seen

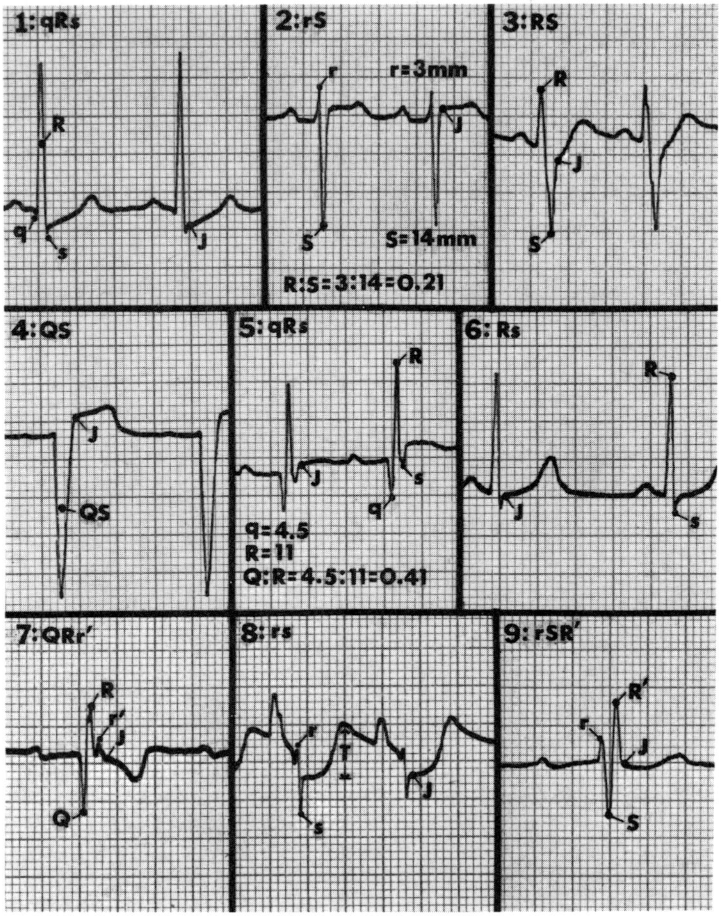

Figure 1–3. Designations of waves and ratios.

following the T wave. Its polarity is normally the same as the preceding T wave. Abnormalities of the U wave are attributed to electrolyte imbalance, drug effects, and myocardial ischemia.

The clinically important ECG intervals are shown in Figure 1–2. The **PR interval** consists of two components, the P wave and the PR segment, and is measured from the beginning of the P wave to the beginning of the QRS complex. The duration of the PR interval is normally from 0.12 to 0.20 second in adults. A PR interval greater than 0.20 second in adults or greater than 0.18 second in children under age 14 constitutes first-degree atrioventricular block.

The **QR interval,** measured from the beginning of the QRS complex to the highest point of the R wave (see Fig. 1–2), is an indirect reflection of ventricular activation time. Its clinical importance and applications are discussed at length in subsequent chapters.

The **QRS interval,** measured from the beginning to the end of the total QRS complex, is normally from 0.05 to 0.10 second in duration. If the QRS interval is 0.12 second or more, an intraventricular conduction delay is present.

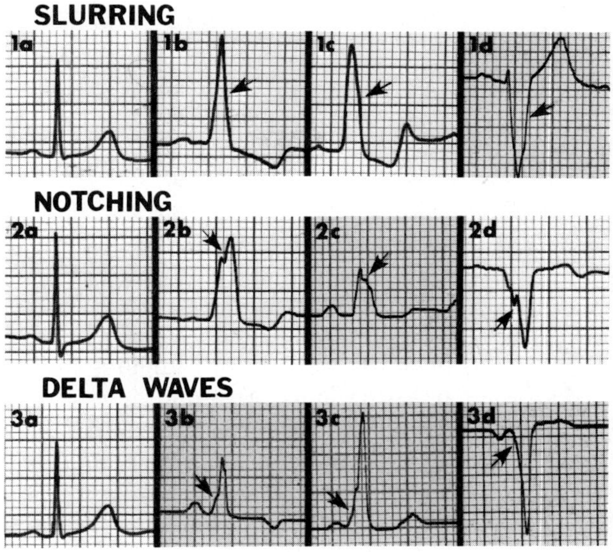

Figure 1–4. Slurring, notching, and delta waves.

The **ST segment** is measured from the end of the QRS complex to the beginning of the T wave (see Fig. 1–2). The junction of the QRS complex and the ST segment is called the **J point.** The J point is illustrated **(J)** in Figure 1–3. The ST segment is normally **isoelectric,** in the same plane as the baseline, but may be normally elevated 1 millimeter in the frontal plane leads and up to 2 millimeters in the horizontal plane leads. Any ST segment depression greater than 0.5 millimeter should be regarded as abnormal. The only exception of clinical importance to the aforementioned guidelines occurs as a normal variant, called **early repolarization,** which is discussed in detail in a subsequent chapter.

The **QT interval** is measured from the beginning of the QRS complex to the end of the T wave (see Fig. 1–2). Prolongation of the QT interval is associated with myocarditis, ischemic heart disease, acute cerebrovascular disease, electrolyte disturbances, congenital syndromes (Romano-Ward; Jervell and Lange-Nielsen), and the use of drugs such as procainamide, quinidine, tricyclic antidepressants, and the phenothiazines. A bizarre form of ventricular tachycardia, **torsade de pointes,** is often preceded by QT interval prolongation (Walter, 1979). The QT interval normally varies with heart rate and to a lesser extent with the sex and age of the subject. The upper limits of the QT interval, adjusted for rate, are shown in Table 1–1.

R:S and Q:R ratios

The sizes of any two deflections relative to each other can be expressed as a ratio. The R:S ratio in lead V1 and the Q:R ratio in various leads have important diagnostic implications, and for this reason it is useful to know how such ratios are determined. The R:S ratio is obtained by measuring the height

Table 1–1. UPPER LIMITS OF THE QT INTERVAL

Rate	QT Interval
40	0.49–0.50 sec
50	0.45–0.46 sec
60	0.42–0.43 sec
70	0.39–0.40 sec
80	0.37–0.38 sec
90	0.35–0.36 sec
100	0.33–0.34 sec
110	0.32–0.33 sec
120	0.31–0.32 sec

of the R wave in millimeters and comparing it with the depth of the S wave in millimeters. An example is shown in panel **2** of Figure 1–3. In this example the R wave height is 3 mm and the S wave depth is 14 mm. The ratio is therefore 3:14, which may be reduced to a single number by division (3/14 = 0.21). The R:S ratio in lead V1 is always less than 1.0 in normal tracings. Causes of increased R:S ratio in this lead are discussed further on.

The Q:R ratio is obtained by measuring the depth of the Q wave and comparing it with the height of the R wave. An example is shown in panel **5** of Figure 1–3. In this case, the depth of the Q wave is 4.5 millimeters and the height of the R wave is 11.0 millimeters. The ratio is reduced to a single number by division (4.5:11.0 = 4.5/11.0 = 0.41). Generally speaking, Q:R ratios greater than 0.25 suggest the presence of myocardial infarction.

Slurring and notching

As shown in Figure 1–4 (panel **1a**), the normal QRS complex is narrow and displays deflections that are clear-cut and crisply inscribed. In the presence of an intraventricular conduction delay the QRS widens and the positive and/or negative deflections tend to drift, a finding known as **slurring.** Slurring of positive complexes **(1b, 1c)** and of a negative complex **(1d)** is illustrated in Figure 1–4.

Notching may be noted on the ascending **(2b)** or descending limb **(2c)** of a deflection, whether it is positive or negative **(2d).** Notches are localized deformities of the QRS complex that do not extend downward or upward to the baseline.

Delta waves

Several preexcitation syndromes produce a localized characteristic deformity of the beginning of the QRS called a **delta wave.** In most cases the delta wave encroaches on the PR segment, with the result that the PR interval is abnormally shortened. Delta waves may appear as fairly discrete humps or as slurring of the initial portion of the QRS complex and may be either positive **(Fig. 1–4, panels 3b, 3c)** or negative **(3d).**

References

Prineas, RJ, et al. **The Minnesota Code Manual of Electrocardiographic Findings.** John Wright, PSG Inc, Boston, 1982, pp 11–42.

Walter, PE. **The Heart, Update I.** McGraw-Hill Book Company, New York, 1979, pp 305–327.

SELF-ASSESSMENT

Multiple Choice

Choose the most appropriate answer.

1. Each millimeter on the horizontal axis of ECG graph paper represents:

   a. 0.04 second elapsed time.
   b. 0.20 second elapsed time.
   c. 0.1 millivolt.
   d. 0.10 millivolt.

2. Cardiac monitoring paper is usually scored across the top at:

   a. 0.04-second intervals.
   b. 0.20-second intervals.
   c. 3-second intervals.
   d. 6-second intervals.

3. The first positive wave of the QRS complex is called:

   a. the P wave.
   b. the Q wave.
   c. the R wave.
   d. the S wave.

4. The second positive wave of the QRS complex is called:

   a. the S wave.
   b. the R wave.
   c. the S′ wave.
   d. the R′ wave.

5. A negative deflection following an R wave is:

   a. a Q wave.
   b. an S wave.
   c. an R′ wave.
   c. an S′ wave.

6. Normal T waves are:

   a. measured from the top of the baseline to the highest point of the written waveform.
   b. sharply pointed.
   c. biphasic.
   d. symmetrical.

7. The duration of the normal PR interval in adults is:

   a. 0.10 to 0.18 second.
   b. 0.11 to 0.19 second.
   c. 0.12 to 0.20 second.
   d. 0.13 to 0.21 second.

8. The J point is:

   a. the beginning of the QRS complex.
   b. the peak of the R wave.
   c. the intersection of the ST segment and the upslope of the T wave.
   d. the intersection of the end of the QRS complex and the beginning of the ST segment.

Practice Strips

Fifteen P-QRS-T complexes are shown below. For each strip, determine (1) the PR interval, (2) the QRS interval, (3) the QT interval, (4) the voltage of the R wave(s) if present, (5) the letter name of the deflections, (6) the polarity of the T waves, and (7) the presence of notching, slurring, or delta waves.

1-1.
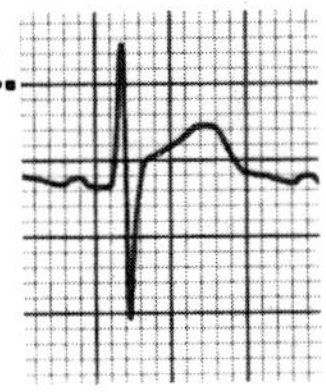

1-2.
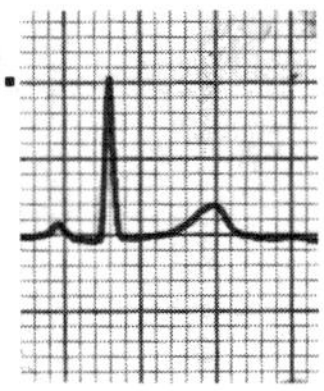

1-3.
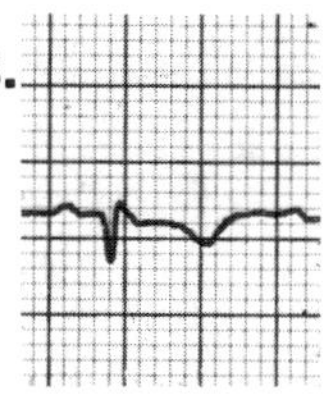

1-4.
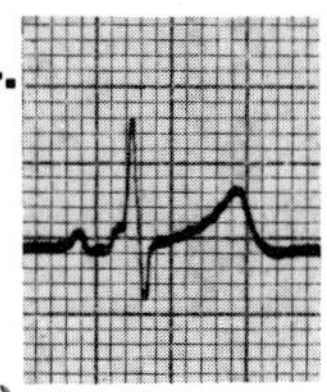

1-5.
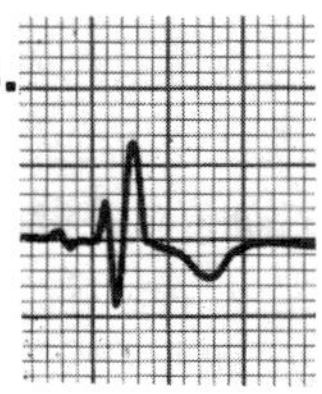

1-6.
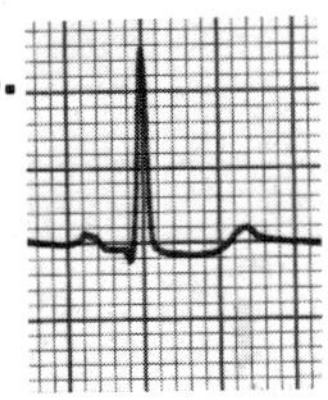

1-7.
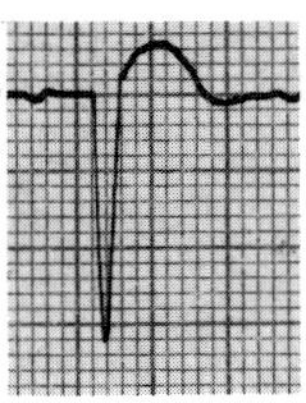

1-8.
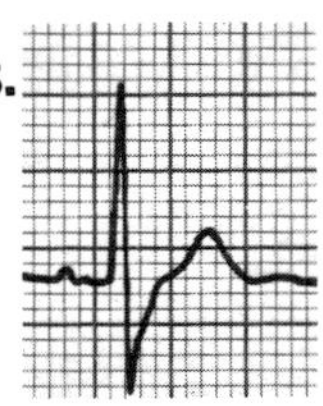

1-9.
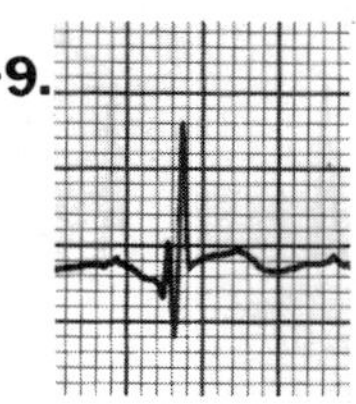

1-10.
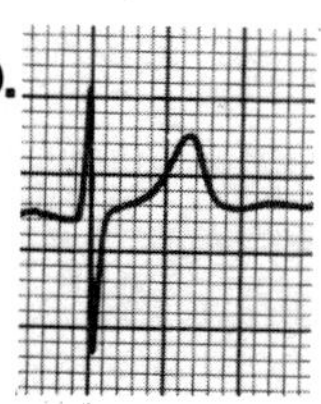

1-11.
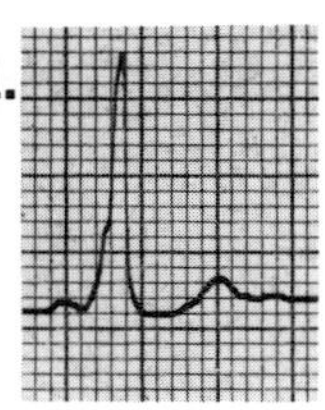

1-12.
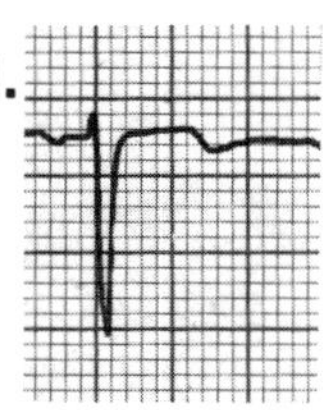

1-13.
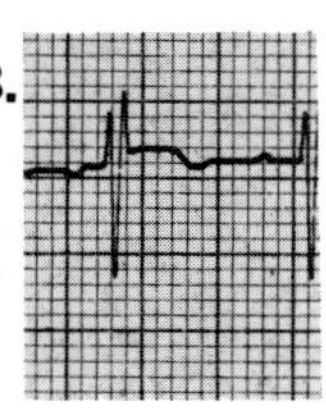

1-14.
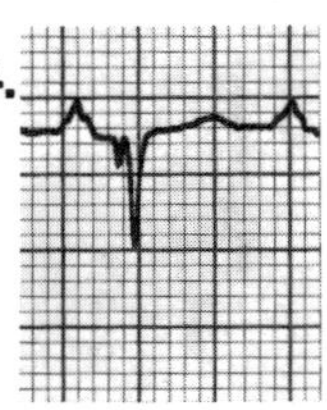

1-15.
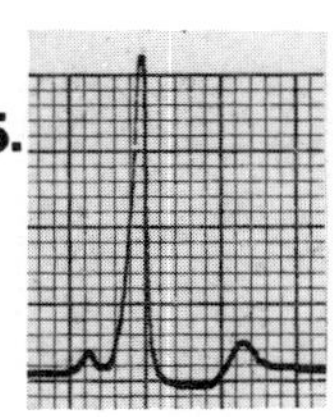

ANSWER KEY

Multiple Choice

1. a
2. c
3. c
4. d
5. b
6. a
7. c
8. d

Practice Strips

1–1. PR 0.12
QRS 0.08
QT 0.36
R = 0.9 mV
RS complex
T wave positive

1–2. PR 0.15
QRS 0.06
QT 0.38
R = 1.1 mV
R complex
T wave positive

1–3. PR 0.14
QRS 0.10
QT 0.38
no R wave
Qr complex
T wave negative

1–4. PR 0.12
QRS 0.12
QT 0.46
R = 0.85 mV
Rs complex
T wave positive
delta wave

1–5. PR 0.14
QRS 0.14
QT 0.42
R waves = 0.9 mV
rSR′ complex
T wave negative

1–6. PR 0.14
QRS 0.08
QT 0.40
R = 1.3 mV
qR complex
T wave positive

1–7. PR 0.20
QRS 0.06
QT 0.44
no R wave
QS complex
T wave negative

1–8. PR 0.14
QRS 0.13
QT 0.38
R = 1.25 mV
RS complex
T wave positive

1–9. PR 0.14
QRS 0.08
QT 0.30
R waves = 1.1 mV
qrsR′ complex
T wave positive

1–10. PR 0.16
QRS 0.08
QT 0.42
R = 0.85 mV
RS complex
T wave positive

1–11. PR 0.10
QRS 0.14
QT 0.44
R = 1.65 mV
R complex
T wave positive
delta wave

1–12. PR 0.16
QRS 0.10
QT 0.42
R = 0.15 mV
rS complex
T wave negative

1–13. PR 0.12
QRS 0.08
QT 0.30
R waves = 0.7 mV
rSr complex
T wave negative

1–14. PR 0.15
QRS 0.10
QT 0.34
no R wave
QS complex
T wave positive

1–15. PR 0.12
QRS 0.14
QT 0.46
R = 2.0 mV
R complex
T wave positive
delta wave

CHAPTER TWO

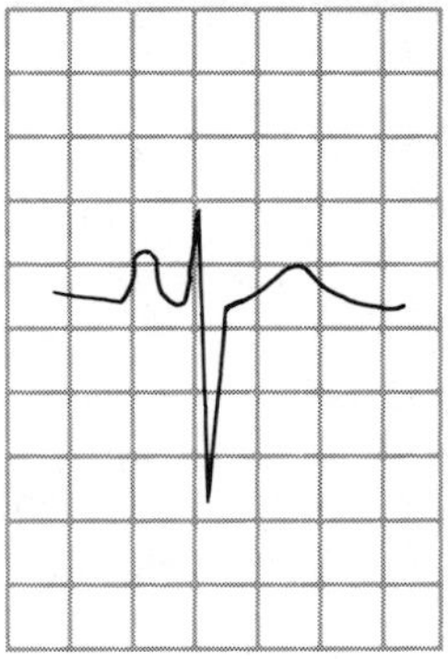

MEAN QRS AXIS DETERMINATION

COGNITIVE GOALS

1. Identify the unipolar and bipolar leads.
2. Describe the derivation of Einthoven's triangle.
3. Define the term **mean cardiac vector.**
4. Define the term **central terminal.**
5. Define the meaning of the letters **a** and **V** in "aVR," "aVL," and "aVF."
6. Describe how the hexaxial system is constructed from the six frontal plane leads.
7. Identify the four quadrants of the hexaxial system and name the leads that form their boundaries.
8. Give the numerical value in degrees of the positive pole of each lead.
9. Give the three rules used to determine the relation of the mean QRS axis to the positive pole of a given lead.
10. Give the criteria for diagnosing normal mean QRS axis.
11. Give the criteria for diagnosing abnormal left mean QRS axis.
12. Give the criteria for diagnosing abnormal right mean QRS axis.
13. Identify the common causes of abnormal left axis deviation.
14. Identify the common causes of abnormal right axis deviation.

The subject of axis determination has acquired a grim reputation in the minds of many students owing to its derivation from vector theory, a conceptually and mathematically challenging body of knowledge concerned with the motion of forces in three-dimensional space. Fortunately, axis determination as practiced in the majority of clinical settings involves a greatly simplified version of vector theory.

Depolarization of the myocardial cells generates millions of tiny electrical forces located in three dimensions. These forces collectively exhibit both magnitude and direction and therefore constitute a **vector.** A vector is a force, in the case of the ECG obviously an electrical force, that has both magnitude and direction. In reality, the electrical forces of the heart move in three dimensions simultaneously and also change direction continuously during the course of each beat. Clearly all these minute electrical forces cannot be considered individually as units. However, the countless individual forces generated by the depolarization of the myocardial cells can be **averaged** together. By averaging all these forces at any given instant during systole, a single net amplitude and direction called the **instantaneous vector** can be obtained. Combining all the instantaneous vectors during systole into a single vector representing the entire depolarization process permits us to obtain the **net** or **mean cardiac vector.** To further simplify the situation, the mean vector may be calculated for only one plane instead of for many. In this way the millions of individual electrical forces generated during depolarization can be reduced to a single vector represented by an arrow moving in a single plane. This net vector represents the mean electrical **axis** of the QRS complex.

The sum of the heart's electrical activity is sensed by electrodes on the body surface. By examining the waveforms recorded from six of these electrodes, the frontal plane leads, the direction or axis can be determined in the frontal plane. Either the direction or the magnitude of the heart's electrical forces can be abnormal. In this chapter we will ignore abnormalities of magnitude and concentrate completely on abnormalities of frontal plane axis.

Frontal plane leads

The six **frontal plane leads** or **limb leads** consist of three **bipolar** or **standard leads** and three **unipolar leads**. The designations of the frontal plane or limb leads are given in Table 2–1, and their derivations are described in the paragraphs that follow.

The standard leads (I, II, III) are called bipolar leads because each records the difference in electrical potential between two limbs. The connections of the bipolar leads are illustrated in Figure 2–1. Lead I connects the right and left arms, with its positive pole and orientation (indicated by the arrow) to the left. Lead II connects the right arm and left leg, and its positive pole and orientation are downward and to the left. Lead III connects the left arm and left leg, and its positive pole and orientation are downward and to the right. The triangle formed by these leads is **Einthoven's triangle,** and the heart is located in its approximate center. The relationship between the voltage of the complexes in the standard leads is summarized by **Einthoven's law,** which states that the net voltage of the complex in lead II will equal the algebraic sum of the voltages of the complexes in leads I and III **(L2 = L1 + L3).**

The unipolar limb leads are aVR, aVL, and aVF. The positive poles are the corners of the Einthoven triangle, and the "negative pole" is the theoretical electrically neutral center of the heart, the **Wilson central terminal** (**CT** in Fig. 2–2). Because the negative point of reference for these leads is the electrically

Table 2–1. FRONTAL PLANE LEADS

Bipolar (Standard)	Unipolar
Lead I	Lead aVR
Lead II	Lead aVL
Lead III	Lead aVF

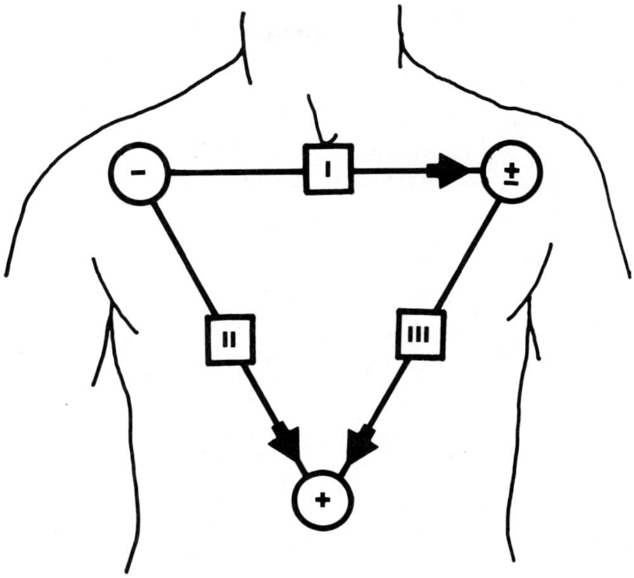

Figure 2–1. The orientation of the bipolar leads.

silent central terminal and a single surface lead, they are called unipolar or **V** leads. The deflections produced by the unipolar leads are ordinarily very small and must be enlarged or **augmented** to make them readable. The designations are broken down in this manner: **R, L,** and **F,** standing for **right** arm, **left** arm, and **foot,** respectively; and **V,** indicating that the leads are unipolar, that the central terminal is the indifferent connection. The letter **a** indicates that the complexes are **augmented** 1.5 times.

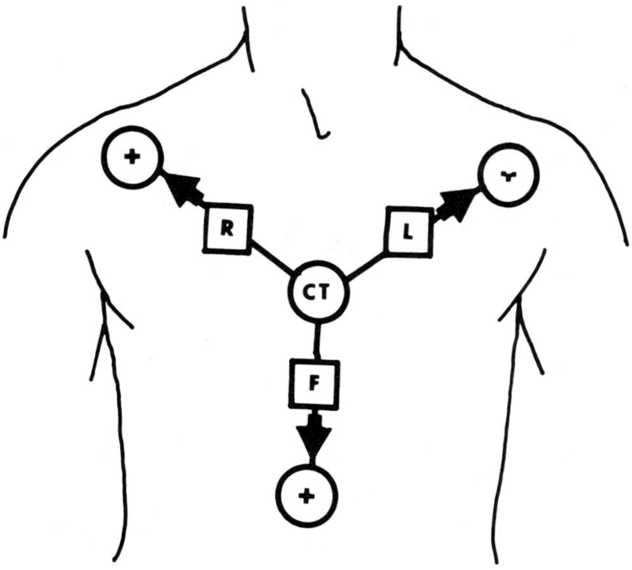

Figure 2–2. The orientation of the unipolar leads.

Construction of the hexaxial system

Axis in the frontal plane is determined by reference to the six frontal plane (limb) leads, I, II, III, aVR, aVL, and aVF. First, however, the limb leads must be arranged to form a reference system. The orientation of the bipolar leads is shown in Figure 2–1. To begin forming the hexaxial reference system, these leads, or **axes,** which are the three sides of the Einthoven triangle, are moved toward each other until they intersect as shown in Figure 2–3. Note that the orientation of the leads, as indicated by the arrows, remains the same. Arranged in this manner, the three bipolar leads divide the precordium into six segments of 60 degrees each (Fig. 2–3).

The next step in the construction of the hexaxial system is the addition of the unipolar leads shown in Figure 2–2. These leads—aVR, aVL, and aVF—are arranged so that they intersect with the bipolar leads. The center point through which all six leads pass is the central terminal, the electrically neutral center of the heart (Fig. 2–4). Note that the orientation of the unipolar leads, indicated by the arrows, remains the same. With the addition of the three unipolar leads, the precordium is now divided into 12 segments of 30 degrees each. All six limb leads or axes now intersect.

Figure 2–5 illustrates the **quadrants of normal and abnormal axis.** Note that leads I and aVF divide the precordium into four quadrants. The positive pole of each of the two leads is indicated by an arrow. The positive poles are the vantage points from which the leads "see" the heart's electrical activity. Lead I is oriented straight to the left; the axis of lead aVF is directed straight downward toward the feet (recall the "F" in aVF is derived from "foot"). When the four quadrants formed by the intersection of leads I and aVF are closed by a circle, each quadrant marks off an arc of 90 degrees (Fig. 2–5).

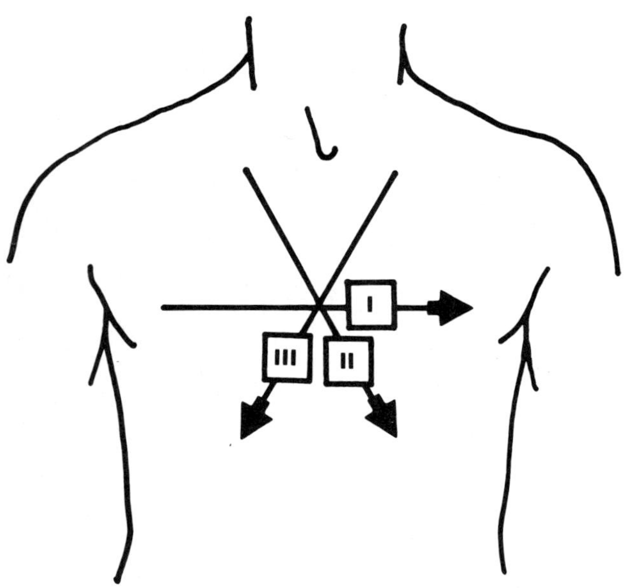

Figure 2–3. The triaxial reference system.

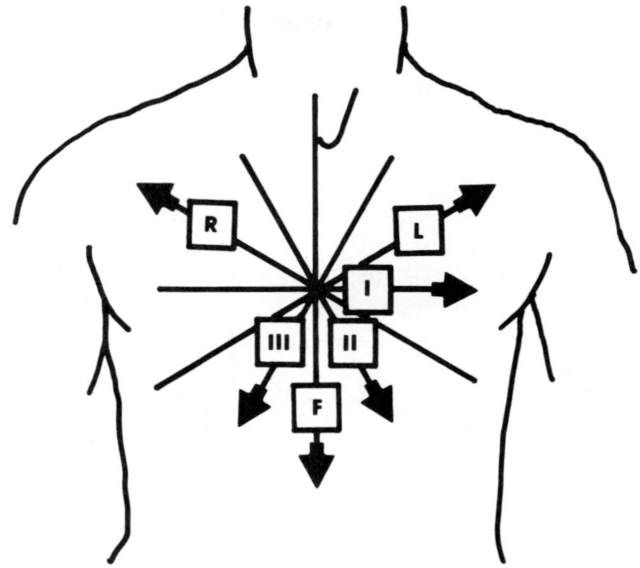

Figure 2–4. The hexaxial reference system.

The quadrant between the positive poles of leads I and aVF is the **quadrant of normal axis** (marked **NA** in Fig. 2–5). The quadrant to the right of the normal axis quadrant is the **quadrant of abnormal right axis** (**ARAD** in Fig. 2–5). Above the quadrant of normal axis is the **quadrant of abnormal left axis** deviation **(ALAD).** The remaining quadrant, marked **IA,** is the **quadrant of indeterminate axis,** sometimes called "no man's land" (Marriott, 1983). Indeterminate axis is considered by most authors to represent extreme right axis deviation.

Further examination of Figure 2–5 reveals that the circle enclosing the

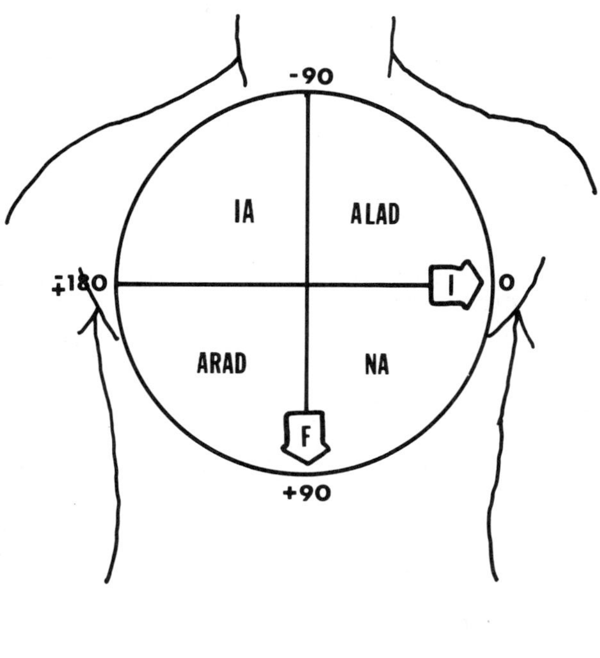

Figure 2–5. The quadrants of the hexaxial system.

four quadrants is divided into **180 positive degrees** below the axis of lead I and **180 negative degrees** above it. Lead I is the dividing line between the positive and negative hemispheres, and the numbering of the degrees conventionally begins at the positive pole of lead I, which is designated **zero.** This arrangement permits axis to be quantified in terms of degrees, with degrees between 0 and +90 representing normal axis, between −1 and −90 representing left axis deviation, and between +90 and +180 representing right axis deviation.

Figure 2–6 develops the hexaxial reference system completely. In this figure all six frontal plane leads are represented and the orientations of the positive poles of the leads are shown by arrows. The numerical value of each lead is also shown. The positive pole of lead II is within the quadrant of normal axis, the positive pole of lead aVL is in the quadrant of abnormal left axis, and the positive pole of lead III is in the quadrant of abnormal right axis deviation. The positive pole of lead aVR, in the quadrant of indeterminate axis, is considered to be within the range of extreme right axis deviation by some authorities.

Before reading the remainder of this chapter, answer the self-assessment questions on page 27. Your answers should be checked against those in the answer key.

In brief, we have established that there are six frontal plane leads and that their axes are combined in such a way that a reference system results. The intersection of leads I and aVF divides the precordium into quadrants of 90 degrees each; the two quadrants above the axis of lead I are numbered in negative degrees and the two quadrants below this axis are numbered in positive degrees.

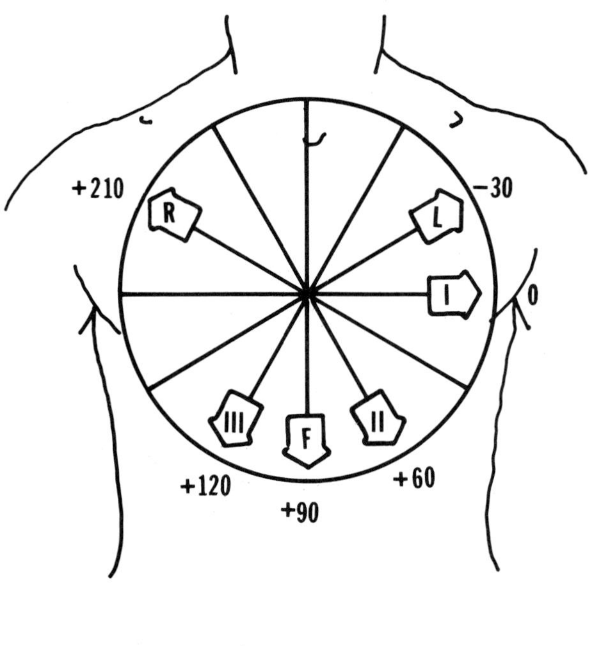

Figure 2–6. The numerical degree designations of the six leads.

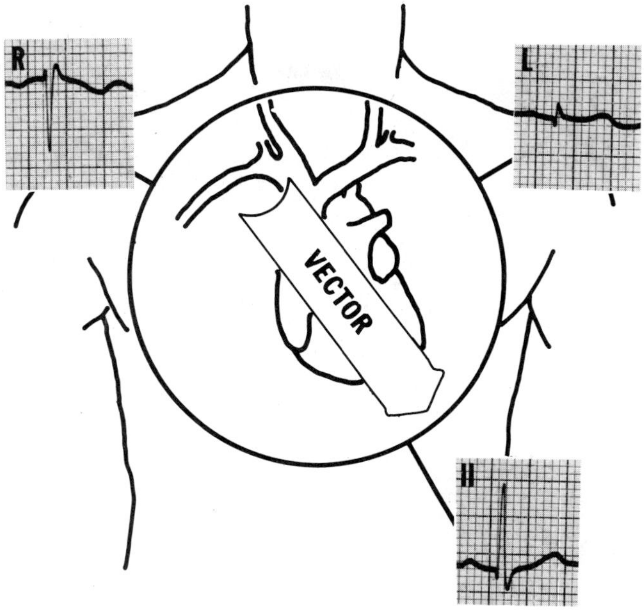

Figure 2–7. The mean vector as seen simultaneously by three leads.

Next we will consider how an individual lead "sees" and records the mean or net cardiac vector and how the QRS complex reflects the amplitude of the vector. Normally the net or overall direction of the heart's electrical forces is **downward and to the left** (Fig. 2–7). Figure 2–7 illustrates three of the frontal plane leads (II, aVR, and aVL) and the complexes they record. These three leads and their complexes demonstrate three essential rules, which must be clearly understood in order to determine axis. The rules, which follow, are simple.

Rule 1: If the heart's electrical forces are *moving away from* the positive pole of a lead, that lead will record a **negative complex.** (In Figure 2–7, the net vector is directed away from lead aVR; therefore, lead aVR records a negative complex.)

Rule 2: If the heart's electrical forces are *moving toward* the positive pole of a lead, that lead will record a **positive complex.** (In Figure 2–7 the net vector is directed toward the positive pole of lead II; therefore, lead II records a positive complex.)

Rule 3: If the electrical forces are *moving perpendicular to* (at a right angle to) the positive pole of a lead, that lead will record a **biphasic** or **flat complex.** When the lead is perpendicular to the orientation of the vector, part of the time the electrical forces are moving toward the positive pole of the lead and part of the time the forces are moving away from it. As the electrode "sees" it, the forces tend to cancel out, resulting in a flattened or biphasic **transition complex.** (In Figure 2–7, lead aVL is perpendicular to the movement of the vector and writes a low amplitude, biphasic transition complex.)

It is imperative that the simple rules described here be clearly understood. As long as the electrical forces are moving toward the positive pole of a lead, an upright, positive complex will be recorded. The orientation of lead II is downward and toward the left (see Fig. 1–1), and when incorporated into the hexaxial reference system it keeps that orientation (see Fig. 2–3). With the reference system complete, lead II is given the numerical designation of +60 degrees (Fig. 2–6). If the mean cardiac vector is directed downward and leftward, it is roughly parallel to the axis of lead II, and lead II will accordingly record a positive QRS complex.

Because the normal net cardiac vector is directed downward and leftward, it travels directly away from the positive pole of lead aVR (see Figs. 2–2 and 2–6). Therefore, on a normal ECG all the complexes (P-QRS-T) in lead aVR are usually negative.

Based on the three rules discussed previously, it is possible to formulate three questions that will assist in determining the axis of the QRS complex:

1. Which lead records the tallest QRS complex? The answer to this question will reveal the lead that the electrical forces are going most directly toward.
2. Which lead records the most negative QRS complex? The answer will reveal the lead the forces are moving most directly away from.
3. Which lead records the smallest or most biphasic (RS) QRS complex? This answer indicates which lead is most nearly perpendicular to the motion of the cardiac vector.

The student will discover that committing the hexaxial reference system to memory both facilitates its use and amplifies its applications. The relationships between the six leads is easier to remember if one considers lead I as an equator (see Fig. 2–6) that divides the system into northern and southern "hemispheres." Continuing the geographic analogy, lead aVF marks the "poles" with the positive pole of aVF at the "south pole" position. The positive pole of lead I is the beginning point for numbering degrees. The positive pole of lead aVF is at the +90 position and the other two standard leads—II and III—are located 30 degrees to either side of +90. Lead II, in the quadrant of normal axis, is at the +60 position and lead III, in the quadrant of right axis deviation, is at +120 degrees.

Recalling the position of the unipolar leads is simplicity itself if it is remembered that the "R" of aVR stands for **right arm.** The positive pole of aVR is therefore at the base of the right arm (+210 degrees if the quadrant of indeterminate axis is considered to represent extreme right axis deviation). The "L" of aVL stands for *left arm* and its positive pole corresponds to the base of the left arm, placing it in the quadrant of left axis deviation. Its numerical value is −30 degrees. Finally, the "F" of aVF stands for **foot,** and the positive pole of aVF is directly downward, toward the feet. The numerical value of aVF is +90 degrees.

Figure 2–8 illustrates normal axis. The relative strength of the net electrical force sensed by each lead is indicated by arrowheads of varying sizes. In this example, the most positive QRS complex, or the tallest R wave, appears in lead II, the positive pole of which is in the quadrant of normal axis. The most nearly flat or equiphasic complex appears in lead aVL because the direction of the

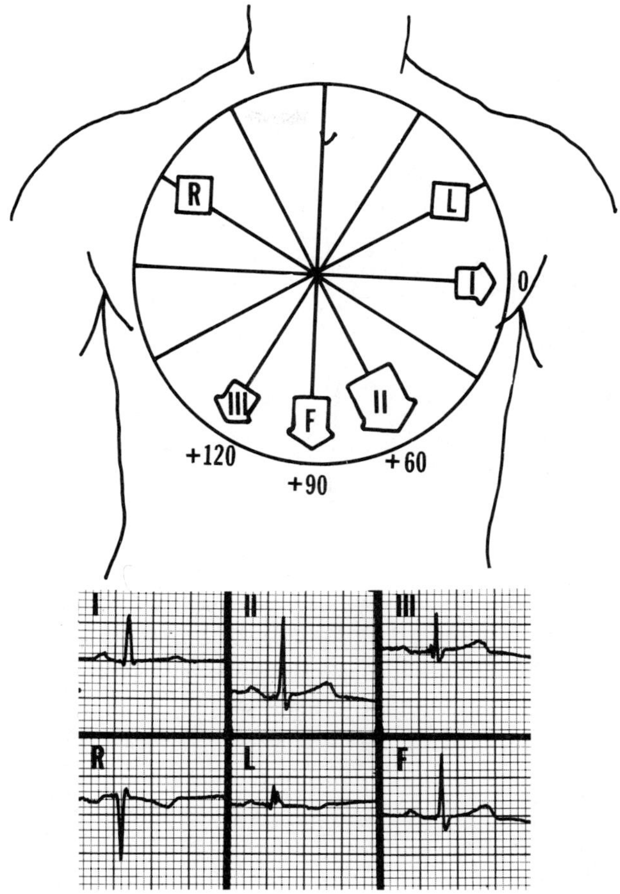

Figure 2–8. Normal axis.

vector is perpendicular to this lead (leads II and aVL form a right angle). The equiphasic complex in aVL represents a transition complex, which marks a zone of transition from predominantly negative complexes to predominantly positive complexes. This zone of transition, which in this case lies in the plane of aVL, is often called the **null plane.** The most negative complex, with the deepest S wave, is in lead aVR because the vector is headed most directly away from this lead. Because the forces are directed toward lead II, all other leads with positive poles in the same hemisphere as that of lead II (leads I, aVF, and III) will also record QRS complexes that are positive to varying degrees.

An example of abnormal left axis deviation is shown in Figure 2–9. The tallest R wave in this case appears in lead aVL because the mean vector is directed upward and leftward toward the positive pole of aVL. The smallest QRS complex appears in lead aVR because the motion of the electrical forces is perpendicular to this lead. Lead aVR now represents the transition zone or null plane. The most negative QRS complex, with the deepest S wave, is in lead III, indicating that the forces are moving most directly away from this lead. Note that **the S wave in lead III is deeper than the R wave in lead aVL is tall.**

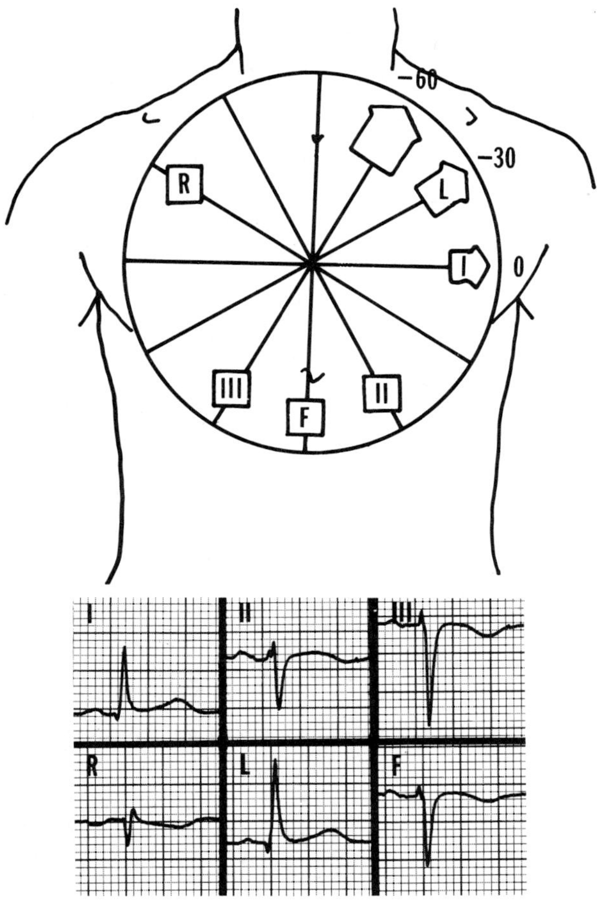

Figure 2–9. Left axis deviation.

This occurs because the net movement of the vector is more directly oriented *away* from lead III than it is *toward* lead aVL (note that the arrowheads are sized to indicate this fact). The axis is further to the left than the positive pole of aVL, in the −60-degree range. Leads I and aVL are both in the hemisphere toward which the electrical forces are moving, and therefore both write positive deflections. Leads II, III, and aVF are in the hemisphere the forces are moving away from and according write basically negative complexes. Lead aVR, in the transition zone, is at right angles to the vector and records a small biphasic complex.

Figure 2–10 shows right axis deviation. The most positive QRS complex, or tallest R wave, is in lead III. The positive pole of lead III is in the quadrant of right axis deviation and has a numerical value of +120 degrees. Negative QRS complexes are noted in leads I and aVL because the vector is moving away from those leads. The most biphasic complex is in lead aVR, which is situated perpendicular to the movement of the electrical forces. The hemisphere into which the vector is moving contains the positive poles of leads II, III, and aVF and all these leads record QRS complexes that are positive to various degrees.

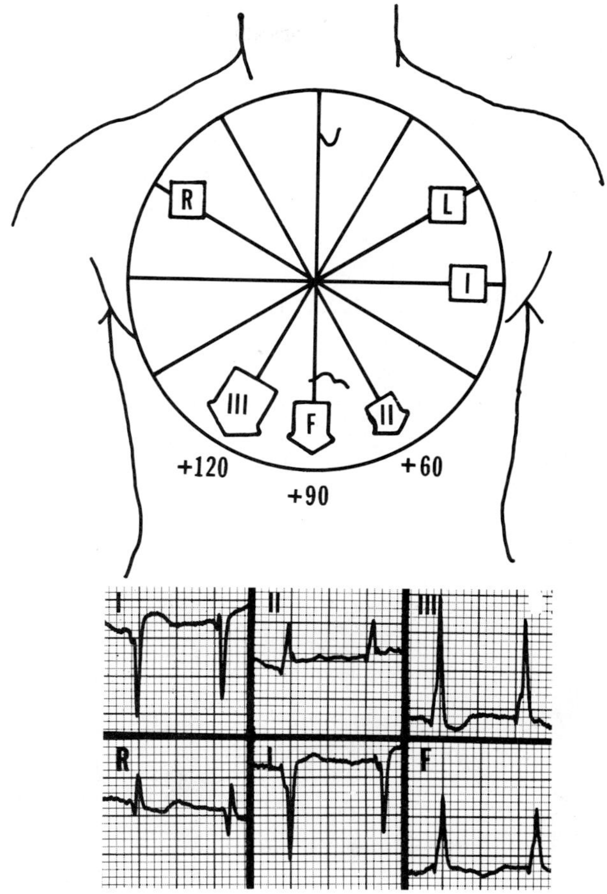

Figure 2–10. Right axis deviation.

Indeterminate axis represents extreme right axis deviation in all but a very few cases. It is occasionally encountered in subjects with congenital heart defects or severe lung disease, or as an expression of left posterior fascicular block. The ECG in Figure 2–11 was recorded from a patient with congenital heart disease. The tallest QRS complex is found in lead aVR (+210 degrees), the deepest S wave in lead II, and the most nearly equiphasic complex in lead III. The vector is directed toward the quadrant of indeterminate axis, or extreme right axis. Because the positive poles of all leads other than aVR and lead III are in the hemisphere opposite the positive pole of aVR, they record predominantly negative complexes. Lead III, which is at right angles to the vector, writes a transition complex.

Vector plotting

In addition to the vector approach to axis calculation, which has been described, an older, more conventional method called vector plotting exists.

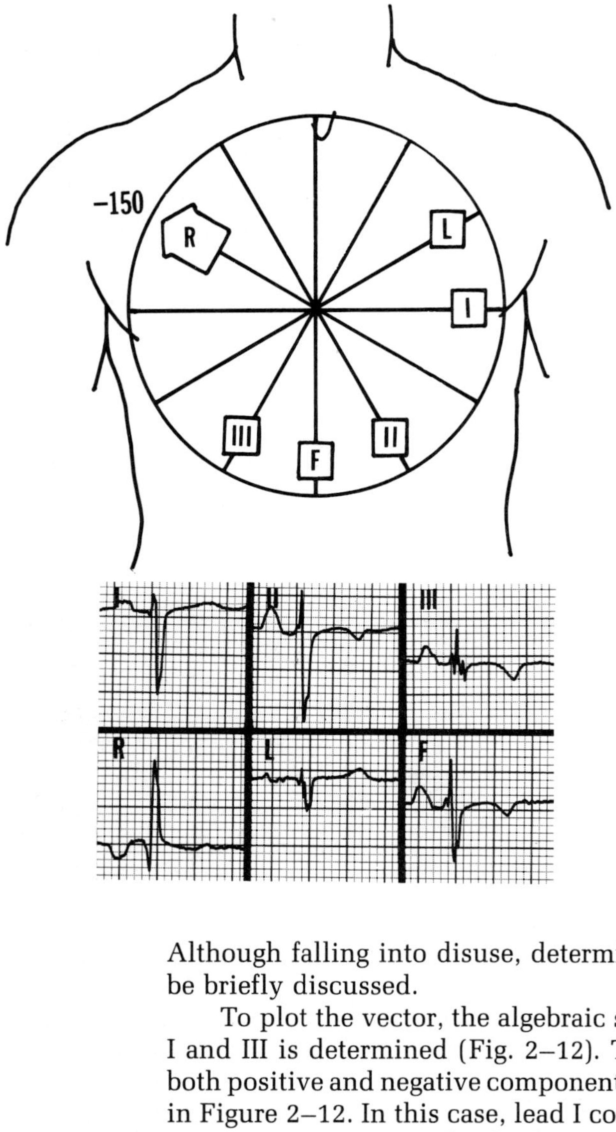

Figure 2–11. Indeterminate (or extreme right) axis deviation.

Although falling into disuse, determination of the vector by this method will be briefly discussed.

To plot the vector, the algebraic sum of the amplitude of the QRS in leads I and III is determined (Fig. 2–12). This may be approximated by measuring both positive and negative components of the QRS and summing them as shown in Figure 2–12. In this case, lead I consists of an R wave 3.5 mm in height and an S wave 2.0 mm in depth; the net positivity is therefore 1.5 mm. In lead III the QRS complex consists of a Q wave 1.5 mm in negative amplitude and an R wave 11.5 mm in positive amplitude. Summing these two values yields a net value of 10.0 mm.

Next the values obtained by algebraic summation of the QRS components are plotted on the respective axes of leads I and III, as shown in Figure 2–12. At the point of 1.5 units of amplitude on the axis of lead I, a perpendicular is drawn. At the point of 10 units of amplitude on the axis of lead III, another perpendicular is drawn and extended until it intersects the perpendicular drawn from the axis of lead I. Finally, a line is drawn from the zero point through the intersection of the two perpendiculars (line with arrow). This line

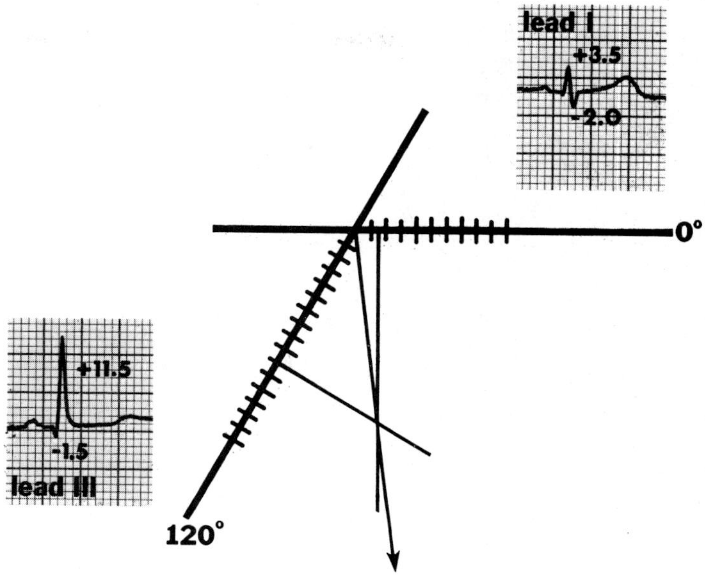

Figure 2–12. The vector plotting approach.

is called the **resultant** and represents the direction of the mean QRS vector. In the case illustrated here, the resultant (vector) has a value of approximately +85 degrees.

This method of estimating the mean QRS vector was mechanical and difficult to teach; required calipers, pencil, graph paper, and straight-edge; and was time consuming (Constant, 1981). The newer vector approach utilizing all six leads as mental points of reference permits almost instant recognition of axis on sight without the encumbrance of the aforementioned instruments.

The essential skill is not to be able to calculate axis to within a single degree, but to recognize abnormalities and changes in axis at a glance. When

Table 2–2. CAUSES OF LEFT AXIS DEVIATION

Diseases of the left bundle branch
Anteroseptal infarction
Lev's disease
Lenègre's disease
Inferior wall infarction
Aberrant ventricular conduction
Severe pulmonary disease
Left anterior fascicular block

Table 2–3. CAUSES OF RIGHT AXIS DEVIATION

Diseases of the left bundle branch
Anteroseptal infarction
Lev's disease
Lenègre's disease
Lateral wall infarction
Aberrant ventricular conduction
Advanced pulmonary disease
Left posterior fascicular block
Right ventricular hypertrophy

possible, axis should be specified in terms of degrees, recognizing that there are as many cases of borderline normal axis as there are cases of borderline normal blood gases or serum electrolytes. Axis deviation is not a diagnosis per se but a supportive finding associated with a large number of conditions, some of which are listed in Tables 2–2 and 2–3.

References

Constant, J. **Learning Electrocardiography,** 2nd ed. Little, Brown and Company, Boston, 1981, p 50.

Marriott, HJL. **Practical Electrocardiography,** 7th ed. Williams & Wilkins, Baltimore, 1983, p 34.

SELF-ASSESSMENT

Multiple Choice—Part I

1. The standard or bipolar leads are:

   a. aVR, aVL, aVF.
   b. I and aVL.
   c. II, III, aVF.
   d. I, II, III.

2. The positive and negative poles of lead I are:

   a. the right shoulder and left leg, respectively.
   b. the left and right arms, respectively.
   c. the left arm and left leg, respectively.
   d. the right and left arms, respectively.

3. The single vector representing the entire depolarization process is:

   a. the QRS complex.
   b. the instantaneous vector.
   c. the mean cardiac vector.
   d. the multidimensional vector.

4. The sides of Einthoven's triangle are formed by leads:

   a. I, II, III.
   b. I, aVL, aVF.
   c. aVR, aVL, aVF.
   d. II, III, aVF.

5. The positive pole of lead II is in:

   a. the quadrant of indeterminate axis.
   b. the quadrant of right axis.
   c. the quadrant of left axis.
   d. the quadrant of normal axis.

6. The six frontal plane leads divide the hexaxial reference system into arcs of:

   a. 15 degrees each.
   b. 30 degrees each.
   c. 60 degrees each.
   d. 90 degrees each.

Multiple Choice—Part II

7. If the main cardiac vector is moving perpendicular to the positive pole of a lead, the lead will record:

   a. a positive complex.
   b. a negative complex.
   c. an equiphasic complex.
   d. a null plane.

8. If the mean cardiac vector is moving toward the positive pole of a lead, the lead will record:

   a. a positive complex.
   b. a negative complex.
   c. an equiphasic complex.
   d. a null plane.

9. In cases of left axis deviation, the tallest R wave will appear in:

   a. lead I.
   b. lead II.
   c. lead aVL.
   d. lead aVF.

10. In the case of right axis deviation, the tallest R wave will appear in:

    a. lead I.
    b. lead III.
    c. lead aVL.
    d. lead aVF.

11. The positive pole of lead II has a numerical value of:

    a. 0 degrees.
    b. −30 degrees.
    c. +60 degrees.
    d. +120 degrees.

12. The positive pole of lead III has a numerical value of:

    a. 0 degrees.
    b. −30 degrees.
    c. +60 degrees.
    d. +120 degrees.

13. The positive pole of lead aVL has a numerical value of:

    a. 0 degrees.
    b. −30 degrees.
    c. +60 degrees.
    d. −60 degrees.

14. The positive pole of lead aVF has a numerical value of:

    a. 0 degrees.
    b. +60 degrees.
    c. +90 degrees.
    d. +120 degrees.

Practice Strips

Determine the mean QRS axis from the frontal plane leads displayed below.

2-1
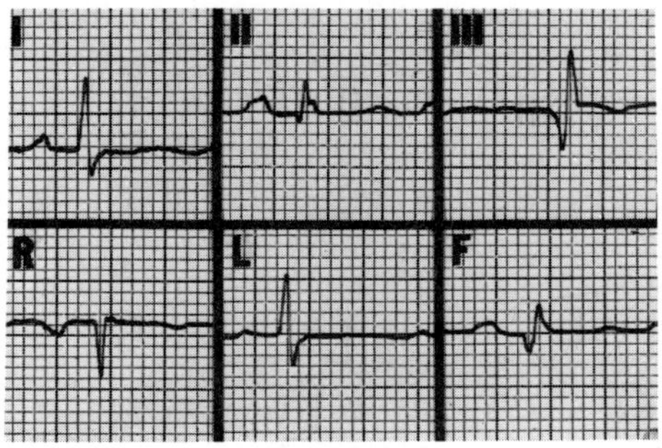

2-2
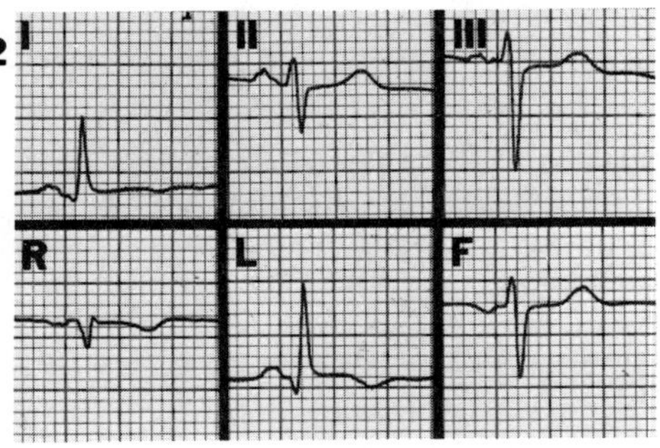

2-3
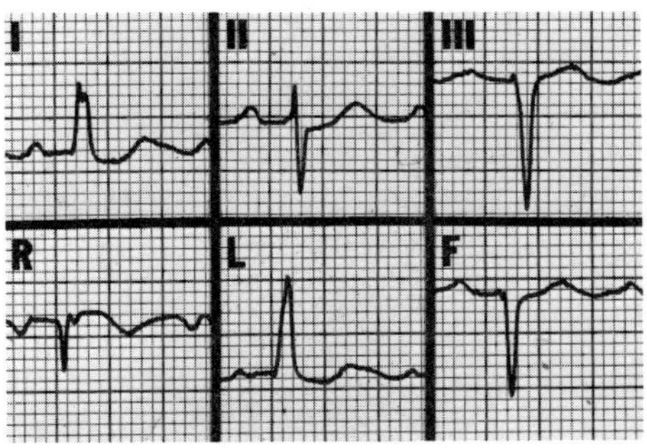

2-4
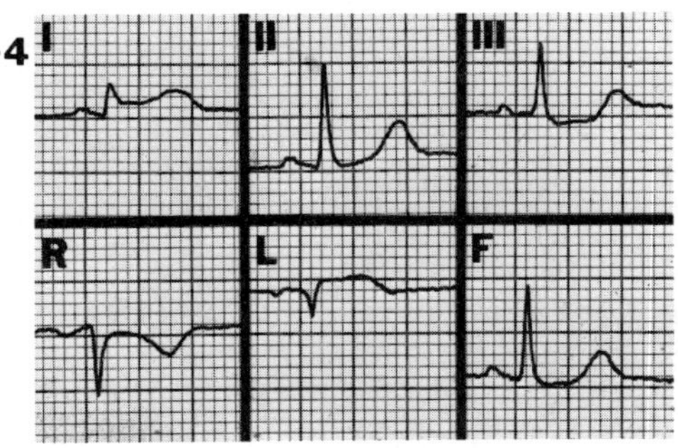

2-5
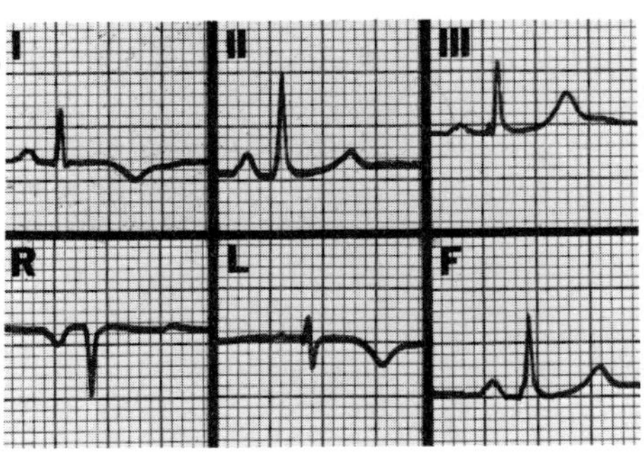

2-6
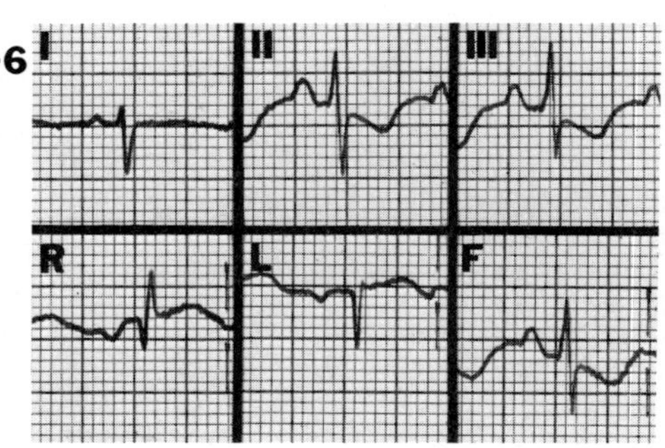

2-7
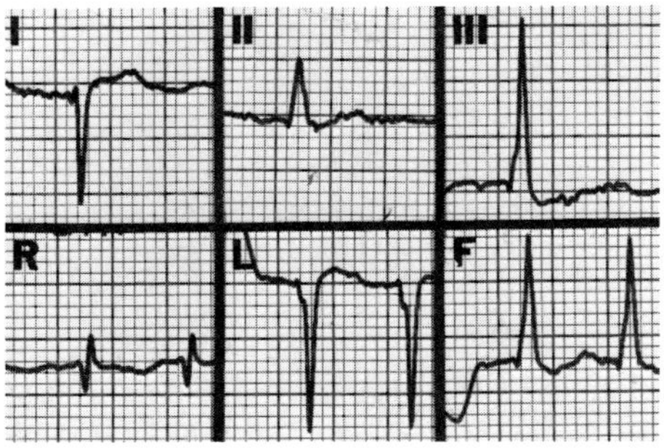

2-8
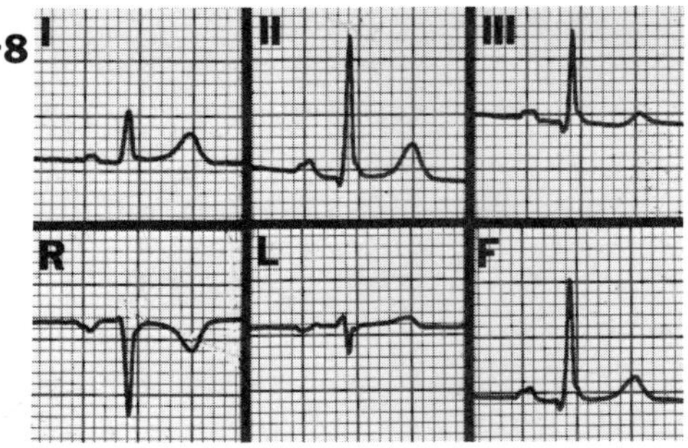

2-9
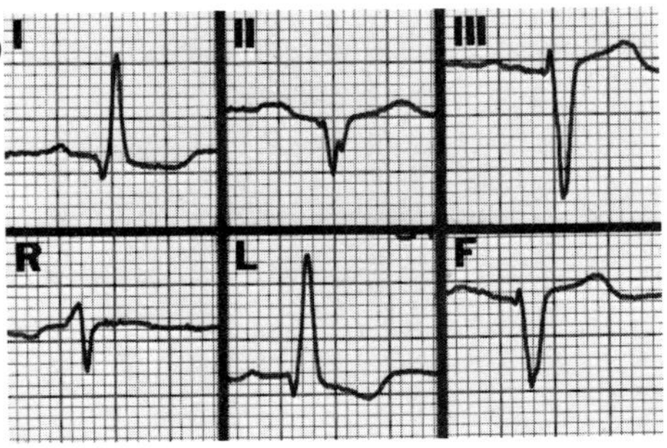

2-10
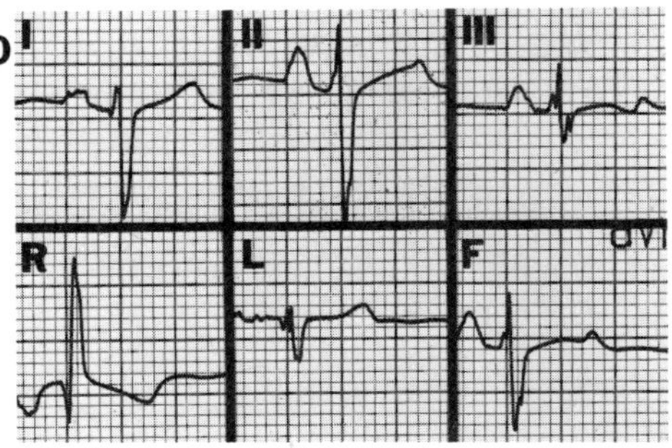

2-11
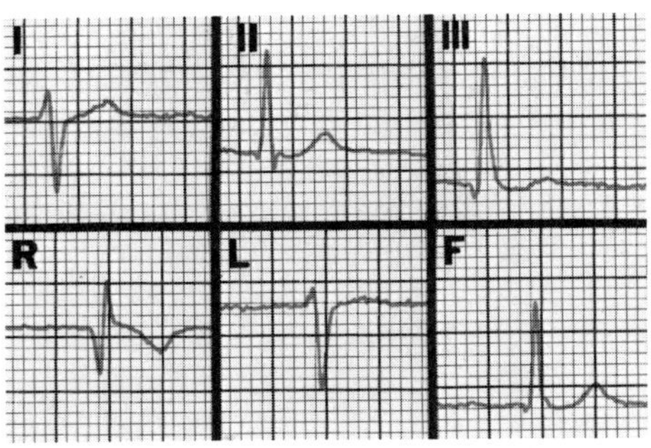

2-12
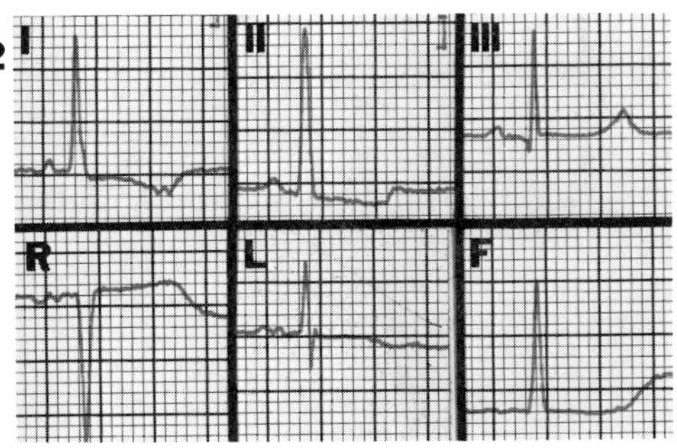

2-13
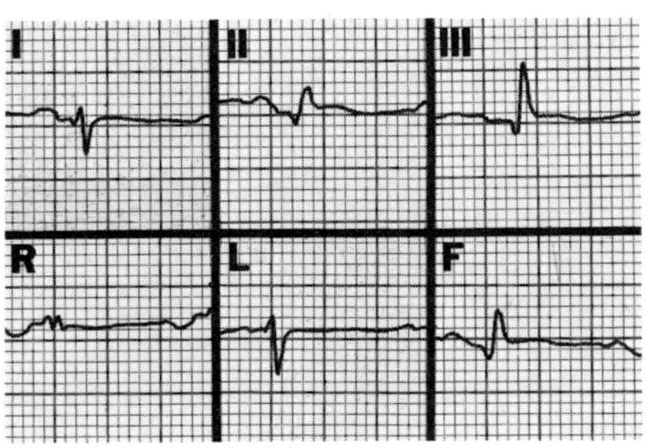

2-14
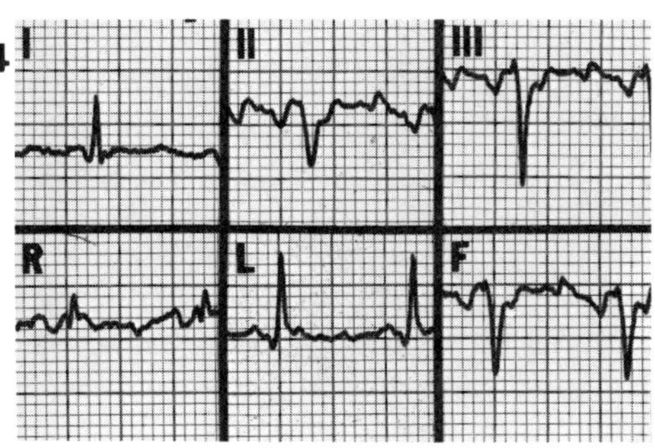

2-15
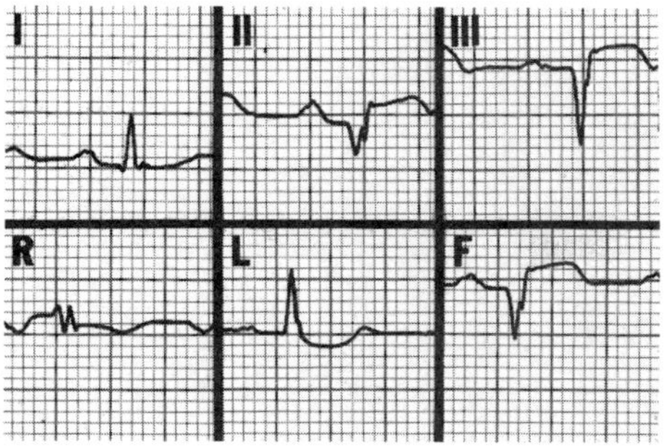

2-16
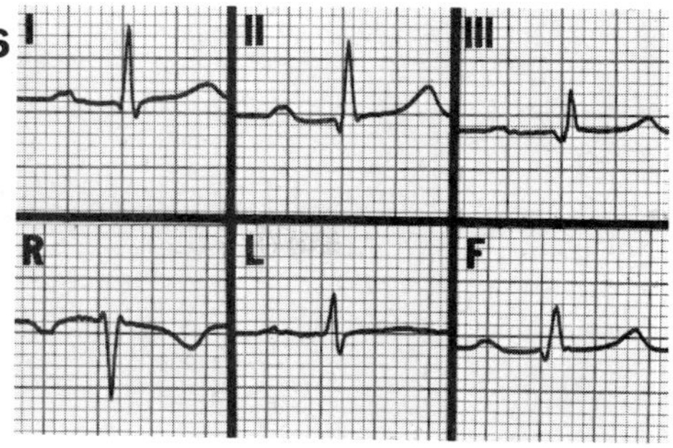

2-17
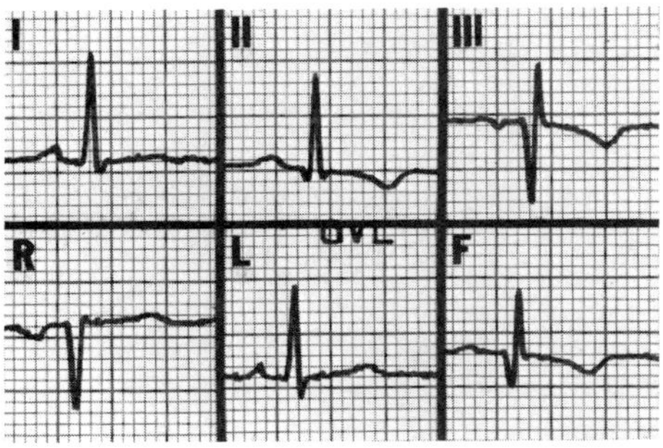

2-18
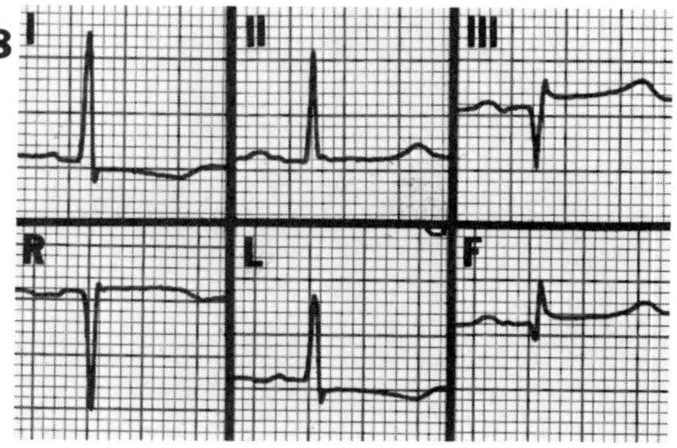

2-19
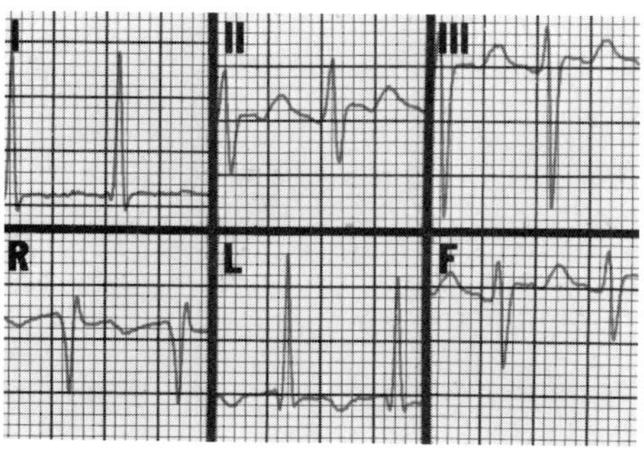

2-20
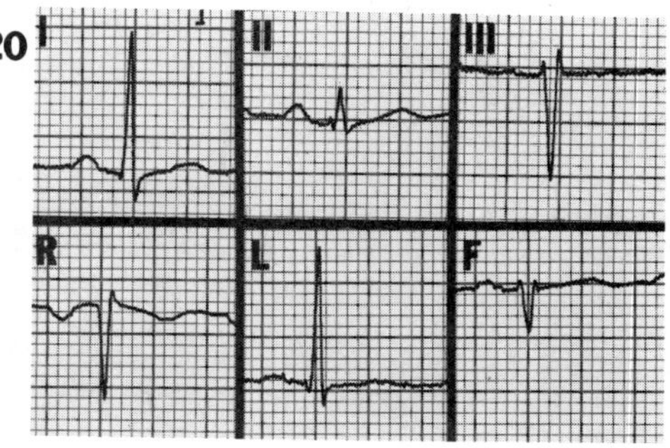

2-21
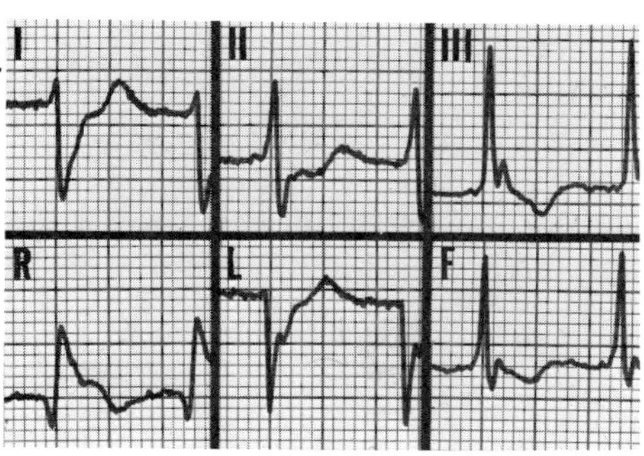

2-22
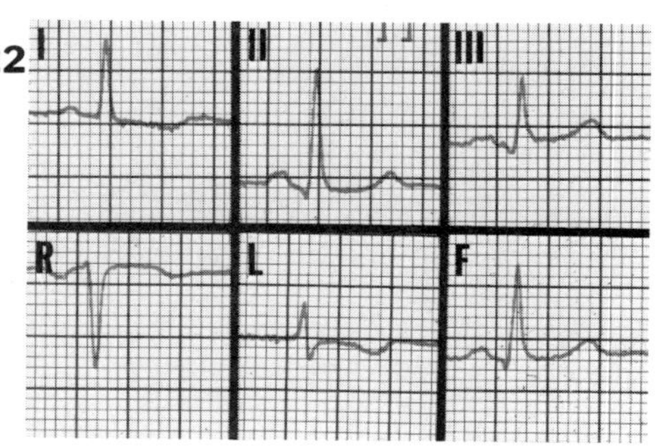

2-23
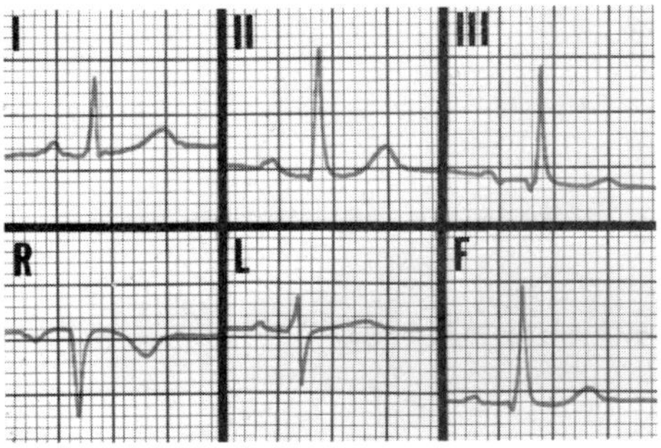

2-24
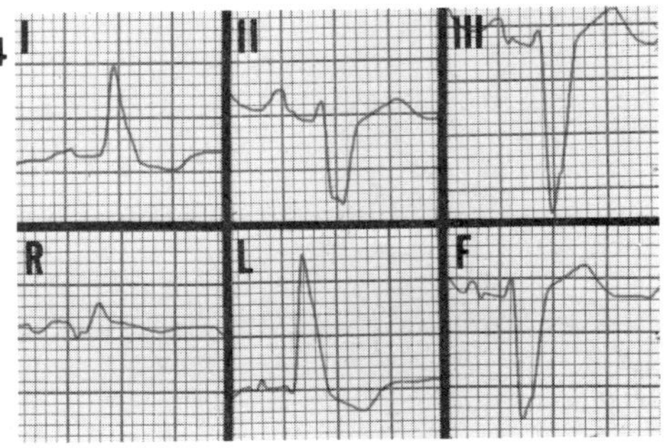

2-25
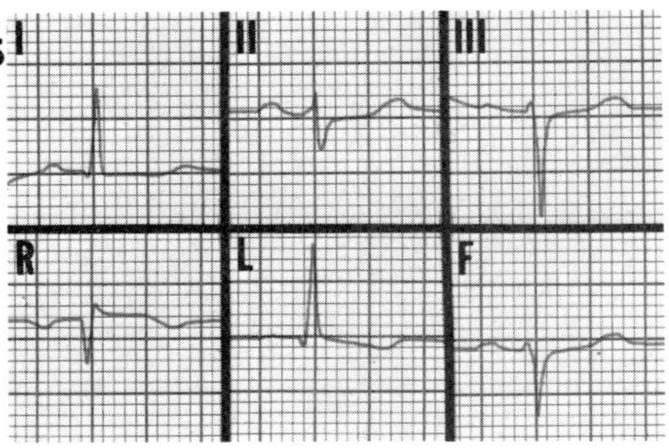

2-26
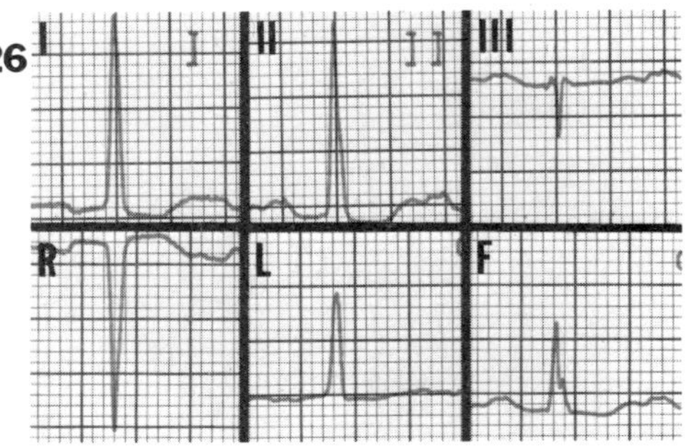

2-27
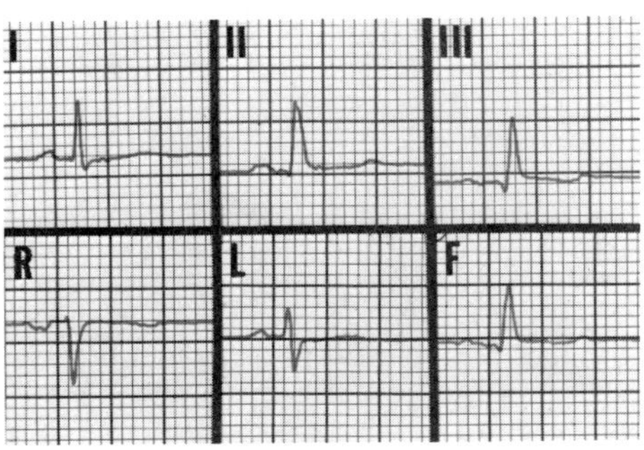

2-28
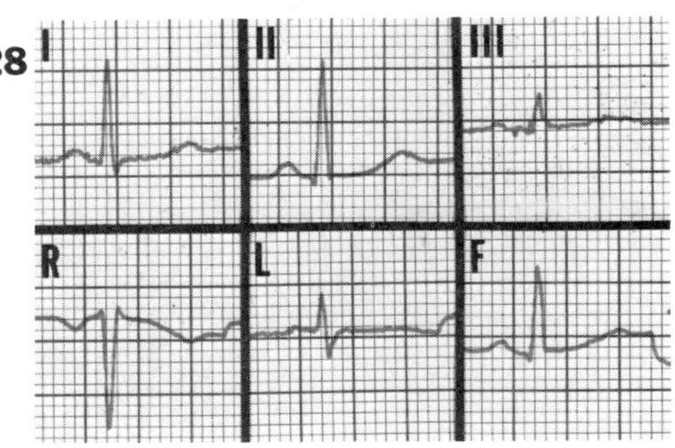

2-29
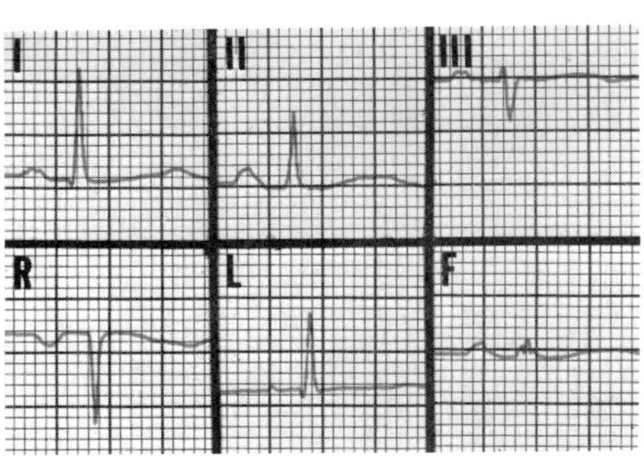

2-30
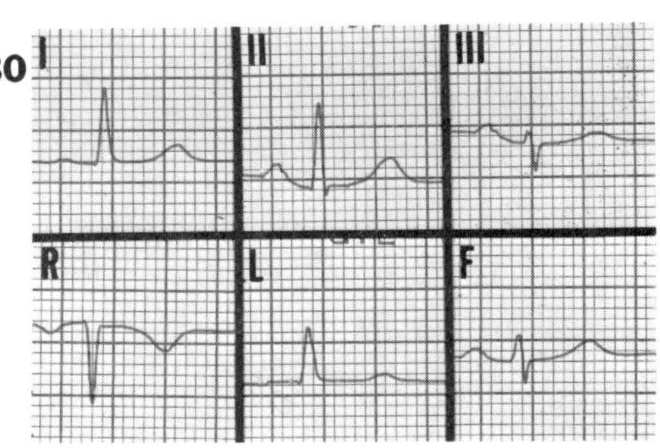

ANSWER KEY

Multiple Choice

1. d
2. b
3. c
4. a
5. d
6. b
7. c
8. a
9. c
10. b
11. c
12. d
13. b
14. c

Practice Strips

Note: The answers for all axis determination problems are given as a range of degrees. Any answer falling within that range should be considered correct.

2–1. Normal axis, +5 to −5 degrees.

2–2. Left axis deviation, −55 to −65 degrees.

2–3. Left axis deviation, −55 to −65 degrees.

2–4. Normal axis, +55 to +65 degrees.

2–5. Normal axis, +55 to +65 degrees.

2–6. Right axis deviation, +145 to +155 degrees.

2–7. Right axis deviation, +115 to +125 degrees.

2–8. Normal axis, +55 to +65 degrees.

2–9. Left axis deviation, −55 to −65 degrees.

2–10. Extreme right axis, +205 to +215 degrees.

2–11. Right axis deviation, +115 to +125 degrees.

2–12. Normal axis, +50 to +60 degrees.

2–13. Right axis deviation, +115 to +125 degrees.

2–14. Left axis deviation, −60 to −70 degrees.

2–15. Left axis deviation, −55 to −65 degrees.

2–16. Normal axis, +25 to +35 degrees.

2–17. Normal axis, 0 to +10 degrees.

2–18. Normal axis, 0 to +10 degrees.

2–19. Left axis deviation, −25 to −35 degrees.

2–20. Left axis deviation, −20 to −30 degrees.

2–21. Right axis deviation, +145 to +155 degrees.

2–22. Normal axis, +55 to +65 degrees.

2–23. Normal axis, +70 to +80 degrees.

2–24. Left axis deviation, −60 to −70 degrees.

2–25. Left axis deviation, −55 to −65 degrees.

2–26. Normal axis, +25 to +35 degrees.

2–27. Normal axis, +70 to +80 degrees.

2–28. Normal axis, +40 to +50 degrees.

2–29. Normal axis, +5 to −5 degrees.

2–30. Normal axis, +25 to +35 degrees.

CHAPTER THREE

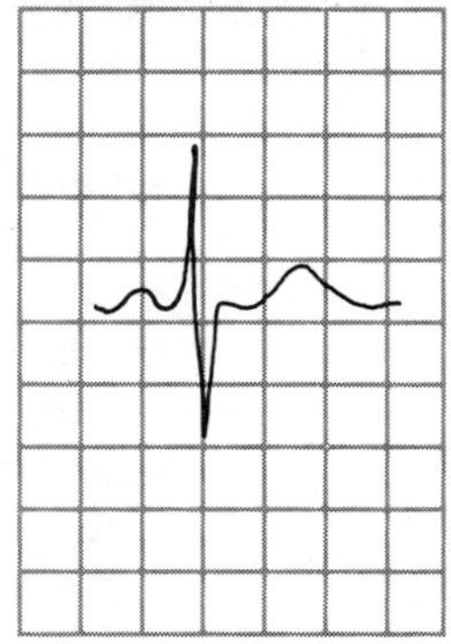

THE NORMAL ECG

COGNITIVE GOALS

1. Name and describe the orientation of each of the horizontal plane leads.
2. Describe the salient features of normal QRS complexes in leads II, aVR, V1, and V6.
3. Define the term **transition zone** and identify its normal location in the precordial leads.
4. Define the term **J point.**
5. Define the terms **right ventricular pattern** and **left ventricular pattern.**
6. Give the diagnostic criteria for low voltage.
7. Give the diagnostic criteria for poor R wave progression.
8. Give the diagnostic criteria for early and late transition.
9. Identify several common causes of low voltage.
10. Identify several common causes of poor R wave progression.
11. Decribe the sequence of normal left ventricular activation and explain how that sequence is related to the instantaneous vectors described in the text.
12. Identify the deflections produced in leads I, aVL, V1, and V6 by left ventricular septal activation.
13. Identify the deflections produced in leads I, aVL, V1, and V6 by depolarization of the anterolateral left ventricular wall.

The goals of this chapter are (1) to introduce the horizontal plane leads, (2) to describe the salient features of the normal 12 lead electrocardiogram, (3) to define transition and low voltage, (4) and to discuss the sequence of ventricular activation and its relationship with the normal QRS complex. These essential goals form a basis for recognizing abnormal tracings and for achieving some insight into the reasons why particular abnormalities occur.

Horizontal plane leads

The **horizontal plane,** or **precordial,** leads are unipolar V leads. The positive electrode is moved across the chest to designated positions, and the indifferent electrode is the Wilson central terminal. Lead **V1** is located in the fourth intercostal space to the right of the sternum, **V2** is in the fourth intercostal space to the left of the sternum, and **V4** is in the fifth intercostal space at the left midclavicular line. Lead **V3** is midway between V2 and V4. Lead **V5** is in the fifth intercostal space at the left anterior axillary line, and **V6** is in the fifth intercostal space, left midaxillary line. The orientation of the precordial V leads is shown in Figure 3–1. Leads V1 and V2 face the right side of the heart, leads V3 and V4 are in the area of the ventricular septum, and leads V5 and V6 face the left ventricle. It can be noted from Figure 3–1 that frontal plane lead I and horizontal plane lead V6 share almost identical orientations. For this reason, the complex recorded in lead I is similar to the complex recorded in lead V6.

Placement of the precordial leads should always be done using the skeletal landmarks described earlier. Misplacement of these leads will result in a defective electrocardiogram that may contain spurious abnormalities.

Features of the normal ECG

Figure 3–2 shows a normal electrocardiogram. Those features of particular importance are numbered for ease of reference. All complexes, P-QRS-T, are normally positive (upright) in lead II (**#1** in Fig. 3–2). The same complexes are all negative (inverted) in lead aVR (**#2** in Fig. 3–2). The mean axis of the tracing is normal; the tallest R wave is in lead II, the only lead with its positive pole in the quadrant of normal axis. Lead V1 is characterized by a small initial **r wave** (**#3**) and a deeper **S wave.** The T wave in V1 (**#4**) may normally be positive, biphasic, or negative. The T waves in leads V2 to V6 are normally positive in adults. The normal T wave begins with a gradually upward sloping proximal limb (**#5**), which then drops back toward the baseline more abruptly

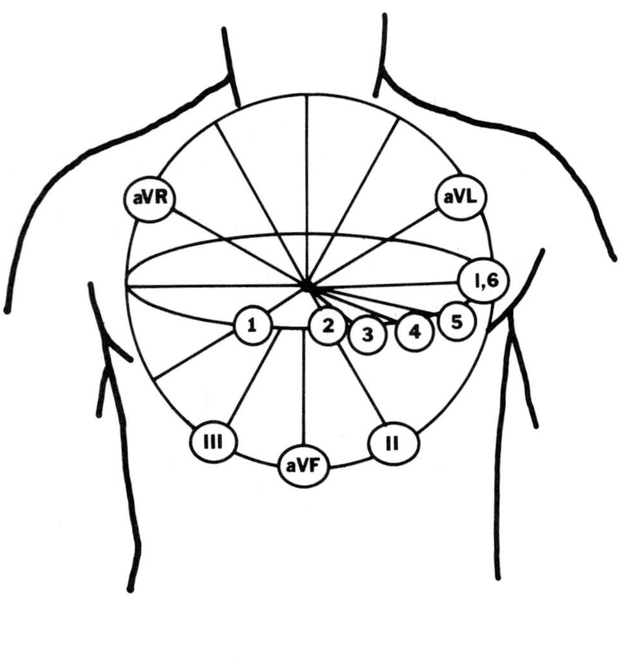

Figure 3–1. The vertical and horizontal planes and their leads.

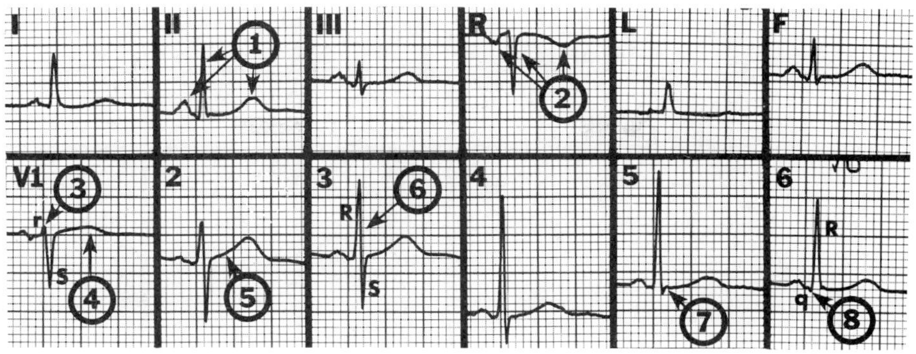

Figure 3–2. Features of the normal electrocardiogram.

in the distal limb. Sharp angles within the proximal limb of the T wave are abnormal and should be regarded with suspicion.

The amplitude of the R waves in the precordial leads normally increases from V1 to V3 until an equiphasic or RS complex is observed. The equiphasic **transition complex** identifies the **transition zone,** which is normally in lead V3 or V4 or between those leads. A transition complex (RS) in lead V1 or V2 indicates **early transition;** an equiphasic complex seen in V5 or V6 represents **late transition.** In Figure 2–2 the most nearly equiphasic complex is seen in lead V3 (**#6**), which displays an RS complex. This indicates that the zone of transition is in V3 or slightly to its right, and is normal. The point at which the ST segment originates from the QRS complex is called the **J point** (**#7**). Further attention to the behavior of the J point will be given in the chapter on myocardial ischemia and infarction.

The QRS complex in lead V6 typically begins with a very narrow **q wave** (**#8**), which is followed by a large **R wave.** The sort of complex usually seen in lead V1, an **rS** complex, is called a "right ventricular pattern" by some authors, and the **qR** pattern usually seen in lead V6 is called a "left ventricular pattern." It should be remembered, however, that any given QRS complex is the sum of all cardiac electrical events and not just those generated immediately beneath the positive pole of a particular lead (Marriott, 1983).

Low voltage is diagnosed when the total of all positive and negative deflections in leads I, II, and III is less than **15 millimeters** (Chung, 1980). The tracing in Figure 3–3 is an example of low voltage. The total height of all complexes in millimeters is indicated in leads I to III (4 + 5 + 4 = 13).

An examination of Figure 3–3 shows that the most nearly equiphasic complex in the precordial leads is in V3 (**RS**). The zone of transition is between leads V3 and V4 and is normal. Further abnormalities noted in this tracing are the inverted T waves in leads II, III, aVF, V5, and V6, and notched P waves, which are noted in nearly all leads.

The QRS complex shown in lead V1 of Figure 3–4 exhibits an **rSr** configuration (**1**), a normal variant found in approximately 5 per cent of the adult population (Burch and DePasquale, 1967). An additional point of interest is

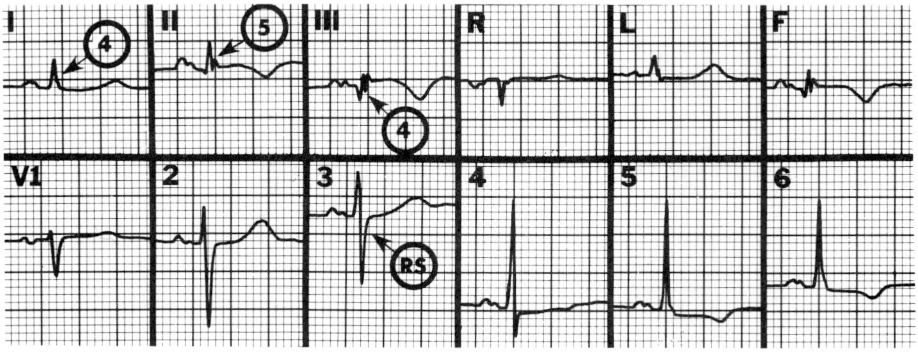

Figure 3–3. Low voltage in the limb leads (I, II, III).

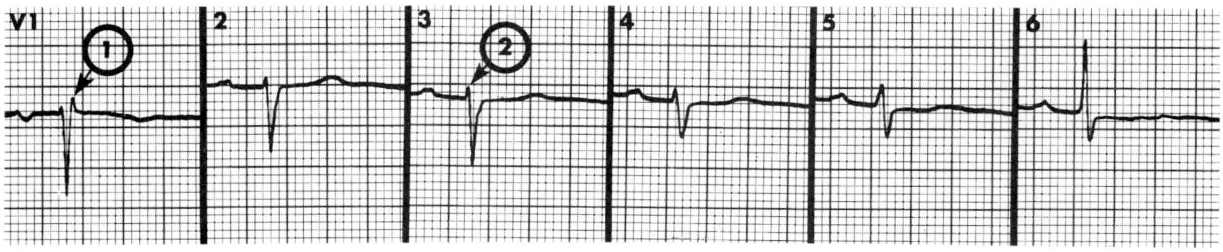

Figure 3–4. Poor R wave progression in the precordial leads.

seen in lead V3 (**2**), in which lead the initial r wave is less than 2 millimeters in height. **If the R wave in lead V3 is less than 2 millimeters tall,** a diagnosis of **poor R wave progression** is made. Tables 3–1 and 3–2 list some of the more common conditions associated with low voltage and poor R wave progression.

Ventricular activation and the QRS complex

In the discussion of mean QRS axis determination, it was mentioned that all the electrical forces that exist in the heart at any given moment during depolarization can be averaged together to obtain an **instantaneous vector.** The instantaneous vector, represented diagrammatically by an arrow, indicates the average **direction** and **amplitude** of the total electrical forces in progress at any instant. A basic understanding of the vector concept permits description of the sequence of ventricular activation in terms of a sequence of instantaneous

Table 3–1. CONDITIONS ASSOCIATED WITH LOW VOLTAGE

Emphysema
Pericardial effusion
Congestive failure
Myocardial infarction
Amyloidosis
Hypothyroidism
Extreme obesity

Table 3–2. CONDITIONS ASSOCIATED WITH POOR R WAVE PROGRESSION

Left ventricular hypertrophy
Anterior myocardial infarction
Emphysema
Left bundle branch block
Misplaced precordial leads

vectors produced as the wave of depolarization spreads through the myocardium. The more important vectors can then be related to the inscription of the deflections of the QRS complex in any lead.

Although the electrical wavefront represented by the instantaneous vector is three-dimensional, the leads employed for obtaining routine ECG tracings record the vector in only two of many possible planes. The bipolar (I, II, III) and unipolar (aVR, aVL, aVF) **limb leads** detect electrical activity in the **frontal** or coronal plane, and the **precordial leads** (V1–F6) detect activity in the **horizontal** or transverse plane. The orientation of these planes and leads is shown in Figure 3–1.

Depolarization of the atrioventricular node, the bundle of His, and the bundle branches produces no deflection on a tracing taken from the body surface because the electrical forces produced are too small to be detected at any distance. Depolarization of the ventricles begins on the surface of the left ventricular septum and results in an initial wave of depolarization that moves **anteriorly** and **rightward.** The initial septal activation generates an instantaneous vector, the **septal vector,** represented by **arrow 1** in Figure 3–5, which illustrates the direction and amplitude of the most important vectors in both the frontal and horizontal planes. Because the net movement of the septal vector is anterior and to the right, it is directed toward lead V1, which correspondingly records a small initial **r wave** in response (**1** in lead V1, Figure 3–5). Because the septal vector is moving away from the laterally oriented leads, they record a small initial **q wave** (**1** in leads I, aVL, V6).

From its septal origin the depolarization process spreads over the lower left and right sides of the septum and begins to penetrate the apical region of the ventricles. This wavefront is represented by an instantaneous vector, **arrow 2** in Figure 3–5, oriented along the long axis of the septum, directed **anteriorly** and **leftward** toward the positive pole of lead II. Because this vector is approximately perpendicular to lead V1, the initial positive deflection in that lead returns to the isoelectric line (**2** in V1). Leads facing anteriorly or leftward or both begin to record a positive deflection (R wave) in response to this vector (**2** in leads I, II, aVL, V6). Lead aVR, which faces away from the net movement of vector 2, begins the inscription of a negative complex (**2** in aVR).

The depolarization wave moves next into the thick anterior and lateral walls of the left ventricle. This phase of myocardial activation is represented by an instantaneous vector (**arrow 3**) moving **leftward, posteriorly,** and **inferiorly.** Those leads facing away from this strong vector will complete the inscription of a deeply negative deflection or S wave (**3** in aVR, V1), while leads facing the movement of this, the **left ventricular vector,** will complete the

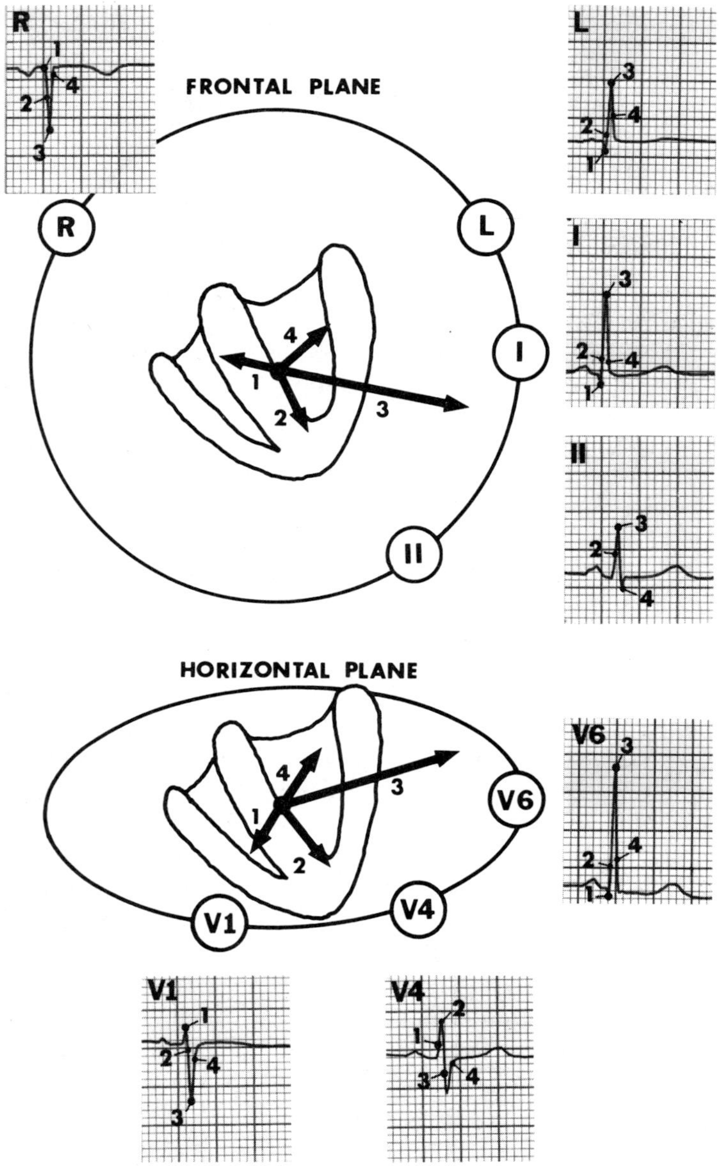

Figure 3–5. Four instantaneous vectors and their contributions to the normal electrocardiogram.

inscription of a tall positive deflection or R wave (**3** in leads I, II, aVL, V6). The horizontal plane (precordial) lead most nearly perpendicular to the net direction of this important vector will write an equiphasic (RS) transition complex (**2–3** in V4).

Activation of the thick basal walls of the ventricles, the base of the left ventricular "cone," marks the completion of the depolarization process and results in a final vector directed **posteriorly, leftward,** and **superiorly.** This vector is represented by **arrow 4.** Leads facing away from the net movement of this vector record the distal limb of a predominant S wave (**4** in aVR and

V1), while those leads facing the movement of vector 4 complete the descending limb of a predominant R wave (**4** in I, aVL, V6) or complete the inscription of a small terminal s wave (**4** in II, V4).

An examination of Figure 3–5 with its representative leads reveals that the small initial r wave in the right precordial leads (V1, V2) and the small initial q wave in the lateral leads (I, aVL, V5, V6) are the result of septal depolarization (vector 1). For this reason, the small q waves, which are normal features in the lateral leads, are often called **septal q waves.**

The deep S waves characteristic of the right precordial leads (V1, V2) and lead aVR of the frontal leads represent powerful forces generated in the thick anterolateral left ventricular wall (vector 3). The precordial transition complex, which is normally found in lead V3 or V4, will be seen in whichever lead is most nearly perpendicular to this major vector. If vector 3 is directed more anteriorly than normal, lead V1 or V2 will be more nearly perpendicular to its net movement and a transition complex will appear in V1 or V2. The result, early transition, reflects **anterior** axis deviation in the horizontal plane. This may occur as a normal variant or may represent a reorientation of electrical forces due to right ventricular hypertrophy. If vector 3 is directed more posteriorly than usual, lead V5 or V6 will then be more nearly perpendicular to its movement and the transition complex (RS) will appear in V5 or V6. The result, late transition, reflects **posterior** axis deviation in the horizontal plane, which may occur as a normal variant or in response to a shift of forces due to left ventricular hypertrophy.

Right ventricular forces are represented in vectors 1 and 2 but are quickly overshadowed by the much greater forces generated in the thicker walls of the left ventricle (vector 3). The four instantaneous vectors selected to represent the sequence of ventricular activation will be invoked again in the following chapter to illustrate the altered sequence due to bundle branch blocks and to explain the typical QRS deformities that result.

References

Burch, GE, DePasquale, NP. **Electrocardiography in the Diagnosis of Congenital Heart Disease.** Lea & Febiger, Philadelphia, 1967, p 57.

Chung, K. **Electrocardiography, Practical Applications with Vectorial Principles,** 2nd ed. Harper & Row, New York, 1980, p 32.

Marriott, JL. **Practical Electrocardiography,** 7th ed. Williams & Wilkins, Baltimore, 1983, p 46–47.

SELF-ASSESSMENT

Multiple Choice

1. The indifferent electrode of the precordial or horizontal plane leads is:

   a. the fifth intercostal space, midclavicular line.
   b. in the same orientation as frontal plane lead I.
   c. the Wilson central terminal.
   d. the fourth intercostal space to the right of the sternum.

2. Leads V1 and V2 predominantly face:

   a. the ventricular septum.
   b. the surface of the left ventricle.
   c. the surface of the right ventricle.
   d. the base of the ventricular cone.

3. The V6 position is in:

   a. the fifth intercostal space, left midclavicular line.
   b. the fourth intercostal space to the left of the sternum.
   c. the fifth intercostal space, left midaxillary line.
   d. the fourth intercostal space to the right of the sternum.

4. The normal "right ventricular pattern" consists of:

   a. an RS complex.
   b. a qR complex.
   c. a QR complex.
   d. an rS complex.

5. An equiphasic (RS) transition complex seen in lead V2 is an indication of:

   a. early transition.
   b. normal transition.
   c. late transition.
   d. transition to the left of normal.

6. Low voltage is diagnosed when the positive and negative components of the QRS complex in leads ______ total less than ______.

   a. aVR, aVL, aVF
   b. I, II, III
   c. V1 to V6
   d. I, aVL

   a. 10 mm
   b. 12 mm
   c. 15 mm
   d. 20 mm

7. Poor R wave progression is diagnosed when the R wave in lead ______ is less than ______ in height.

a. V1
b. V2
c. V3
d. V4

a. 1 mm
b. 2 mm
c. 3 mm
d. 4 mm

8. The T wave in lead V1 may normally be ______ in adults.

a. positive only
b. positive or biphasic
c. negative or biphasic
d. positive, biphasic, or negative

9. The limb leads (I, II, aVR, aVL, aVF) detect electrical activity in the ______ plane and the precordial leads (V1 to V6) detect electrical activity in the ______ plane.

a. frontal
b. null
c. horizontal
d. transition

a. horizontal
b. frontal
c. null
d. transition

10. All the electrical forces which exist in the heart at any given moment during depolarization can be averaged together to obtain a single:

a. mean QRS axis.
b. positive deflection.
c. instantaneous vector.
d. transition complex.

11. Depolarization of the left ventricular septum results in the inscription of ______ in lead V1 and the inscription of ______ in leads I and aVL.

a. a small initial r wave
b. a small initial q wave
c. a transition (RS) complex
d. an S wave

a. a small initial q wave
b. a small initial r wave
c. a transition (RS) complex
d. an R wave

12. Depolarization of the anterior and lateral left ventricular wall results in the inscription of ______ in lead V1 and the inscription of ______ in leads V5 and V6.

a. a tall R wave
b. a deep S wave
c. a Q wave
d. a transition (RS) complex

a. a tall R wave
b. a deep S wave
c. a Q wave
d. a transition (RS) complex

13. If an electrode in any plane or lead records a transition (RS) complex, the electrical forces sensed by that electrode are:

a. moving toward the electrode.
b. ignored for the purpose of axis calculation.
c. assigned a numerical value to zero degrees.
d. moving perpendicularly (at a right angle) to the lead.

14. The normal "left ventricular pattern" consists of:

a. a qR complex.
b. an rS complex.
c. an RS complex.
d. a Q wave.

Practice Strips

Determine the axis, zone of transition, voltage, and R wave progression in the ECGs that follow. Identify the arrhythmias when applicable.

3-1.

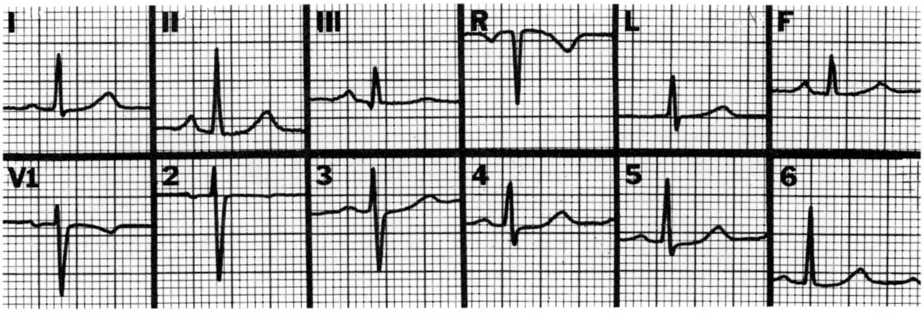

3-2.

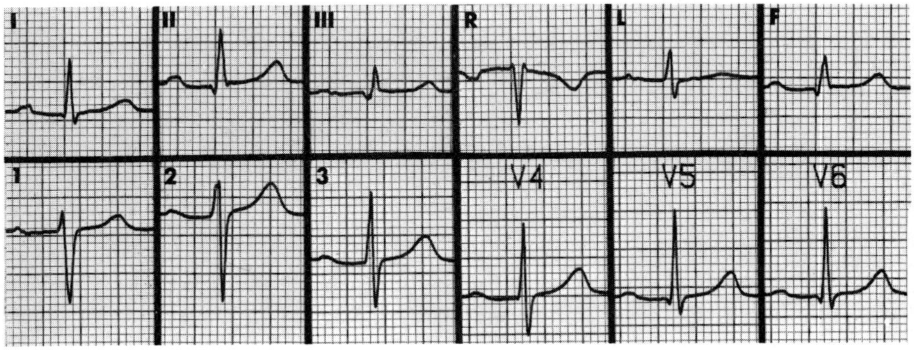

3·3.

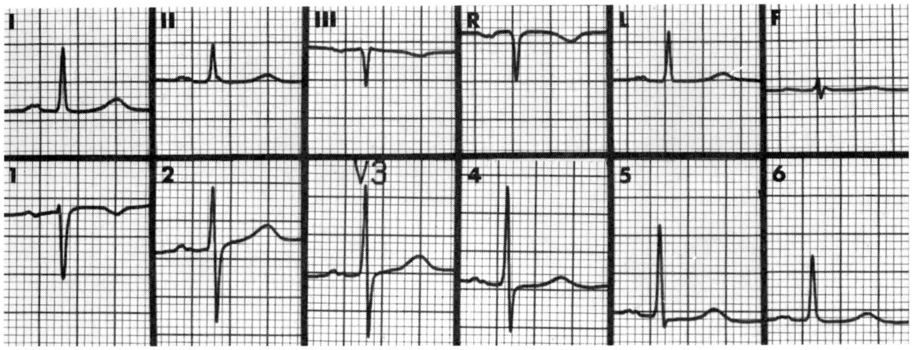
I
II
III
R
L
F
1
2
V3
4
5
6

3·4.

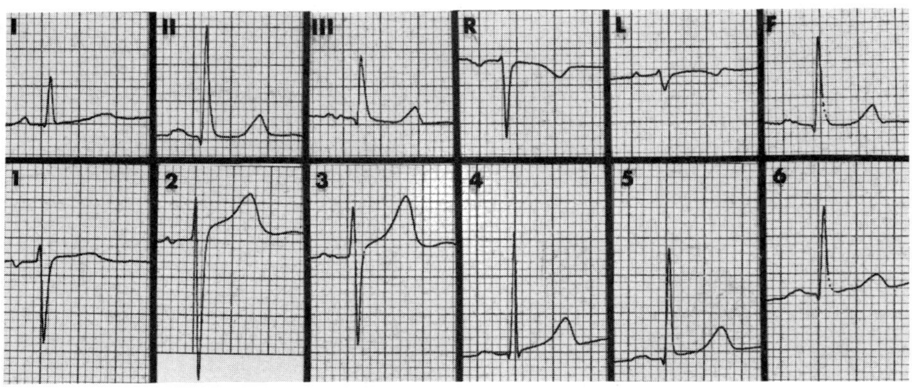
I
II
III
R
L
F
1
2
3
4
5
6

3·5.

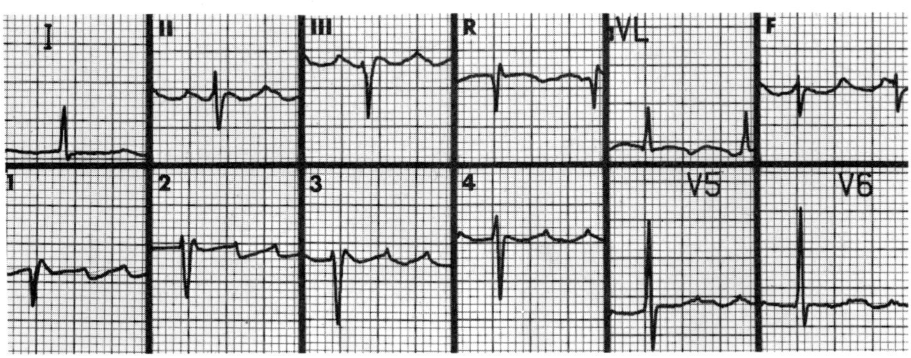
I
II
III
R
aVL
F
1
2
3
4
V5
V6

3·6.

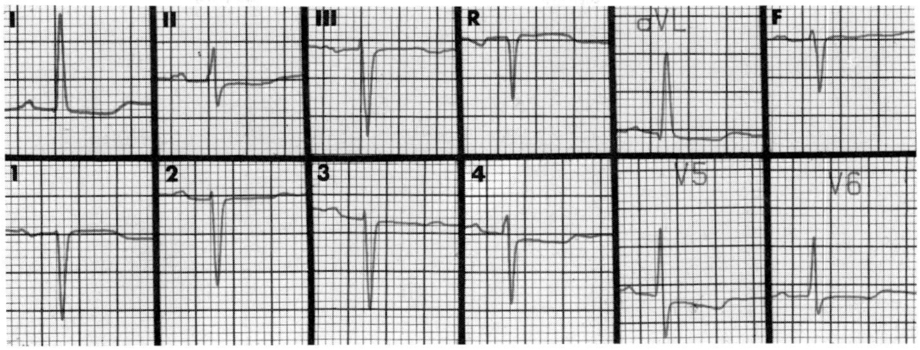
I
II
III
R
aVL
F
1
2
3
4
V5
V6

3·7.

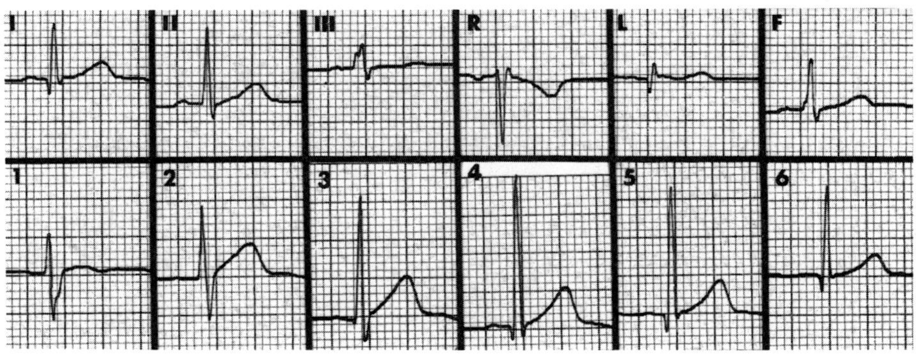
I
II
III
R
L
F
1
2
3
4
5
6

3·8.

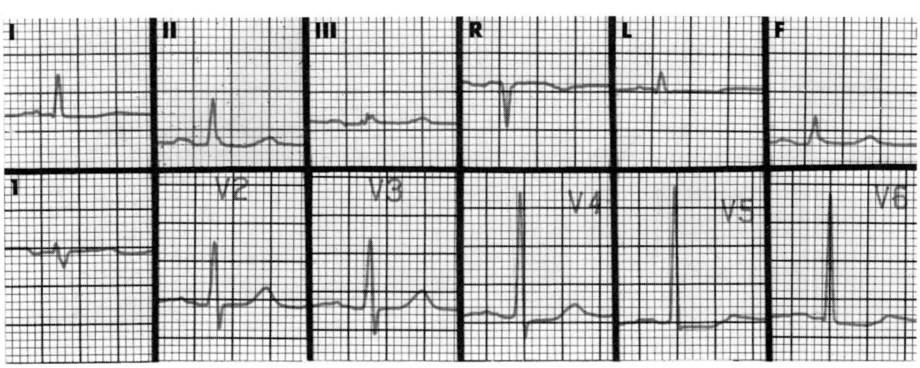
I
II
III
R
L
F
1
V2
V3
V4
V5
V6

3-9.

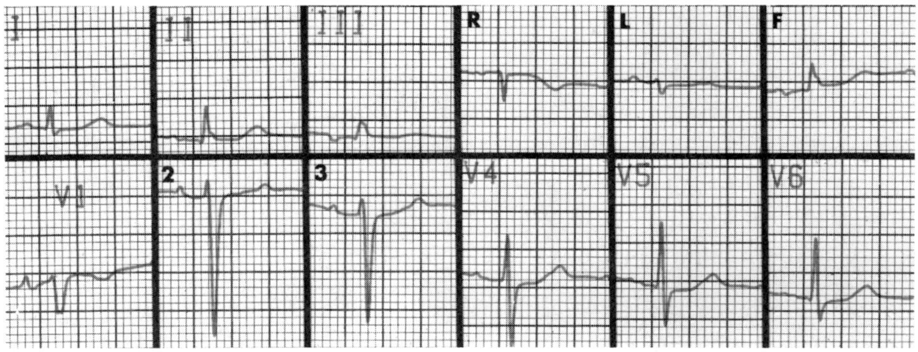
I
II
III
R
L
F
V1
2
3
V4
V5
V6

3-10.

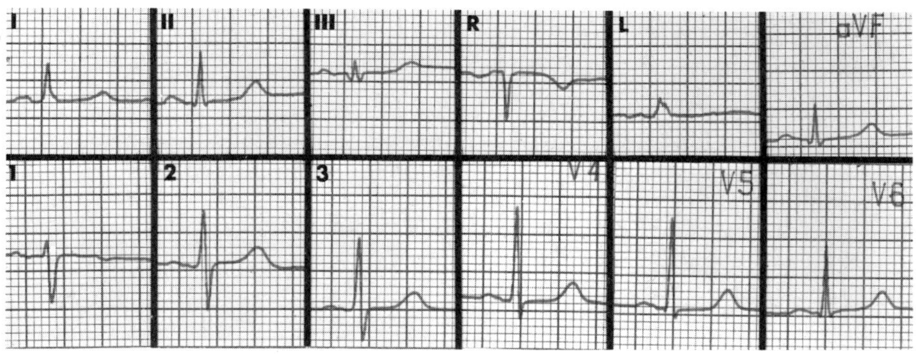
I
II
III
R
L
aVF
1
2
3
V4
V5
V6

3-11.

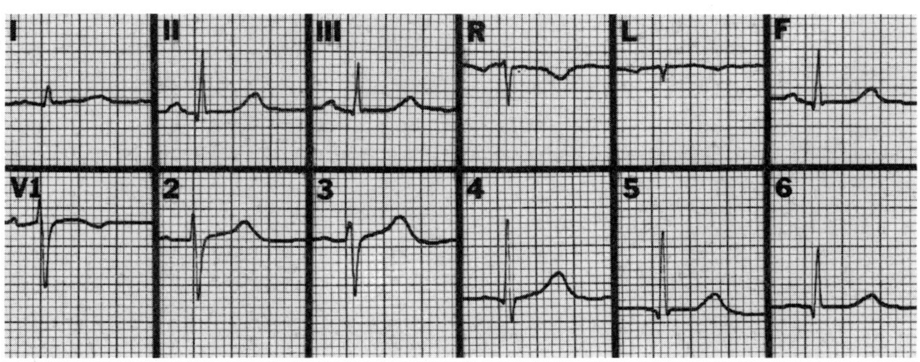
I
II
III
R
L
F
V1
2
3
4
5
6

3-12.

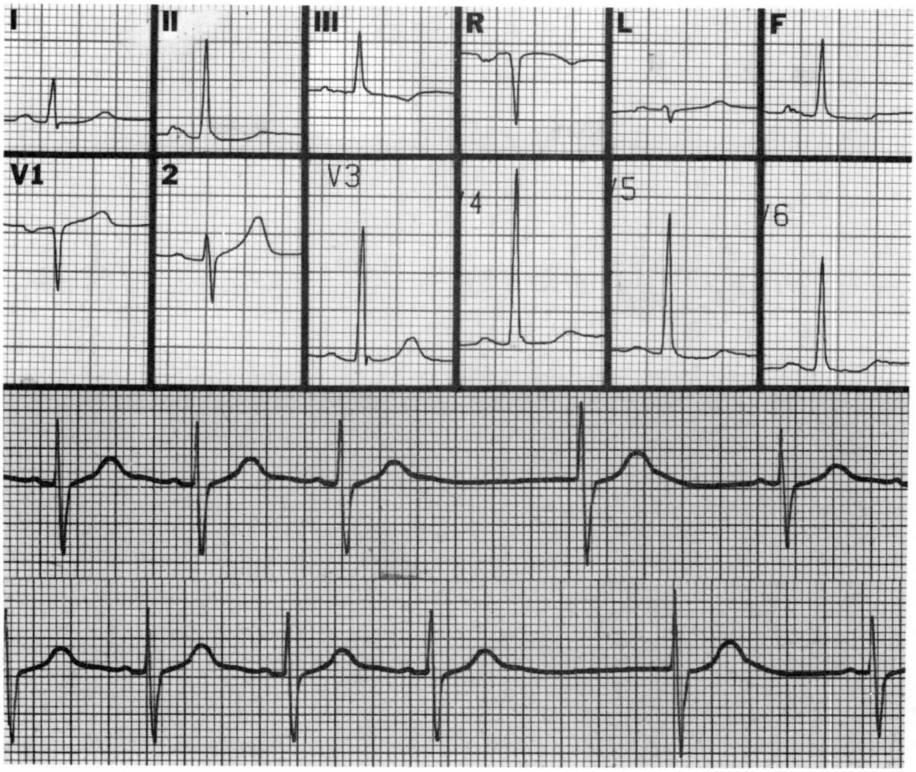

3-13.

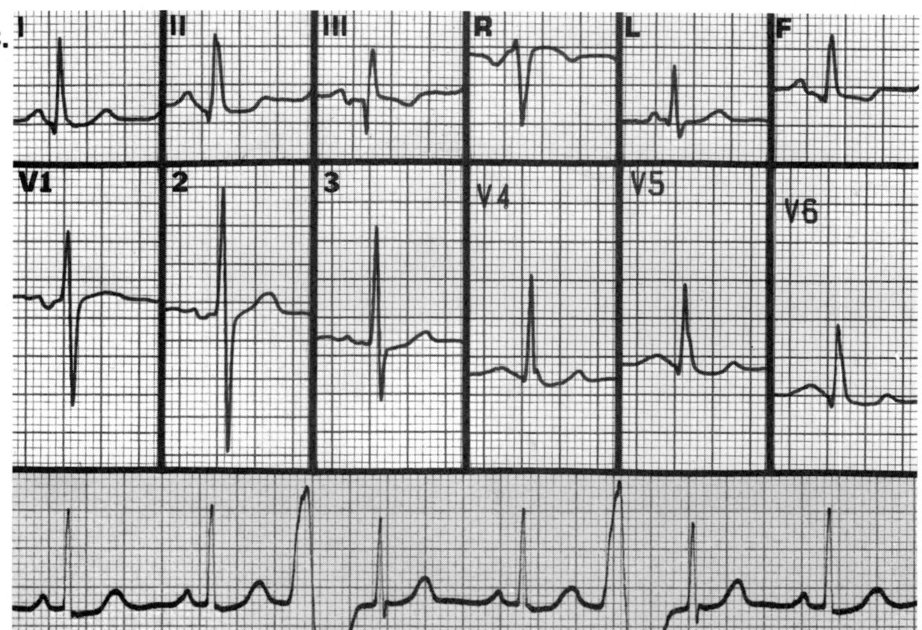

3-14.

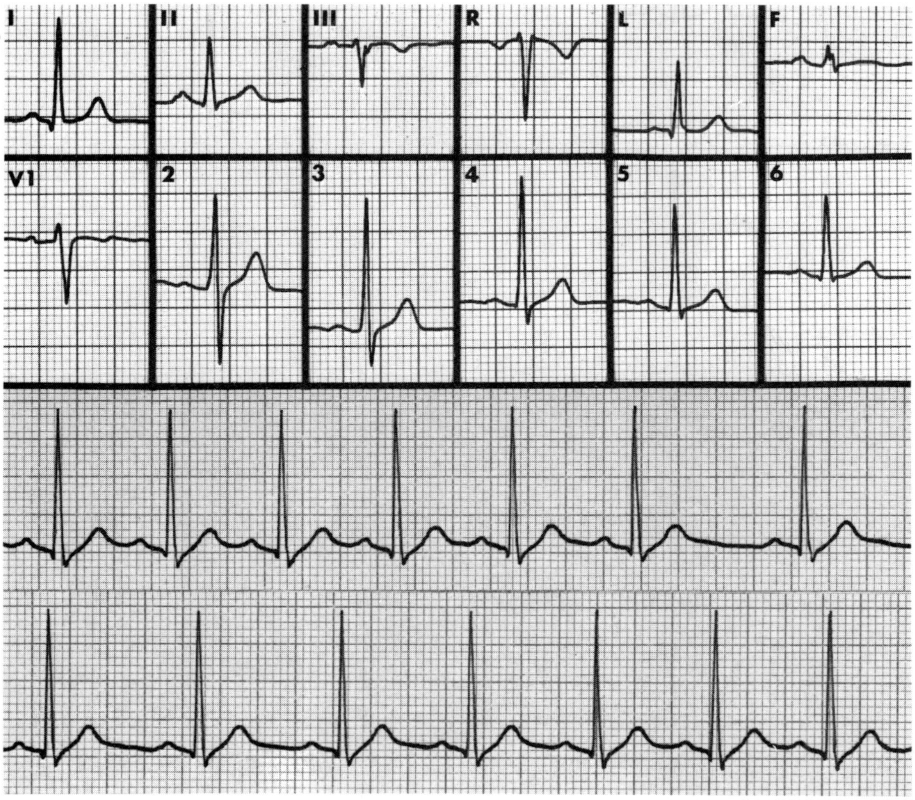

3-15.

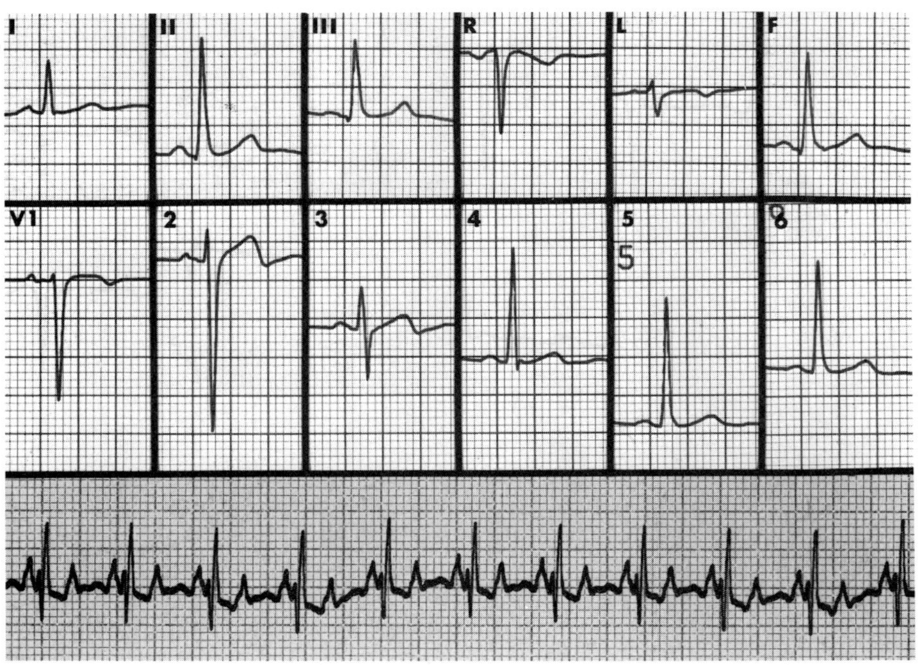

ANSWER KEY

Multiple Choice

1. c
2. c
3. c
4. d
5. a
6. b, c
7. c, b
8. d
9. a, a
10. c
11. a, a
12. b, a
13. d
14. a

Practice Strips

3–1. Normal axis, +45 to +55 degrees.
Normal transition, between V3 and V4.
Normal voltage and normal R wave progression.

3–2. Normal axis, +25 to +35 degrees.
Normal transition, between V2 and V3.
Normal voltage and normal R wave progression.
First-degree AV block (PR 0.24).

3–3. Normal axis, +5 to −5 degrees.
Normal transition, between V2 and V3.
Normal voltage and normal R wave progression.

3–4. Normal axis, +65 to +75 degrees.
Normal transition, between V3 and V4.
Normal voltage and normal R wave progression.

3–5. Left axis deviation, −50 to −60 degrees.
Late transition, V4 to V5.
Normal voltage and poor R wave progression.
Atrial flutter.

3–6. Late axis deviation, −10 to −20 degrees.
Late transition, between V4 and V5.
Normal voltage and poor R wave progression.
Biphasic T waves in leads V4 to V6.

3–7. Normal axis, +55 to +65 degrees.
Early transition, between V1 and V2.
Normal voltage and normal R wave progression.

3–8. Normal axis, +30 to +40 degrees.
Early transition, between V1 and V2.
Low voltage (12.5), normal R wave progression.

3–9. Normal axis, +55 to +65 degrees.
Late transition, V4 to V5.
Low voltage (12.0), poor R wave progression.

3–10. Normal axis, +55 to +65 degrees.
Early transition, V1 to V2.
Normal voltage, normal R wave progression.

3–11. Normal axis, +55 to +65 degrees.
Normal ECG.

3–12. Normal axis, +55 to +65 degrees.
Normal ECG.
Sinus rhythm, 79/minute, sinoatrial block with junctional escape beats.

3–13. Normal axis, +45 to +55 degrees.
Early transition, V2.
Sinus rhythm, 80/minute, interpolated premature ventricular complexes.

3–14. Normal axis, +5 to +15 degrees.
Early transition, V2.
Marked sinus arrhythmia, 65 to 100/minute.

3–15. Normal axis, +65 to +75 degrees.
Biphasic T waves in V2 and V3, otherwise unremarkable.
Atrial tachycardia, 250/minute with 2:1 atrioventricular conduction.

CHAPTER FOUR

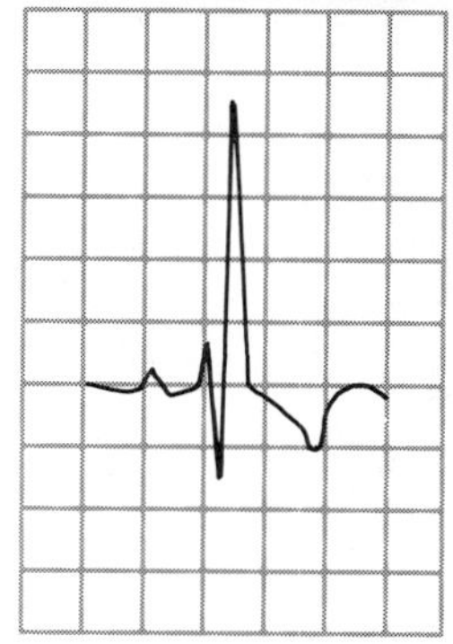

INTRAVENTRICULAR CONDUCTION DEFECTS

COGNITIVE GOALS

1. Name the major parts of the fibrous skeleton of the heart and describe its relationship to the distal conduction system.
2. Name the distal fascicles of the conduction system and identify the main source of blood supply for each.
3. Define the terms **fascicular block** and **bundle branch block.**
4. Give the diagnostic criteria for left anterior fascicular block.
5. Give the diagnostic criteria for left posterior fascicular block.
6. Discuss the correlation of fascicular block by ECG with the results of histopathologic studies of the left bundle branch.
7. Give the diagnostic criteria for right bundle branch block.
8. Give the diagnostic criteria for left bundle branch block.
9. Define the term **multifascicular block** and give at least two examples of expected ECG findings.
10. Describe how the criterion of total waveform area is used to determine the relative negativity or positivity of a QRS deflection.
11. Describe the essential pathology of Lenègre's disease.
12. Describe the essential pathology of Lev's disease.

The fibrous skeleton of the heart

The fibrous skeleton of the heart is a complex body of connective tissue that serves to anchor the atrial and ventricular muscle bundles and to secure the cusps of the atrioventricular and semilunar valves. Because it is intimately related to various parts of the distal conduction system, a basic grasp of its anatomy is essential to an understanding of the pathology of several important forms of atrioventricular and intraventricular block.

Each of the four heart valves is surrounded by a ring of fibrous tissue, the **annulus,** which serves as a line of attachment for the fixed edges of the valve cusps. The contiguous annuli are connected to each other by dense tissue (Fig. 4–1). The mitral and aortic annuli are fused at their left point of contact by a small triangular area of tissue, the **left fibrous trigone** (**lft** in Fig. 4–1). The

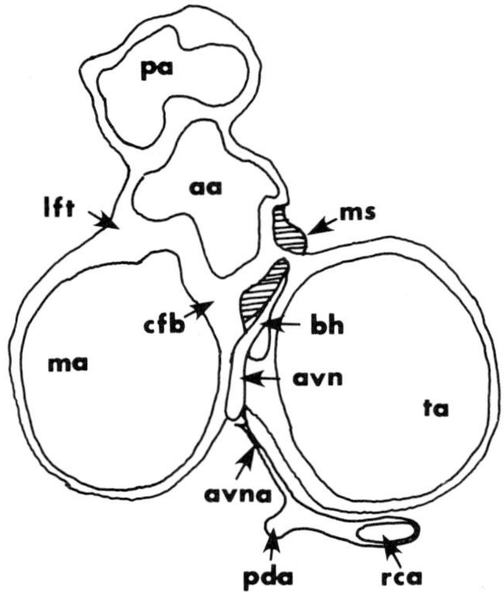

Figure 4–1. The fibrous skeleton of the heart. aa = aortic annulus; avn = AV node; avna = AV nodal artery; bh = bundle of His; cfb = central fibrous body; lft = left fibrous trigone; ma = mitral annulus; ms = membranous septum; pa = pulmonic annulus; pda = posterior descending artery; rca = right coronary artery; ta = tricuspid annulus.

mitral, tricuspid and aortic annuli are fused at their mutual point of contact by another core of connective tissue, the **right fibrous trigone** or **central fibrous body (cfb).**

An extension of the central fibrous body and part of the aortic annulus projects downward as the **membranous intraventricular septum (ms),** a thin, tough partition that separates the upper parts of the ventricular chambers. The membranous septum is continuous below with the much thicker summit of the muscular interventricular septum.

There is a very close association between the fibrous skeleton and the conduction system. The atrioventricular node is situated against the mitral annulus, and the bundle of His penetrates the central fibrous body, passes downward in the posterior edge of the membranous septum, and branches into the left and right bundle branches at the summit of the muscular septum. The fascicles of the left bundle branch are closely adjacent to the aortic annulus and the summit of the muscular septum. Congenital deformities of the valves, great vessels, and atrial or ventricular septa are accompanied by derangements of the fibrous skeleton and sometimes by conduction disturbances. Pathologic changes in the central skeleton caused by the stress of systemic hypertension or valvular disease are also associated with a significant increase in the incidence of distal conduction disturbances (Lev, 1964; Bharati, 1976).

The distal conduction system

The atrioventricular node (of Tawara) is situated in the lower atrial septum adjacent to the annulus of the mitral valve. Resting above the septal leaflet of the tricuspid valve, anterior to the ostium of the coronary sinus, it is supplied by the **nodal branch** of the right coronary artery in 90 per cent of subjects and by a corresponding branch of the circumflex in the remaining 10 per cent (Hurst et al, 1982.)

The **atrioventricular bundle** (of His) begins at the distal artrioventricular node, penetrates the midportion of the central fibrous body, and descends in the posterior margin of the membranous septum to the summit of the muscular septum. The posterior and septal fascicles of the left bundle branch arise as a continuous sheet from the His bundle along the crest of the septum. At its terminus, the His bundle bifurcates to form the anterior fascicle of the left bundle branch and the single slender fascicle of the right bundle branch. In about half of the population there is a dual blood supply to the bundle of His derived from the **nodal branch** of the right coronary artery and the **first septal perforating branch** of the left anterior descending artery (see Fig. 5–3). In the remainder, the His bundle is supplied by the posterior descending branch of the right coronary artery alone (Hurst, 1982).

The **right bundle branch** arises at the bifurcation of the His bundle, its fibers diverging from those of the anterior fascicle of the left bundle branch. The right bundle branch, a long, slender fascicle, travels within the muscle of the ventricular septum or immediately beneath the endocardium to the base of the anterior papillary muscle. The blood supply of the right bundle is derived from both the **nodal branch** of the right coronary artery and the **first septal perforator** of the anterior descending artery in about 50 per cent of the population and from the first septal perforator alone in the rest (Schlant and Hurst, 1972).

The initial portion of the **left bundle branch** is related to the noncoronary and right coronary cusps of the aortic valve. Its fibers fan out from the length of the His bundle along the crest of the muscular septum and are organized into three recognized fascicles.

The **left anterior fascicle** of the left bundle branch, the longest and thinnest of the fiber tracts, diverges from the rest to reach the base of the anterior papillary muscle of the mitral valve. This fascicle receives its blood supply from the **septal perforating branches** of the left anterior descending artery. Anatomically and physiologically the left anterior fascicle and the right bundle branch are bilateral complements of each other: they are structurally similar, share a common blood supply, and are the two fascicles most likely to block (Hurst et al, 1982; Krickler and Goodwin, 1975).

The **middle** or **centroseptal fascicle** arises from the angle between the anterior and posterior fascicles of the left bundle branch or occasionally from one or both of the other fascicles. Numerous interconnections are known to exist between the three major fascicles. In an elegant study, Durrer and associates found that left ventricular activation started simultaneously in three widely separate areas on the left ventricular endocardial surface (Durrer et al, 1970). It is believed that these three islands of initial excitation correspond to the distribution of the three main fascicles of the left bundle branch. With the recognition of a third, septal, fascicle in the left bundle, the distal conduction system is now widely regarded as **quadrifascicular** rather than trifascicular in nature (Hecht et al, 1973; Krikler and Goodwin, 1975; Mandel et al, 1980; Marriott, 1983; Massing and James, 1976; Uhley, 1972, 1979; Wellens, Lie and Janse, 1976).

The **left posterior fascicle** is a short, fan-shaped tract of fibers that is directed toward the base of the posterior papillary muscle. Its blood supply is derived from both the **nodal branch** of the right coronary artery and the **septal perforating branches** of the left anterior descending artery in 50 per cent of subjects and from the nodal branch alone in the remainder.

Electrocardiographic criteria and anatomic correlations

Certain ECG patterns emerge when relative or absolute conduction loss occurs in either or both of the main bundle branches or in the fascicles of the left bundle branch. These ECG patterns are called **bundle branch blocks** and **fascicular blocks,** respectively. The diagnostic criteria for the bundle branch and fascicular blocks are described in detail subsequently.

Left anterior fascicular block

Conduction delay or loss in the anterior fascicle of the left bundle branch (**LAFB** in Fig. 4–2), the most common of the intraventricular conduction defects, reorients the normal mean vector upward and to the left, resulting in left axis

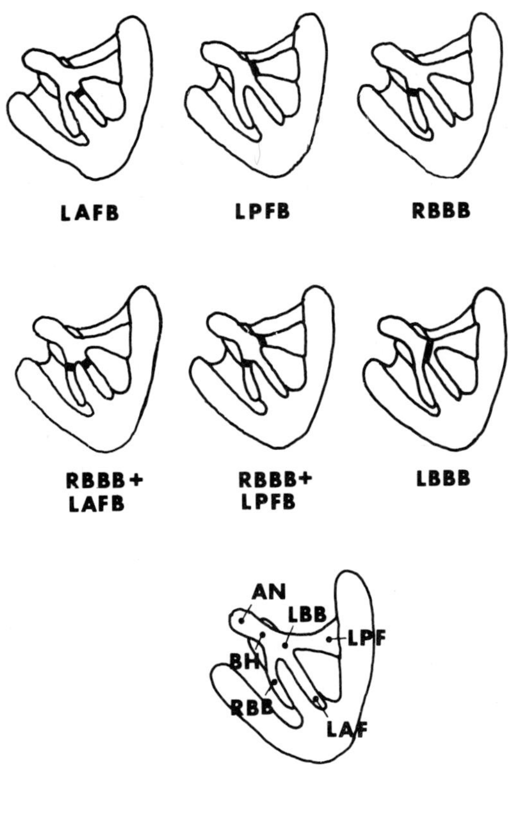

Figure 4–2. Fascicular and bifascicular blocks. AN = atrioventricular node; BH = bundle of His; LAF = left anterior fascicle; LAFB = left anterior fascicular block; LPF = left posterior fascicle; LPFB = left posterior fascicular block; LBB = left bundle branch; LBBB = left bundle branch block; RBB = right bundle branch; RBBB = right bundle branch block.

deviation (−30 to −90 degrees) and certain characteristic changes in the QRS complex. Small initial **r waves** and deep, terminal **S waves** appear in the inferior leads, II, III, and aVF (**3** and **4** in Fig. 4–3). Small **q waves** followed by tall **R waves** are noted in the lateral leads I and aVL (**1** and **2** in Fig. 4–3). Notching is sometimes observed in the terminal part of the QRS complex in aVR **(5)**, and the small initial Q waves, or septal Q waves, normally seen in leads V5 and V6 are often replaced by S waves **(7)**. Late transition or poor R wave progression, or both, are other features commonly noted in cases of left anterior fascicular block **(6)**.

Attempts to correlate the ECG criteria for left anterior fascicular block (LAFB) with observable lesions found postmortem in the left anterior fascicle have not met with any consistent success. Investigators have established that the ECG finding of LAFB indicates disease in the left bundle branch, sometimes in the anterior radiations of the left bundle branch prior to its division into fascicles (Bharati et al, 1976), in the anteriorly directed fibers of the anterior and septal fascicles, or in all three main fascicles of the left bundle (Demoulin and Kulbertus, 1972; Demoulin, Simar, and Kulbertus, 1975; Entman et al, 1967; Hecht et al, 1973; Rosen et al, 1973; Rossi, 1976). In a recent histopathologic study of eleven hearts done by Nakaya, Hiraga and Mori, LAFB was found to correlate with "widely distributed" lesions of the anterior and mid-septal portions of the left bundle branch. In all cases the left bundle branch was found to be a widely splayed, fanlike structure (Nakaya et al, 1987). The preponderance of available evidence suggests that attempts to draw an exact correlation between the electrocardiographic entity of LAFB and disease confined to the anatomic left anterior fascicle are unwarranted (Hurst et al, 1982; Marriott, 1983).

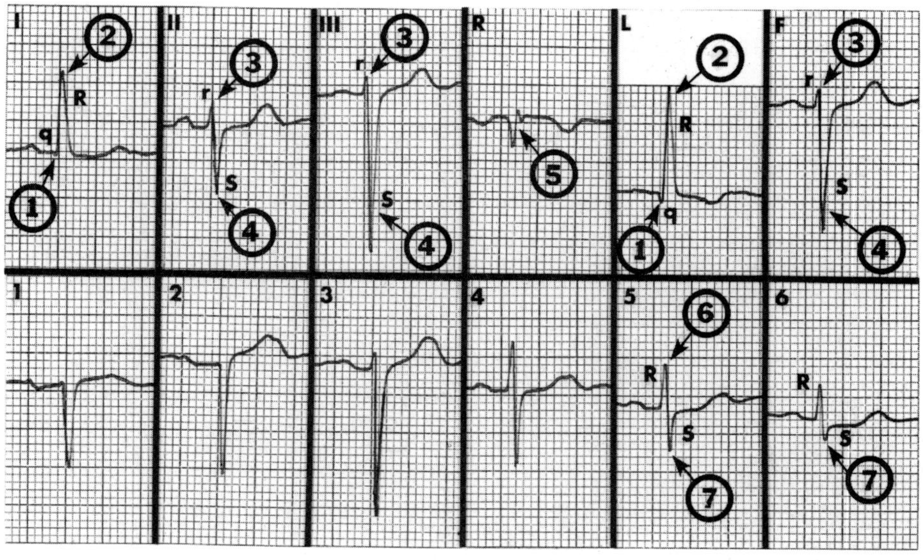

Figure 4–3. The electrocardiogram of left anterior fascicular block.

Left posterior fascicular block

Isolated conduction delay or loss in the left posterior fascicle (**LPFB** in Fig. 4–2), the least common of the intraventricular conduction defects, reorients the mean cardiac vector downward and to the right (+100 to +180 degrees). The typical resulting changes in the QRS complex consist of small initial **r waves** (**1** in Fig. 4–4) and deep **S waves** (**2** in Fig. 4–4) in the lateral leads I and aVL, and small initial **q waves (3)** and tall **R waves (4)** in the most inferior leads, III and aVF. LPFB almost always occurs in conjunction with right bundle branch block as in the case illustrated in Figure 4–4. Owing to its relative rarity and the fact that fewer histopathologic correlative studies have been done on this lesion, the exact criteria for LPFB are somewhat arbitrary. For example, some authorities accept a mean axis of +90 degrees as evidence of LPFB (Chou, 1986).

Attempts to correlate the ECG pattern of LPFB with discrete lesions of the left posterior fascicle have been essentialy unsuccessful. It is established that lesions found in the left bundle branch at necropsy do not correspond with the lesions that would have been predicted on the basis of ECGs taken during life (Rosen et al, 1973). Several studies have found a correlation between LPFB and severe obstructive lesions of the left anterior descending and right coronary arteries, with lesions of the posterior radiations of the left bundle branch, or with lesions of the main body of the left bundle before its division into fascicles (Demoulin and Kulbertus, 1979; Rizzon et al, 1975). In the setting of acute myocardial infarction, LPFB implies extensive, often complete, necrosis of the ventricular septum. Not surprisingly, occluding lesions of both the right and anterior descending coronary arteries are documented causes (Becker, Lie, and Anderson, 1978; Demoulin and Kulbertus, 1979; Nimetz et al, 1975; Rizzon et al, 1975). In a recent study in which transient LPFB during myocardial ischemia and infarction was correlated with angiographic findings, Sclarovsky and his

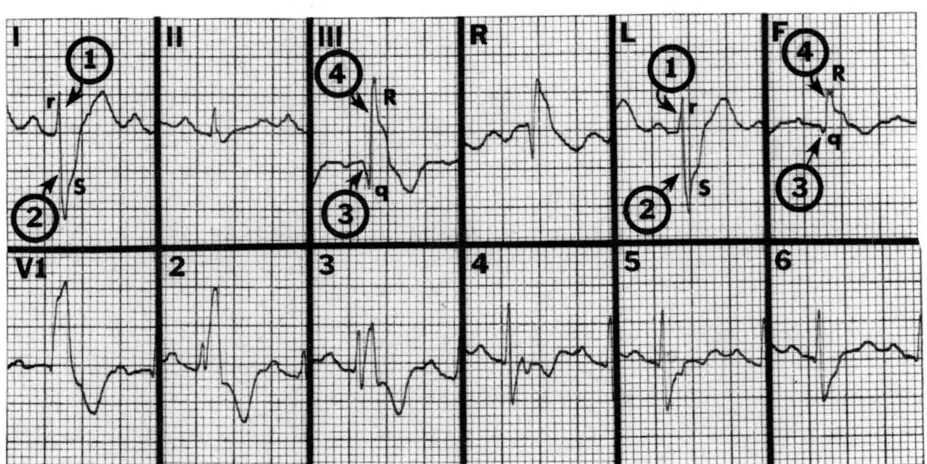

Figure 4–4. The electrocardiogram of left posterior fascicular block.

associates consistently documented significant right coronary artery stenosis in addition to severe left anterior descending artery blockage (Sclarovsky et al, 1986).

The criteria for fascicular blocks are given in Table 4–1. Many authors still use the older term "hemiblock" to describe fascicular block patterns. Because the older term seems to imply "half a block" (Marriott, 1983), appropriate terminology only if the left bundle branch is conceived of as divided into two equal halves, it has not been employed in this text (Uhley, 1972, 1979).

Right bundle branch block

Right bundle branch block results in certain characteristic deformities of the QRS complex, which include (1) **QRS prolongation** to 0.12 second or more; (2) the appearance of an **rSR′ pattern** in the right precordial leads, particularly V1 and V2; (3) a **wide S wave** in the lateral leads I, aVL, V5, and V6; and (4) an **increased ventricular activation time** in the right precordial leads. The mean QRS axis may be normal or may be deviated leftward or rightward, particularly when the right bundle branch block coexists with left fascicular blocks, as is frequently the case.

The ECG pattern of right bundle branch block (RBBB) is illustrated in Figure 4–5. The QRS duration is prolonged to 0.14 second, the right percordial leads

Table 4–1. DIAGNOSTIC CRITERIA FOR CONDUCTION DEFECTS

Left Anterior Fascicular Block (LAFB)
qR complexes in I and aVL
rS complexes in II, III, aVF
Left axis deviation (−30 to −90 degrees)
Left Posterior Fascicular Block (LPFB)
rS complexes in I and aVL
qR complexes in II, III, aVF
Right axis deviation (+95 to +220 degrees)
Right Bundle Branch Block (RBBB)
rSR′ pattern in V1
Slurred, wide S waves in I, aVL, V5, and V6
Inverted T wave in V1
Prolonged VAT in V1 (greater than 0.035 second)
QRS duration 0.12 second or more
Left Bundle Branch Block (LBBB)
rS or QS in V1
No Q waves in I, aVL, or V6
R wave in I, aVL, V6 (usually notched or slurred)
Inverted T wave in V6
Prolonged VAT in V6 (greater than 0.045 second)
QRS duration 0.12 second or more
Bilateral Bundle Branch Block (BBBB)
Mobitz type II 2nd-degree block
Alternating right and left bundle branch block
Nonspecific Intraventricular Conduction Delay (NSIVCD)
QRS duration 0.12 second or more
QRS morphology that does not meet the criteria for right or left bundle branch block

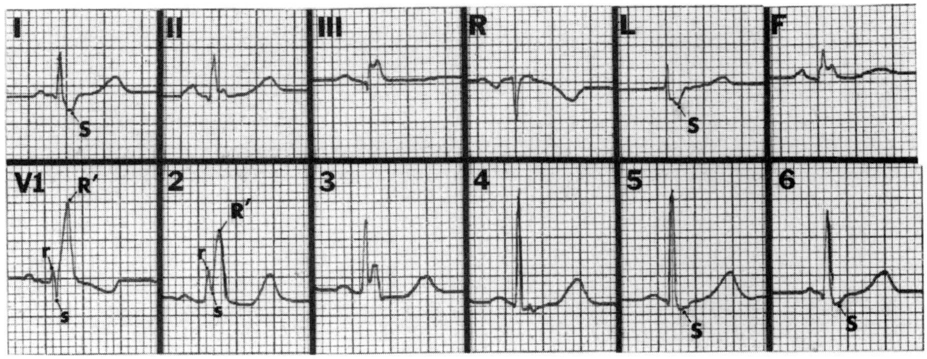

Figure 4–5. The electrocardiogram of right bundle branch block.

(V1, V2) exhibit an rSR′ configuration, and the lateral leads (I, aVL, V5, V6) display the typical widened, slurred terminal S waves. The second R wave in lead V1 is normally taller than the primary R wave, but the complex in V1 is variable and may assume the shape of a widened, notched single R wave. In cases of septal infarction, the initial small R wave is lost and an abnormally wide **qR** complex results in lead V1. The T wave in V1 is normally inverted in RBBB due to the abnormal sequence of ventricular depolarization.

Increased ventricular activation time (VAT) in the right precordial leads reflects delayed or absent conduction in the right bundle branch. The ventricular activation time is reflected by the **QR** interval, measured from the beginning of the QRS complex to the lowest point of the S wave in lead V1 in cases of normal intraventricular conduction, or from the beginning of the QRS complex to the peak of the R′ (R prime) wave in cases of RBBB. The normal QR interval does not exceed 0.035 second in lead V1. In cases of RBBB, the QR interval (VAT) is often delayed to 0.07 second or more (Friedman, 1977). Figure 4–6 shows both a slightly prolonged QR interval (0.04 second) and a markedly prolonged QR interval (0.11 second) typical of RBBB.

Extensive damage to the right bundle branch as determined by histopathologic studies correlates very well with the RBBB pattern on the ECG. However, an RBBB **pattern** cannot be taken to prove that the **anatomical** right bundle branch is totally incapable of impulse transmission (Bharati et al, 1976; Wu et al, 1974).

Ventricular activation in right bundle branch block

Because the integrity of the left bundle branch is undisturbed, ventricular activation begins normally in the case of RBBB, starting from the surface of the middle third of the left ventricular septum. The electrical forces generated by initial septal activation are directed **anteriorly** and **rightward** and produce a normal **septal vector** (**arrow 1** in Figure 4–7). The septal vector, which is responsible for the small initial **r wave** in lead V1, is lost in the event that

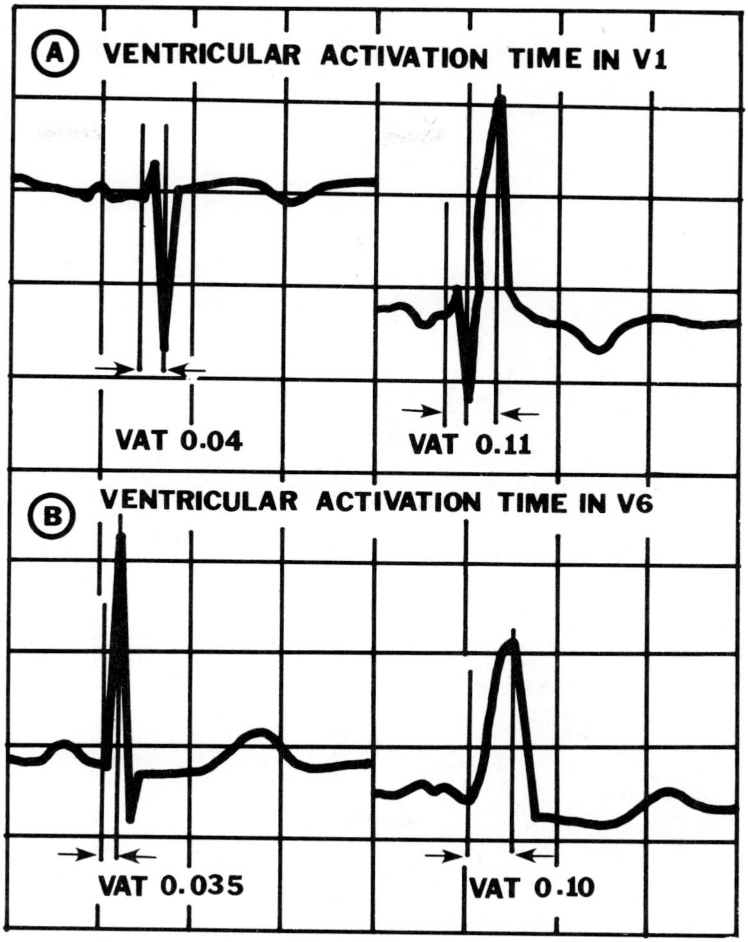

Figure 4–6. Ventricular activation times in bundle branch block.

RBBB is associated with septal infarction. As in the case of normal intraventricular conduction, the septal vector, moving rightward, produces a small initial **q wave** in the left lateral leads I and V6.

Because there is no block in the left bundle branch, activation of the left ventricular muscle mass occurs next. The electrical forces produced by the **left ventricular vector** are directed **leftward** and **posteriorly** (**arrow 2** in Fig. 4–7) and produce a small **s wave (2)** in lead V1 and tall R waves in the left lateral leads I, II, and V6. The height of the R wave in the frontal plane leads reflects the net QRS axis in those leads, which is frequently abnormal owing to concomitant left fascicular block.

Slow conduction through the septal myocardium eventually results in right ventricular septal activation. The **right septal vector (arrow 3)** is directed **rightward** and **anteriorly** and is reflected on the surface ECG by the upstroke of the R′ wave in lead V1 and the beginning of the wide, slurred terminal S wave in the left lateral leads I, aVL, V5, and V6.

A fourth instantaneous vector, represented by **arrow 4** in Figure 4–7, results

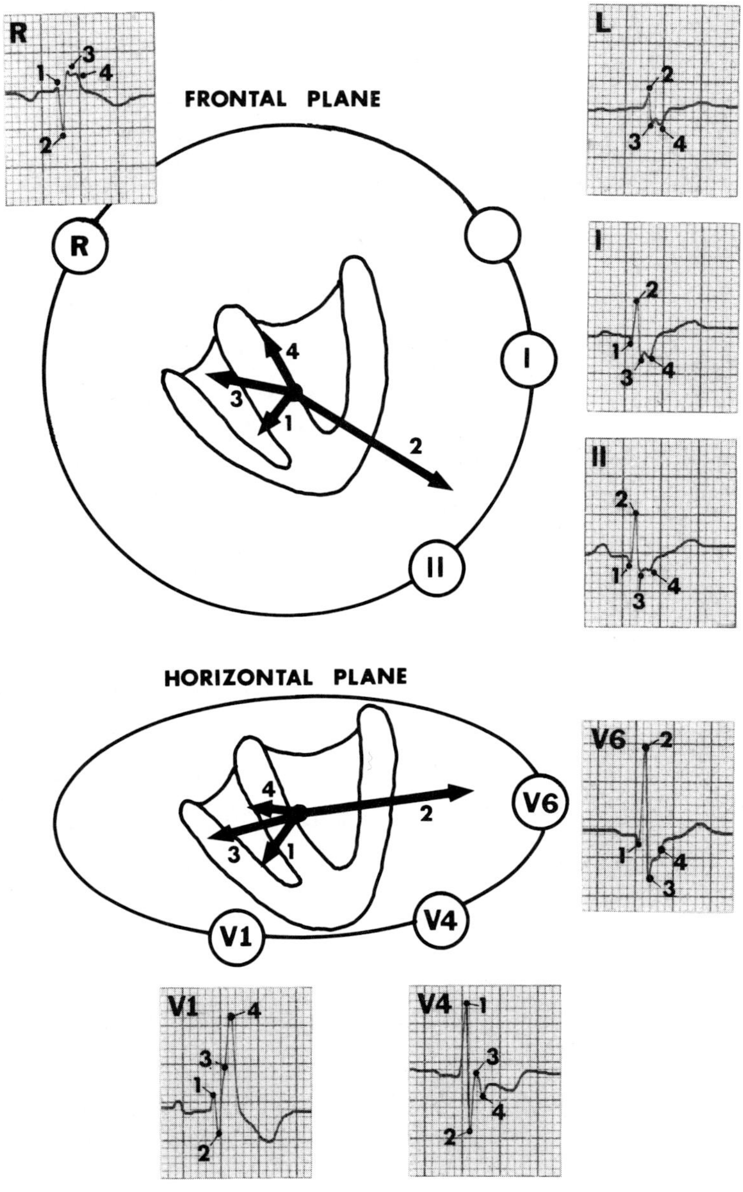

Figure 4–7. Four instantaneous vectors and their contributions to the electrocardiogram of right bundle branch block.

from activation of the right ventricular free wall and the right ventricular outflow tract (crista supraventricularis). Oriented **rightward** and **anteriorly,** these forces result in the inscription of the peak of the R′ wave in lead V1 and the terminal portion of the slurred terminal S wave in the left lateral leads I, aVL, and V6.

Leads overlying the transition zone in the horizontal plane may record a polyphasic RSr′s′ complex like the one illustrated in lead V4 of Figure 4–7. The T wave, like that of V1, is inverted. The initial septal forces (vector 1) are responsible for the R wave, left ventricular activation (vector 2) is reflected by the S wave, and the succeeding R′ and S′ waves represent right ventricular septal (vector 3) and free wall (vector 4) activation respectively.

Left bundle branch block

The ECG criteria for left bundle branch block (LBBB) include (1) **QRS prolongation** to 0.12 second or more; (2) a broad, slurred **S wave** in the right precordial leads (V1, V2); (3) a broad **R wave,** which often displays notching and slurring, in the left lateral leads I, aVL, V5, and V6; (4) **ST** and **T wave displacement** in the direction opposite the polarity of the QRS complex; and (5) **prolonged ventricular activation time.** In complete forms of LBBB, Q waves are absent in the left lateral leads I, aVl, V5, and V6.

The ECG pattern of left bundle branch block is shown in Figure 4–8. The QRS complex is abnormally wide (0.12 second); the QRS complex in the right precordial leads (V1, V2) consists of a small initial **r wave** followed by a wide, slurred **S wave;** the left lateral leads (I, aVL, V5, V6) exhibit wide **R waves** marked by prominent slurring and/or notching; and the ST segments and T waves are displaced in the direction opposite the QRS polarity.

Increased ventricular activation time in the left precordial leads (V5, V6) reflects delayed or absent conduction in the left bundle branch. Prolonged ventricular activation time in lead V6, reflected by a QR interval greater than 0.045 second, is illustrated in Figure 4–6, panel **B,** which shows both a normal left ventricular complex (VAT = 0.035 second) and complex typical of LBBB (VAT = 0.10 second).

Several studies have concluded that a pattern of LBBB does not always indicate total loss of conduction in the left bundle branch (Unger et al, 1968; Wu et al, 1974). As in the case of LPFB, the finding of LBBB has been shown to correlate with advanced obstructive lesions of the right coronary and left anterior descending coronary arteries, with diffuse degenerative changes in the

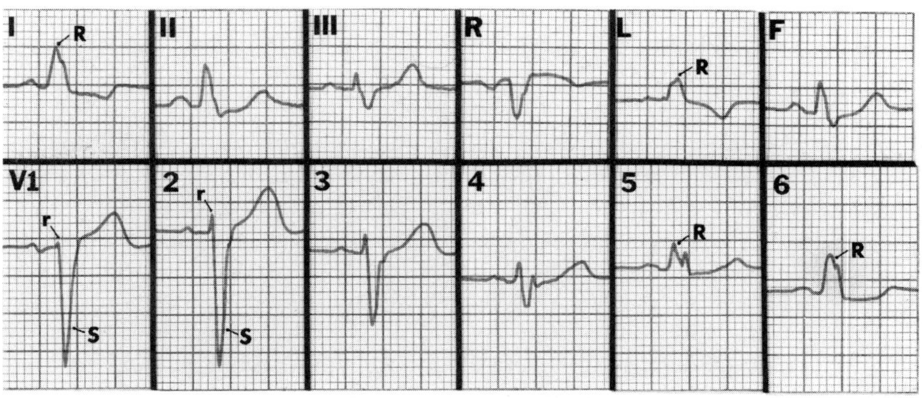

Figure 4–8. The electrocardiogram of left bundle branch block.

distal fascicles of the left bundle, and with complete interruption of the left bundle branch at its orgin on the crest of the septum (Dalen and Alport, 1981; Hurst et al, 1982; Rosen et al, 1973; Unger et al, 1968). Data obtained from the Framingham study indicate that LBBB combined with left axis deviation beyond −30 degrees predicted a higher prevalence of cardiac enlargement and clinical evidence of congestive heart failure and coronary artery disease. The presence of left atrial abnormality by ECG identified patients with high blood pressure, and hypertensive cardiomyopathy was felt to be the leading cause of LBBB in this group (Schneider et al, 1985). In the data released from the Coronary Artery Surgical Study (CASS), which studied cases of chronic LBBB, its presence predicted a 30 per cent average decrease in left ventricular ejection fraction and was found to contribute strongly to the risk of sudden cardiac death, probably secondary to ventricular arrhythmias (Freedman et al, 1987).

Ventricular activation in left bundle branch block

In the case of right bundle branch block, initial septal activation is normal, beginning on the middle third of the left septal surface. In the case of left bundle branch block, the sequence of activation is totally deranged and activation begins on the right septal surface, producing an initial vector (**arrow 1** in Fig. 4–9) that is directed **anteriorly** and **leftward.** This instantaneous vector may result in small positive deflections in the right precordial leads (**1** in V1) and contributes to the beginning of the upstroke of the R wave in the left lateral leads I, V5, and V6.

The second instantaneous vector **(arrow 2),** representing depolarization of the lower septum, is directed **leftward** and **posteriorly.** It produces the downstroke of the S wave in the right precordial leads (**2** in V1) and the ascending limb of the QRS complex in the left lateral leads I, aVL, V5 and V6. As septal depolarization continues, a third vector **(arrow 3)** is generated. This vector is reflected by the notching or slurring at the peak of the R wave in the left lateral leads.

Activation of the left ventricular free wall and base of the left ventricle produces a fourth, final vector **(arrow 4),** directed **leftward** and **posteriorly,** which is responsible for the descending limb of the R wave in the left lateral leads and for the ascending limb of the S wave in the right precordial leads. This vector may be directed extremely posteriorly in the horizontal plane, with the result that leads I and aVL record the expected upright R wave morphology, but leads V5 and V6 record a biphasic RS or transition complex. Some authorities believe that the depolarization wave is able to enter the distal parts of the conduction system, having bypassed the blocked areas of the left bundle branch, and that extreme left, or very rarely right, axis deviation represents concomitant left anterior or posterior fascicular block.

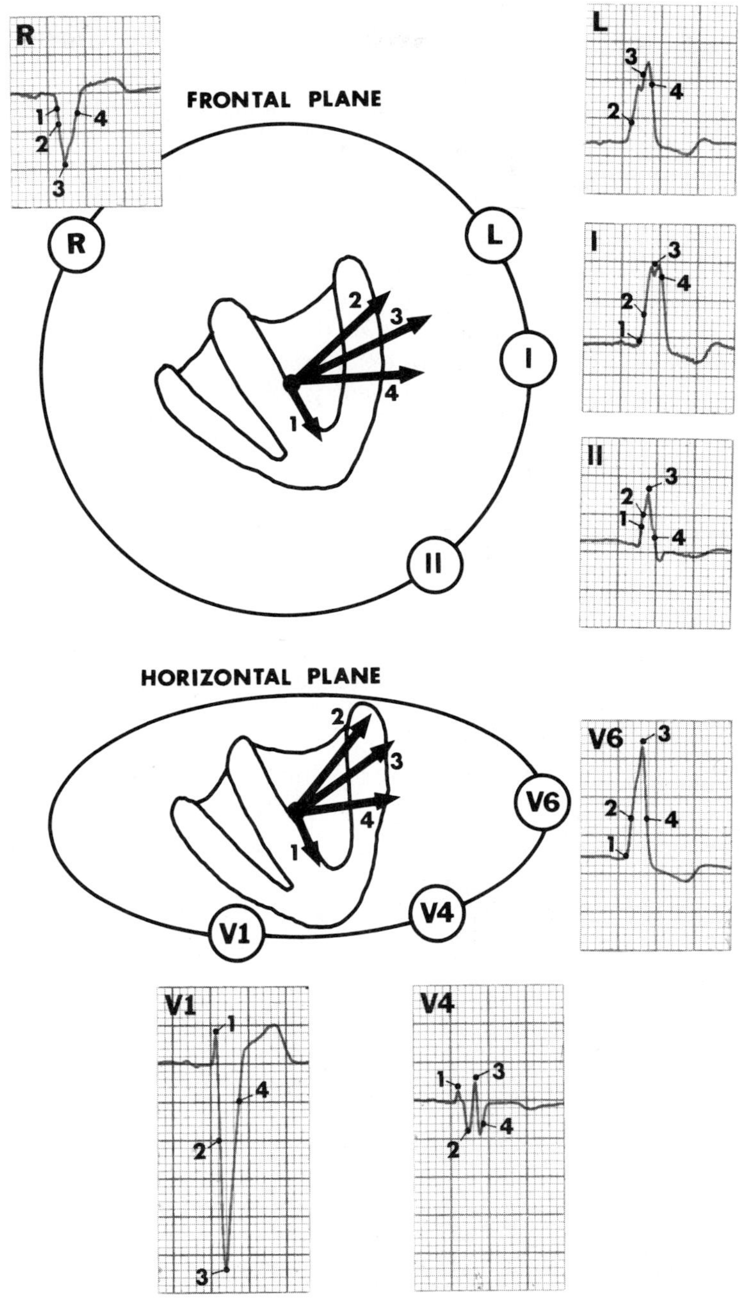

Figure 4–9. Four instantaneous vectors and their contributions to the electrocardiogram of left bundle branch block.

Multifascicular block

Obviously, block need not be confined to a single fascicle or to only one of the bundle branches. In fact, combinations of blocks are fairly common. The most frequently encountered form of multifascicular block is right bundle branch block and left anterior fascicular block (RBBB + LAFB in Fig. 4–2). The least common is right bundle branch block and left posterior fascicular block (RBBB + LPFB). The latter combination may present certain diagnostic difficulties, particularly if the axis deviation is very far to the right.

Figure 4–10 illustrates an example of RBBB and LPFB. Five of the six frontal plane leads—I, II, III, aVR, and aVL—have been enlarged for ease of visualization. The characteristic features of RBBB are obvious: the QRS complex is abnormally wide (0.16 second) and the expected morphologies are present—an rSR′ complex is present in lead V1 and a wide, slurred S wave is noted in the left lateral leads I, aVL, V5, and V6. Leads I and aVL exhibit rS complexes, which at first glance may appear equiphasic since the **height** of the r wave in lead I, 4 mm, is equal to the **depth** of the S wave. However, closer examination clearly shows that the S waves in leads I and aVL are much wider than the R waves and correspondingly enclose a much greater **total area.** Using the total area enclosed within a wave, rather than its height, as the criterion for judging its negativity or positivity, it is immediately obvious that the R wave of lead III is much more positive than the Q wave is negative, even though the waves are essentially equal in height. The most equiphasic lead is lead II; therefore, the net axis is oriented at right angles to lead II, toward leads III and aVR, and away from leads I and aVL. The net vector is therefore about +160 degrees and the tracing meets the criteria for RBBB and LPFB.

Block in both bundles may occur simultaneously or alternately. Mobitz

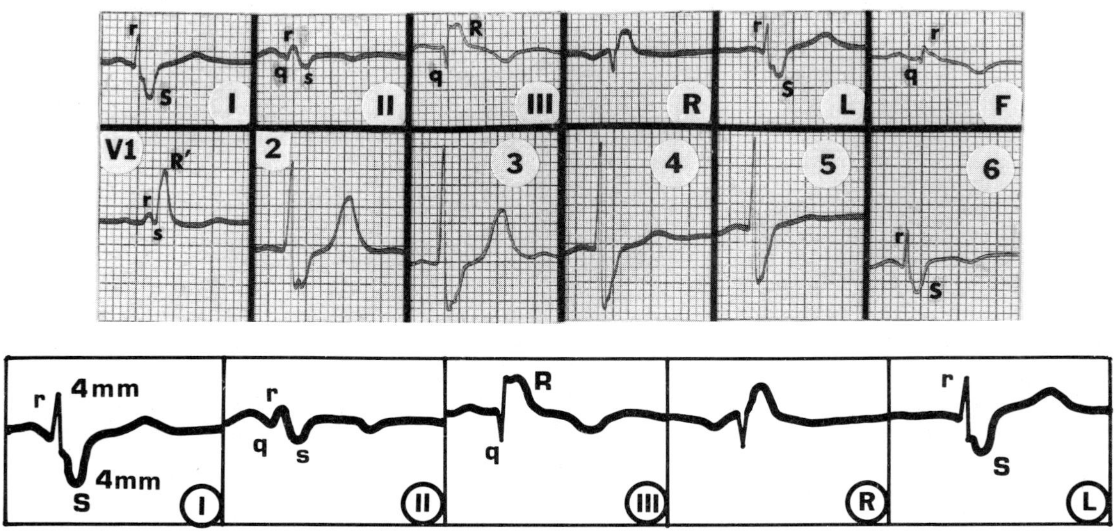

Figure 4–10. Calculating the axis in a case of right bundle branch block and left posterior fascicular block.

type II second-degree block is an example of simultaneous bilateral bundle branch block. Alternative patterns of RBBB and LBBB permit a firm diagnosis of bilateral bundle branch block (BBBB). Bundle branch block with first-degree AV block sometimes represents complete block in one bundle and delayed conduction through the other. A complete evaluation of bilateral bundle branch disease often requires His bundle electrograms (HBE). The interested reader is referred to recent excellent discussions (Puech, 1975; Narula and Shantha, 1980).

Nonspecific intraventricular conduction delay

Nonspecific intraventricular conduction delay (NSIVCD) is a term reserved for those intraventricular conduction deficits that exhibit abnormally wide QRS complexes (0.12 second or more) but do not conform to the morphologic criteria for bundle branch blocks. The morphology of the QRS complexes in the precordial leads is often bizarre and frequently polyphasic (panel **D** in Fig. 4–11), but may present typical fascicular blocks in the frontal plane leads. Various examples of NSIVCD are illustrated in Figure 4–11.

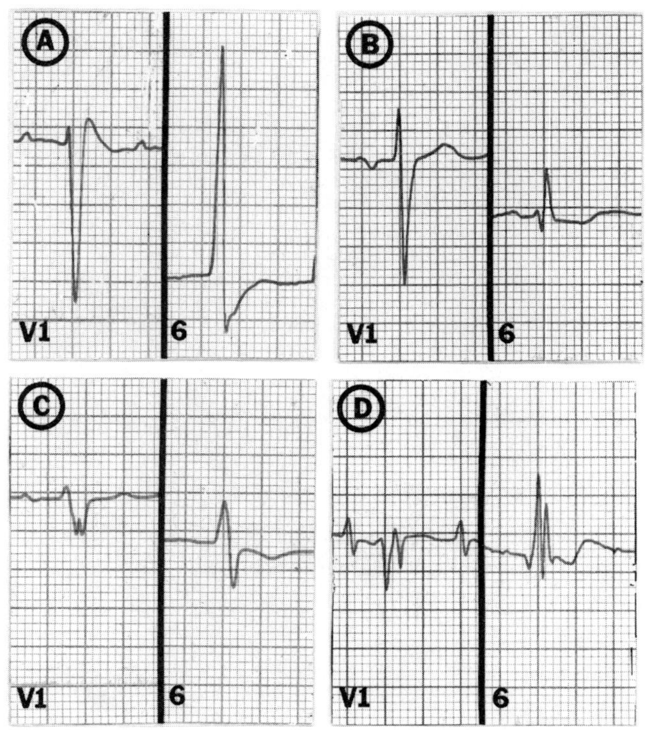

Figure 4–11. Examples of nonspecific intraventricular conduction delay (NSIVCD).

Etiologies of intraventricular conduction defects

There are many etiologies of fascicular and bundle branch block, but three account for the vast majority in the North American population. The most common cause of intraventricular block is ischemic heart disease with its various sequelae, particularly myocardial infarction. This etiology is discussed at length in the following section.

A common cause of block in the aged population is a diffuse sclerodegenerative process that usually involves all the distal fascicles to some extent but tends to spare the adjacent working myocardium. This syndrome, called **Lenègre's disease,** may take place in the presence of normal coronary arteries and is not widely thought to be related to ischemia. It may represent a part of the aging process and is sometimes called "gray hair of the conduction system." Atrioventricular block and signs of sinus node dysfunction may also be present in addition to distal conduction deficits (Lenègre, 1964).

Calcification of the central fibrous body or the valvular annuli, or both, often accompanies rheumatic valvular disease or the degenerative changes that occur in response to the added stress of systemic hypertension or congenital deformity such as bicuspid aortic valve. Calcification of the fibrous skeleton may impinge upon or invade the His bundle or bundle branches and produce serious atrioventricular and bundle branch block. This process is called **Lev's disease** (Lev, 1964, 1974; Lev and Bharati, 1975, 1981).

References

Becker, AE, Lie, KI, and Anderson, RH. **Br Heart J** 40:773–782.

Bharati, S, et al. **Am J Cardiol** 38:508–518, 1976.

Chou, T-C. **Electrocardiography in Clinical Practice,** 2nd ed. Grune & Stratton, New York, 1986, pp. 129–130.

Dalen, JE, and Alper, JS. **Valvular Heart Disease.** Little, Brown & Company, Boston, 1981, pp. 184–185, 210, 303.

Demoulin, JC, and Kulbertus, HE. **Br Heart J** 34:807–814, 1972.

Demoulin, JC, and Kulbertus, HE. **Am J Cardiol** 44:1083–1088, 1979.

Demoulin, JC, Simar, LJ, and Kulbertus, HE. **Am J Cardiol** 36:751–756, 1975.

Durrer, D, et al. **Circulation** 41:899–912, 1970.

Entman, ML, et al. **Am Heart J** 74:202–207, 1967.

Freedman, RA, et al. **J Am Coll Cardiol** 10:73–80, 1987.

Friedman, HH. **Diagnostic Electrocardiography and Vectorcardiography,** 2nd ed. McGraw-Hill, New York, 1977, p. 190.

Hecht, H, et al. **Am J Cardiol** 31:232–244, 1973.

Hurst, JW, et al. **The Heart,** 5th ed. McGraw-Hill, New York, 1982, pp 35–37, 43–44, 510–513, 540, 869.

Krikler, DM and Goodwin, JF. **Cardiac Arrhythmias, the Modern Electrophysiologic Approach.** WB Saunders, Philadelphia, 1975, pp. 22–24.

Lenègre, J. **Prog Cardiovasc Dis** 6:409–444, 1964.

Lev, M. **Prog Cardiovasc Dis** 6:317–326, 1964.

Lev, M. **Am J Med** 37:742–748, 1964.

Lev, M. **Circulation** 50, 1974, pp 479–486.

Lev, M, and Bharati, S. **Arch Intern Med** 135:405–410, 1975.

Lev, M and Bharati, S. **The Heart, Update IV.** McGraw-Hill, New York, 1981, pp 7–17.

Mandel, WJ, et al. **Cardiac Arrhythmias, Their Mechanism, Diagnosis and Management.** JB Lippincott, Philadelphia, 1980, pp 30–32.

Marriott, HJL. **Practical Electrocardiography,** 7th ed. Williams & Wilkins, Baltimore, 1983, pp 84–97.

Massing, GK, and James, TN. **Circulation** 53:609–621, 1976.

Nakaya, Y, Takashi, H, and Mori, H. **Am J Cardiol** 69:95–98, 1987.

Narula, OS, and Shantha, N. **In** Mandel, WJ (ed). **Cardiac Arrhythmias, Their Mechanism, Diagnosis and Management.** JB Lippincott, Philadelphia, 1980, pp 437–453.

Nimitz, AA, et al. **Am Heart J** 90:439–444, 1975.

Puech, P. **In** Krikler, DM, and Goodwin, JF (eds). **Cardiac Arrhythmias, the Modern Electrophysiologic Approach.** WB Saunders, Philadelphia, 1975, pp 81–115.

Rizzon, P, et al. **Br Heart J** 37:711–720, 1975.

Rosen, KM, et al. **Am J Cardiol** 32:783–793, 1973.

Rossi, L. **Br Heart J** 38:1304–1311, 1976.

Schlant, RC, and Hurst, JW. **Advances in Electrocardiography.** Grune & Stratton, New York, 1972, pp 183–220.

Schneider, JF, et al. **Am J Cardiol** 55:1332–1338, 1985.

Sclarovsky, S, et al. **J Am Coll Cardiol** 8:27–31, 1986.

Uhley, HN. **Am J Cardiol** 30:919–920, 1972.

Uhley, HN. **Am J Cardiol** 43:643–646, 1979.

Unger, PN, et al. **Am Heart J** 76:486–497, 1968.

Wellens, HJJ, Lie, KI, and Janse, MJ. **The Conduction System of the Heart, Structure, Function and Clinical Application.** Lea & Febiger, Philadelphia, 1976, pp 287–295.

Wu, D, et al. **Am J Cardiol** 33:583–589, 1974.

SELF-ASSESSMENT

Multiple Choice

1. The most common form of multifascicular block is:

   a. right bundle branch block and left posterior fascicular block.
   b. right bundle branch block alternating with left bundle branch block.
   c. right bundle branch block and left anterior fascicular block.
   d. left bundle branch block.

2. The typical configuration of the QRS complex in V1 in left bundle branch block (LBBB) is:

   a. rSR′
   b. RS
   c. qR
   d. rS or QS

3. The ring of tissue that serves to anchor the fixed edges of the atrioventricular and semilunar valves is called:

   a. the annulus.
   b. the right fibrous trigone.
   c. the tendon of Todaro.
   d. the central fibrous body.

4. The bundle of His penetrates the ______ and descends to the summit of the muscular septum in the posterior edge of the ______.

   a. membranous septum
   b. central fibrous body
   c. mitral annulus
   d. left fibrous trigone

   a. membranous septum.
   b. aortic annulus.
   c. central fibrous body.
   d. left fibrous trigone.

5. Notching and slurring of the QRS complex is typically noted in leads ______in cases of ______.

   a. I, aVL, V6
   b. II, III, aVF
   c. aVR, aVL, aVF
   d. V3, V4

   a. right bundle branch block.
   b. normal conduction.
   c. left anterior fascicular block.
   d. left bundle branch block.

6. Left anterior fascicular block results in left axis deviation, ________complexes in leads I and aVL, and ________complexes in leads III and aVF.

a. qR	a. rSR′
b. rS	b. qR
c. RS	c. rS
d. rSR′	d. RS

7. The most reliable method for determining the positivity or negativity of a deflection is to estimate:

   a. the height or depth of the wave.
   b. the mean cardiac vector.
   c. the instantaneous vector.
   d. the total area enclosed by the wave.

8. In about 50 per cent of the population, the blood supply to the bundle of His is derived from:

   a. the AV nodal artery and the ramus branch.
   b. the AV nodal artery and the circumflex branch.
   c. the AV nodal artery and the first septal perforating branch.
   d. the AV nodal artery and the conus branch.

9. The left bundle branch divides into ________fascicles in the majority of cases, making the distal conduction system ________in nature.

a. two	a. monofascicular
b. three	b. bifascicular
c. four	c. trifascicular
d. five	d. quadrifascicular

10. Attempts to correlate the fascicular block patterns on the ECG with discrete anatomical lesions in the fascicles these patterns supposedly represent have been:

    a. consistently successful.
    b. untried to date.
    c. largely unsuccessful.
    d. inconclusive.

Practice Strips

Determine the axis and any abnormalities that appear in the electrocardiograms that follow.

4-1.

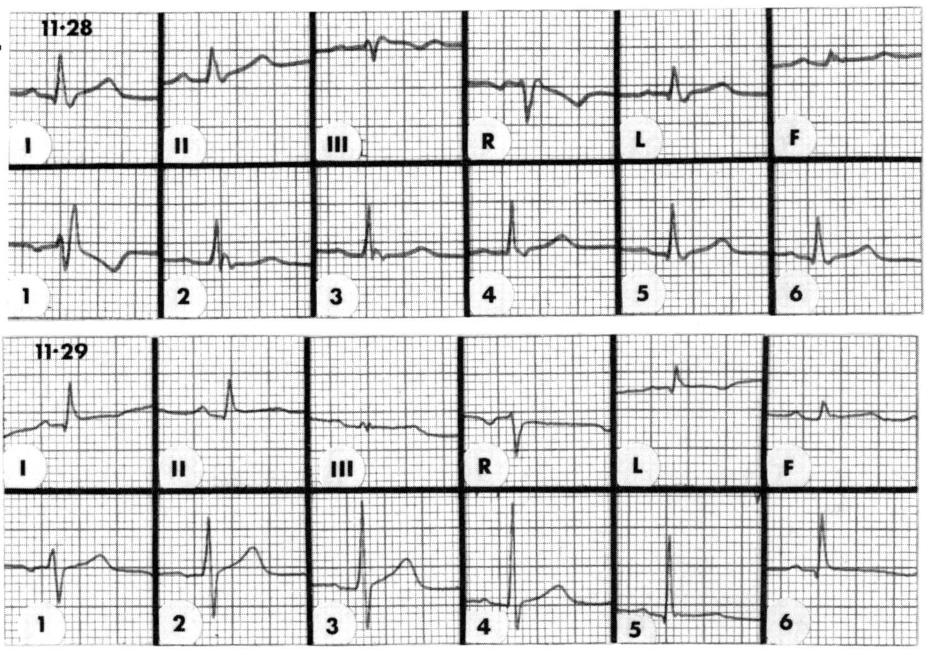

4-2.

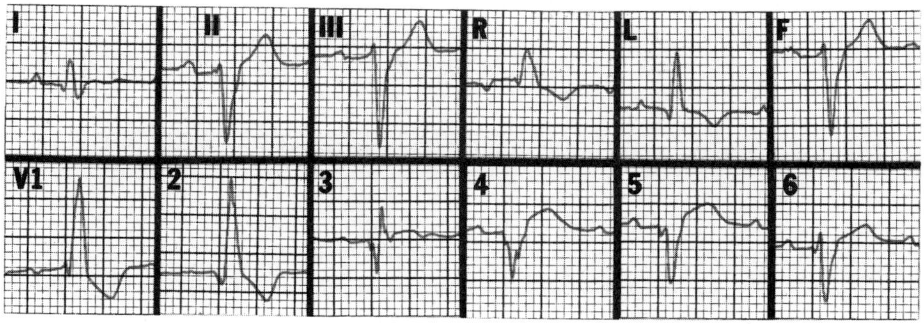

4-3.

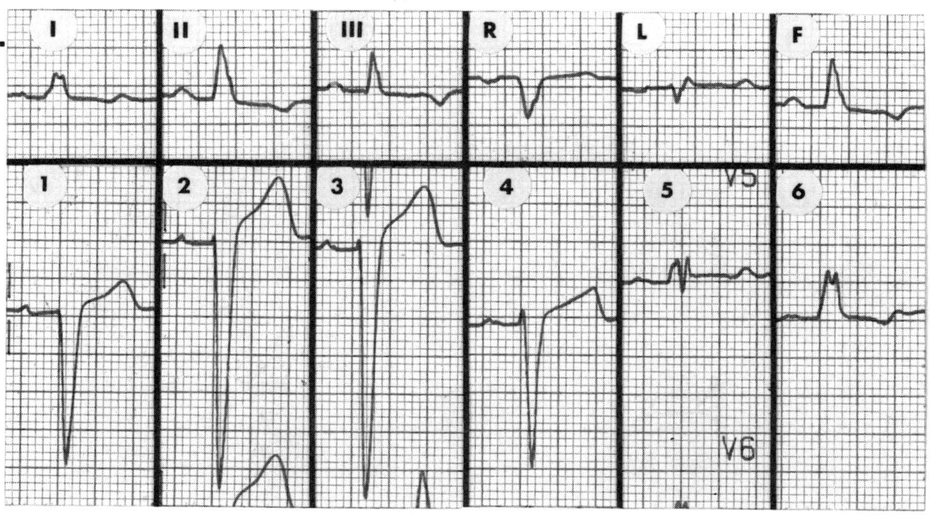

4-4.

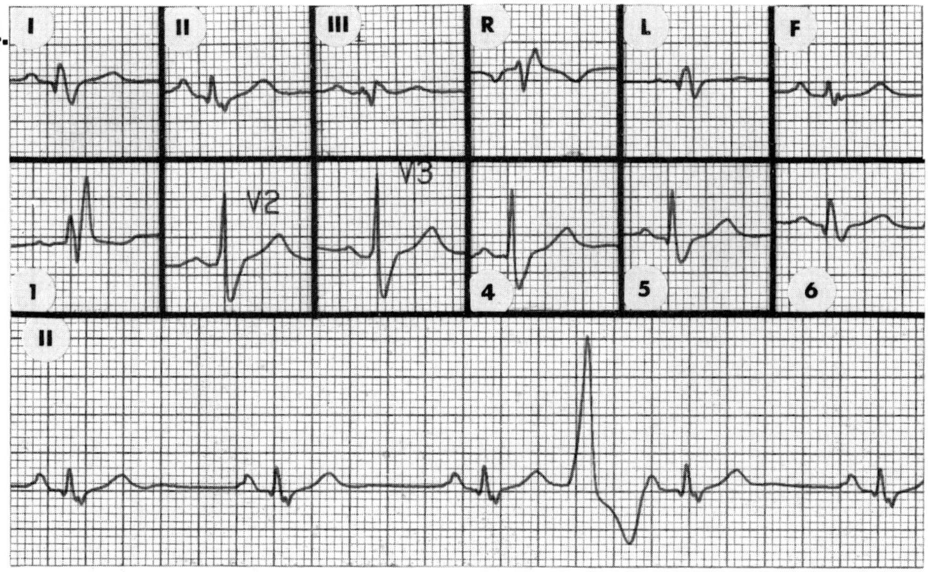

4-5.

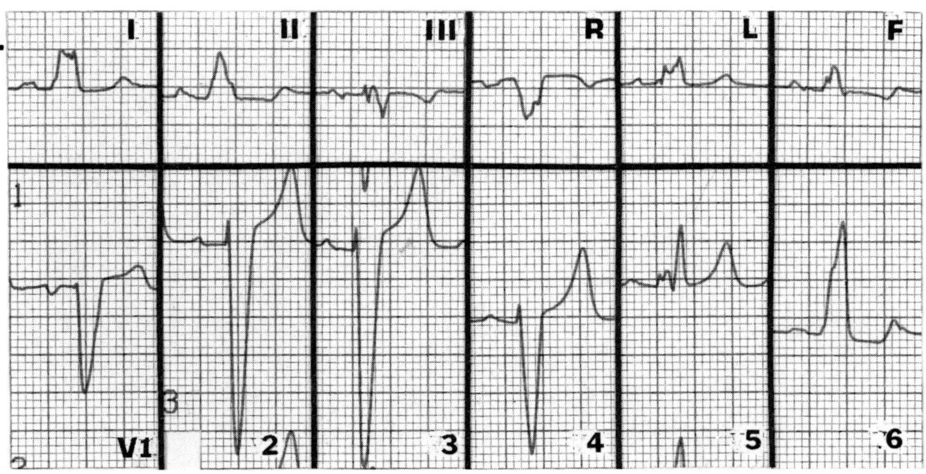

4-6.

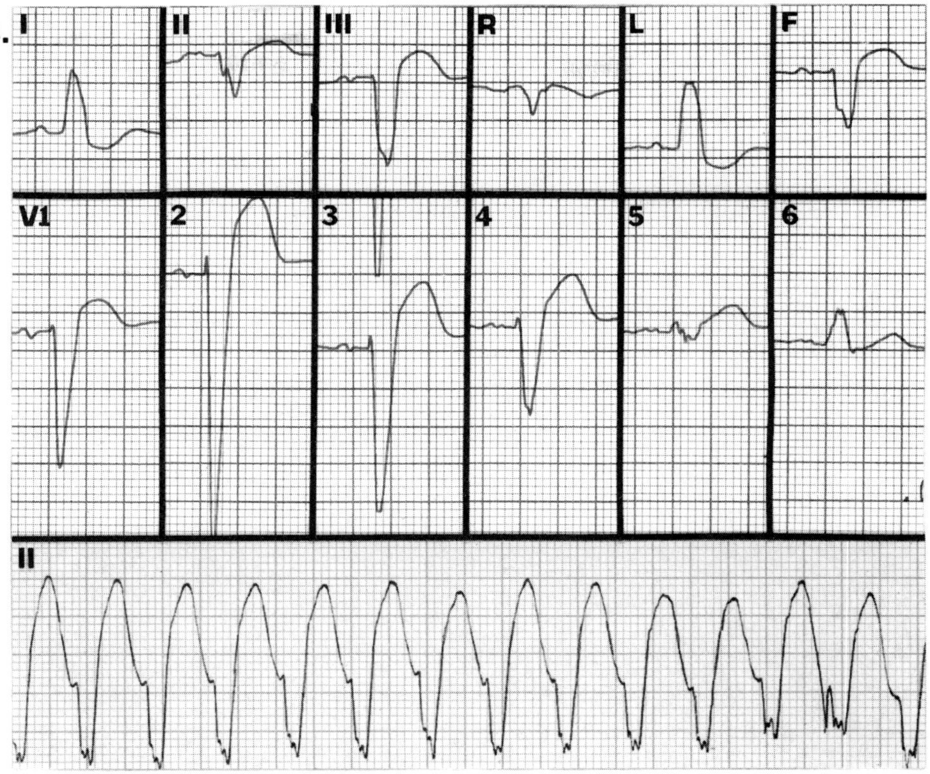

4-7.

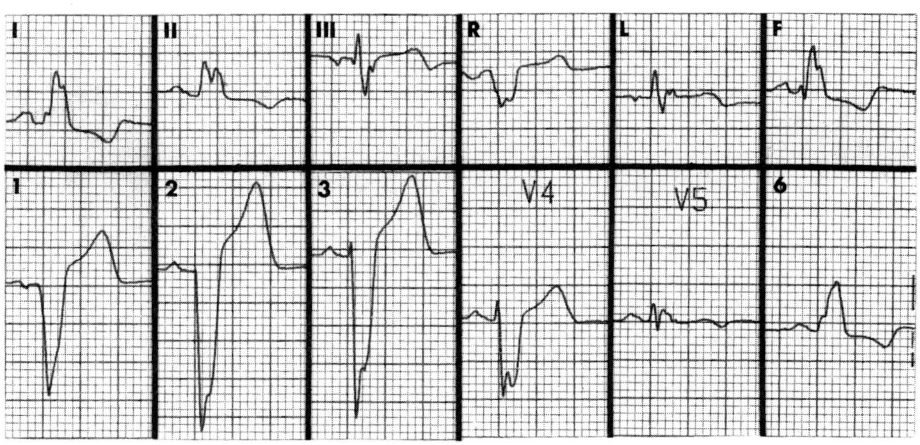

4-8.

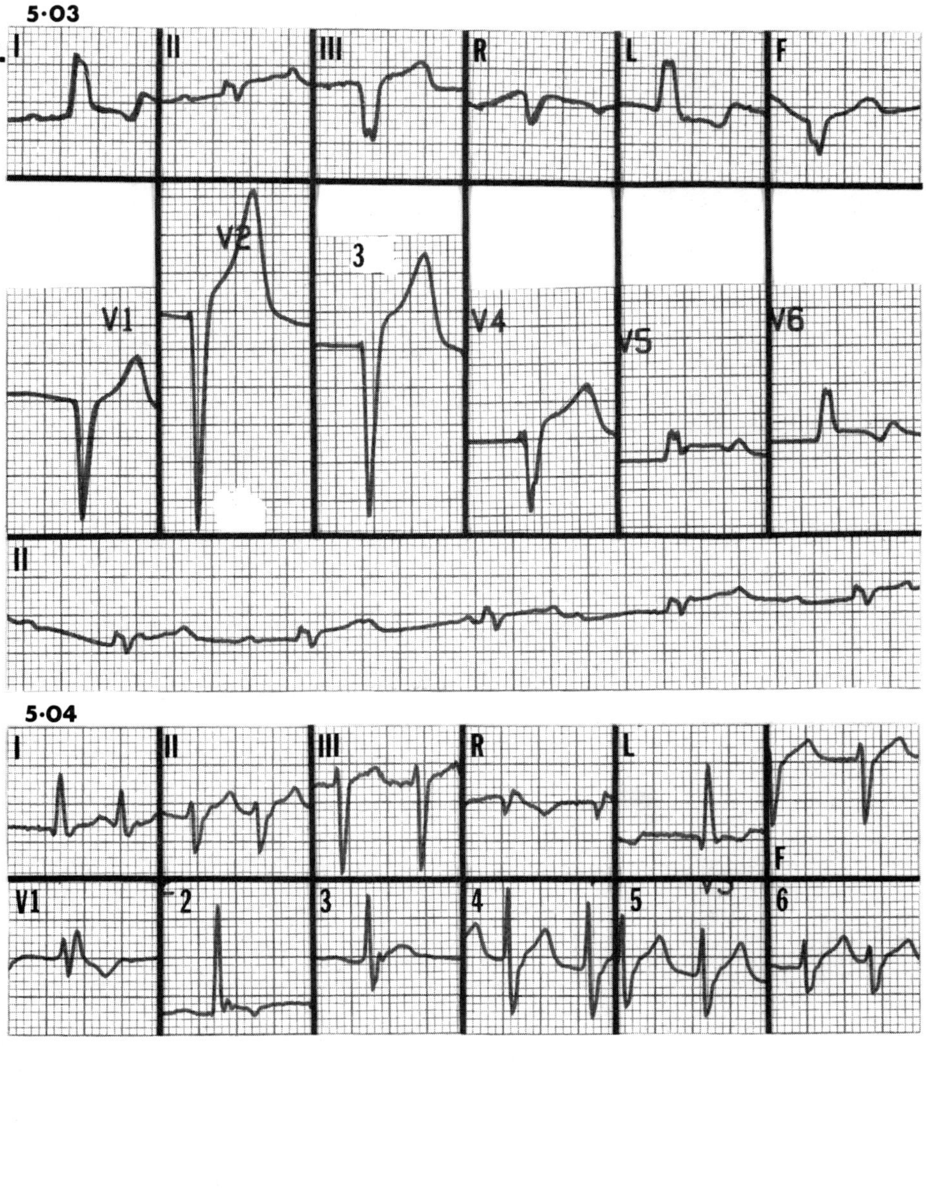

4-9.

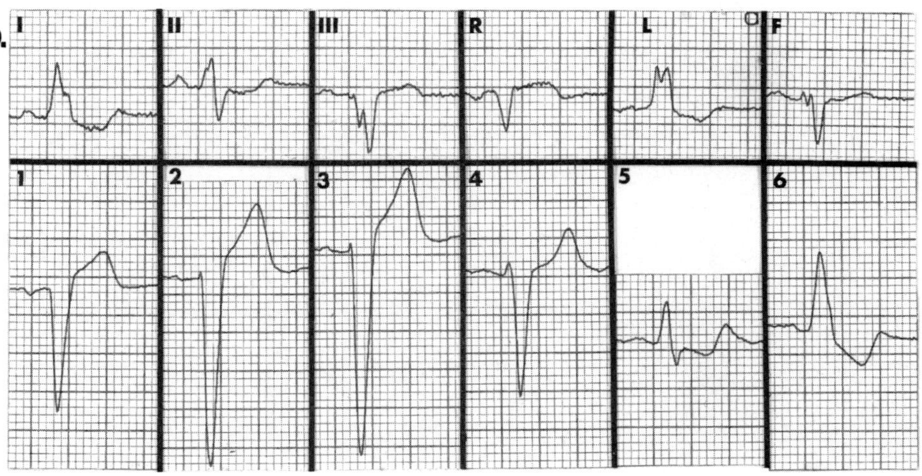

4-10.

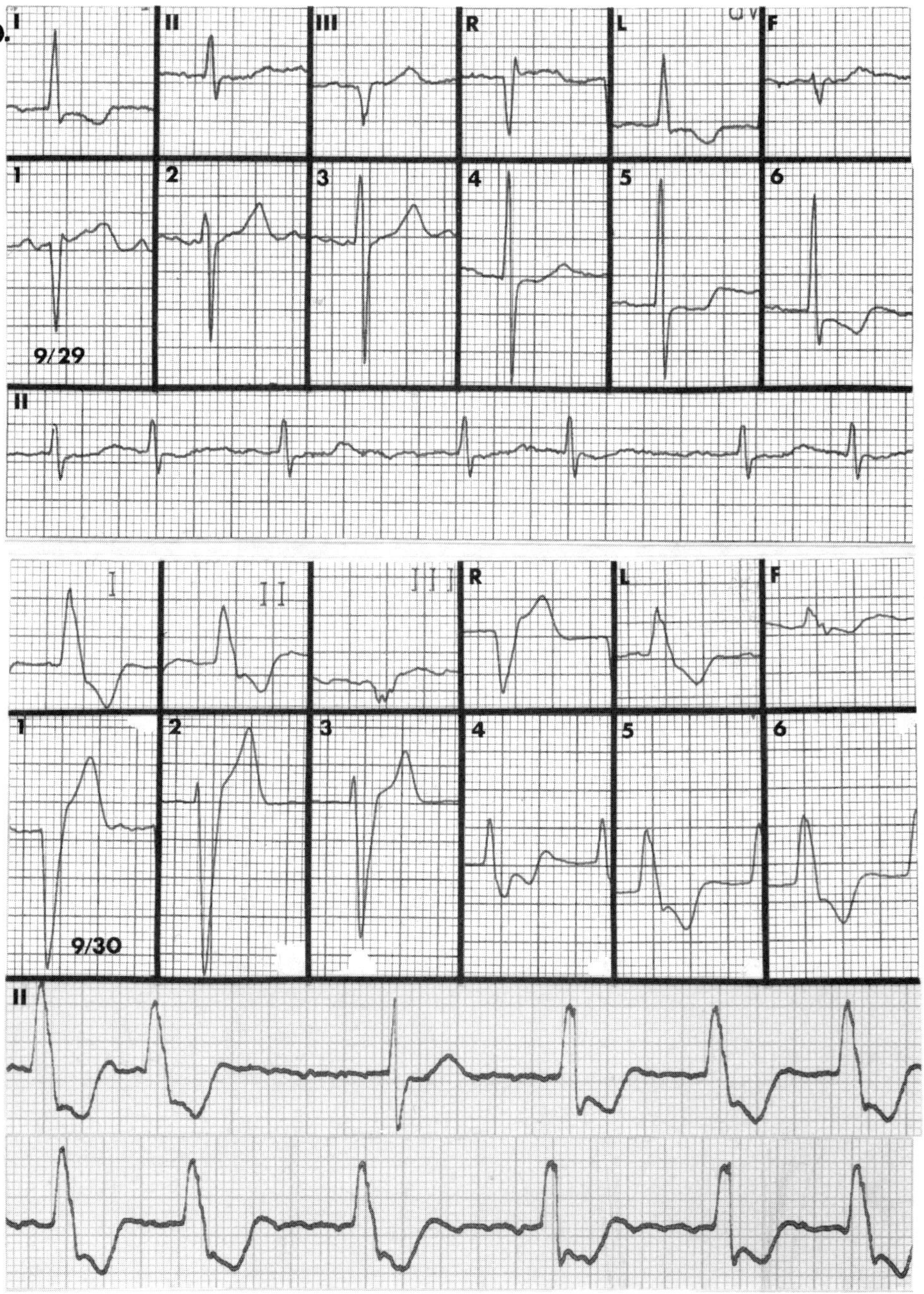

4-11.
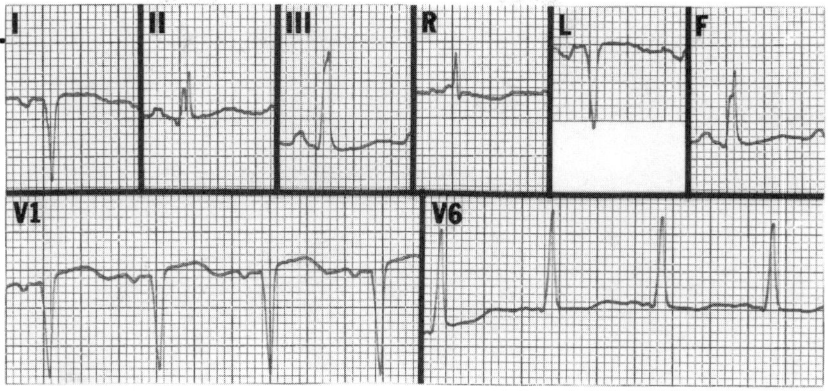

4-12.
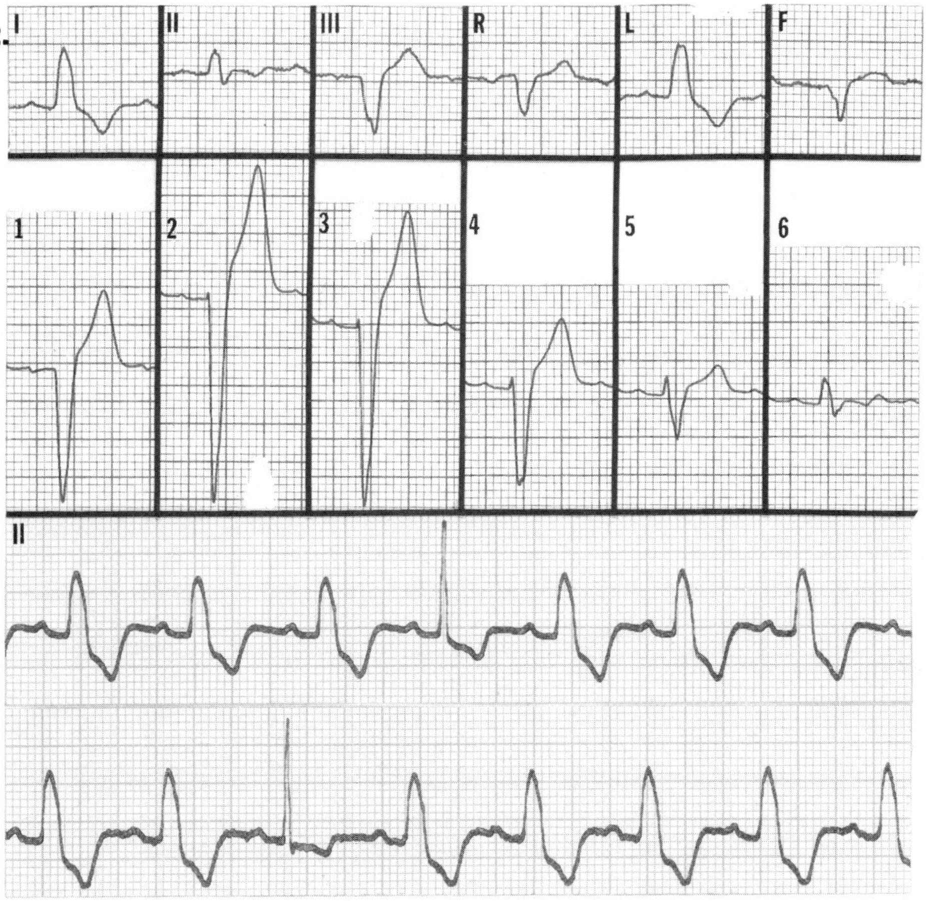

4-13.

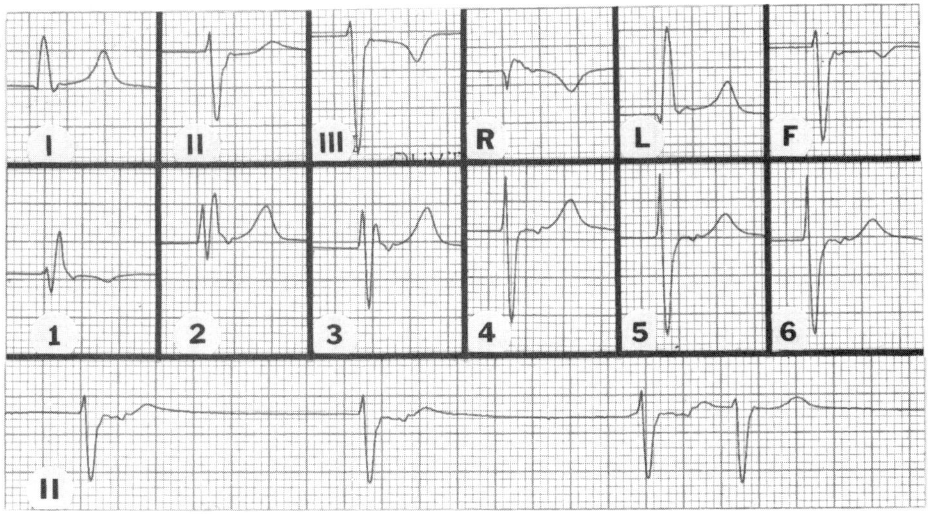

4-14.

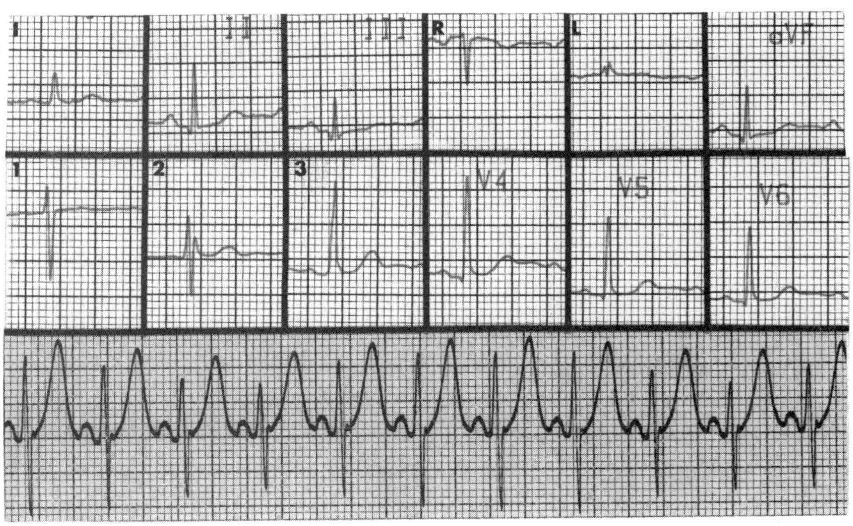

4-15.

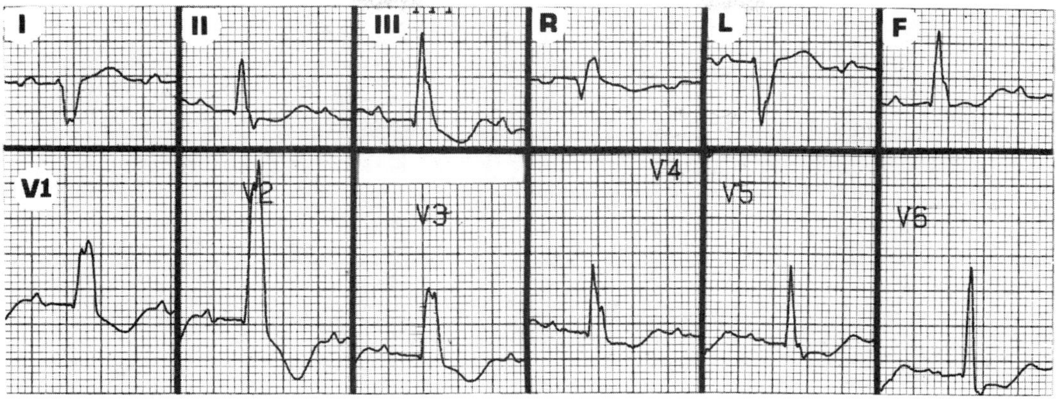

4-16.

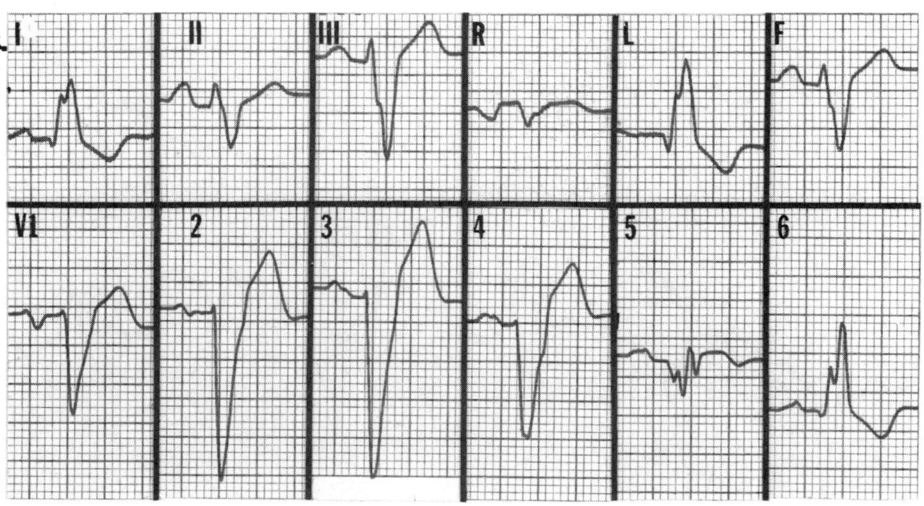

4-17.

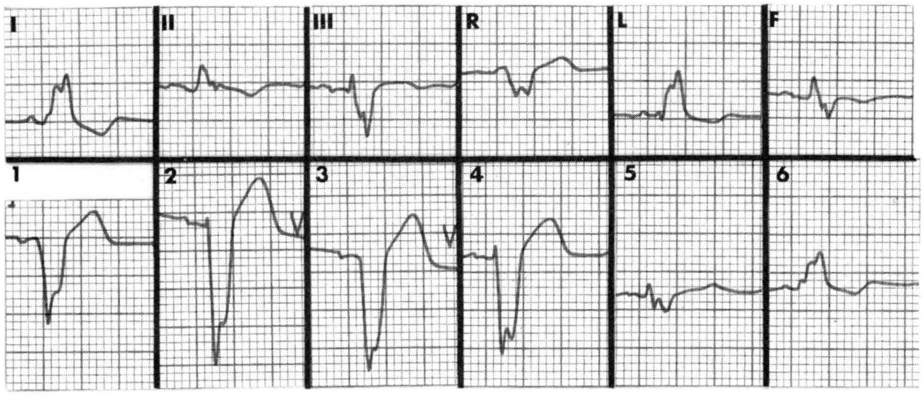

4-18.

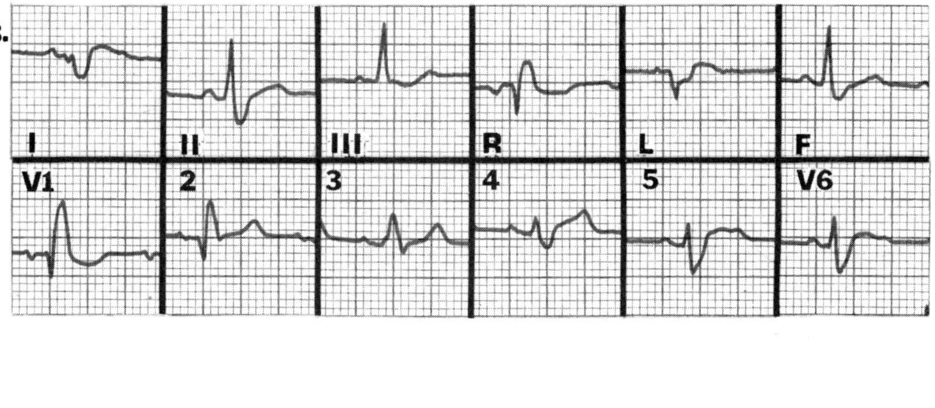

4-19.

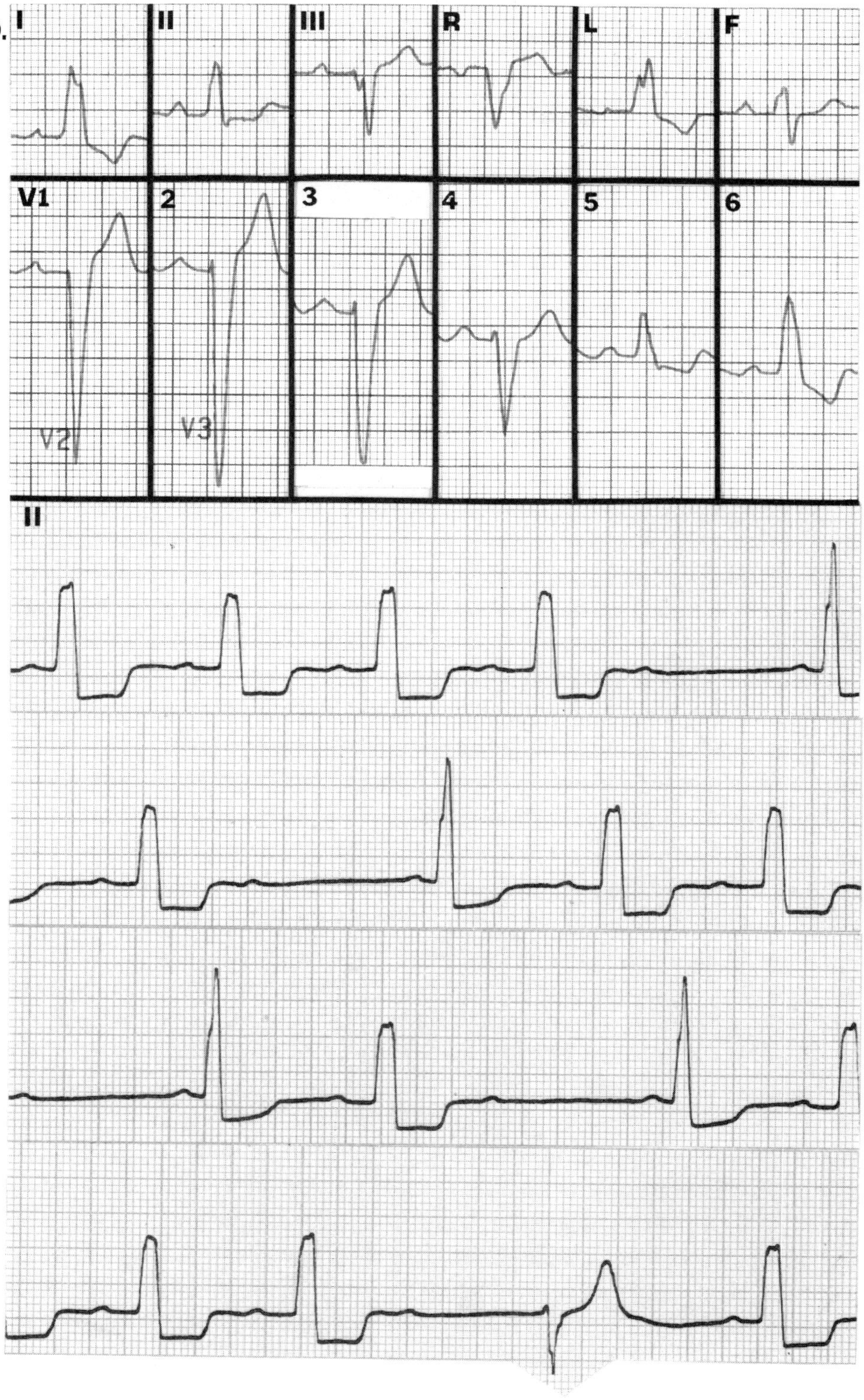

4-20.

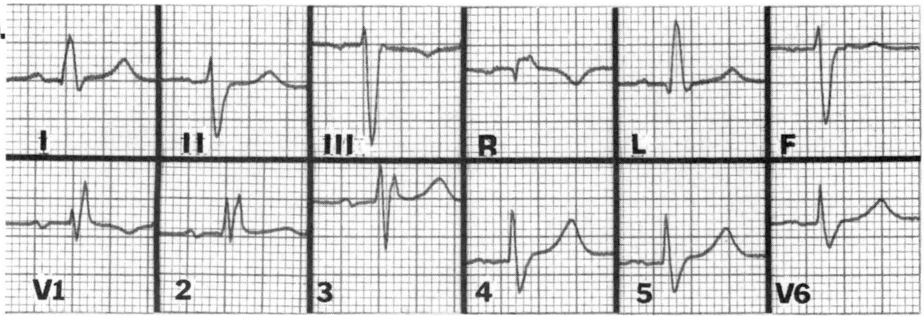

4-21.

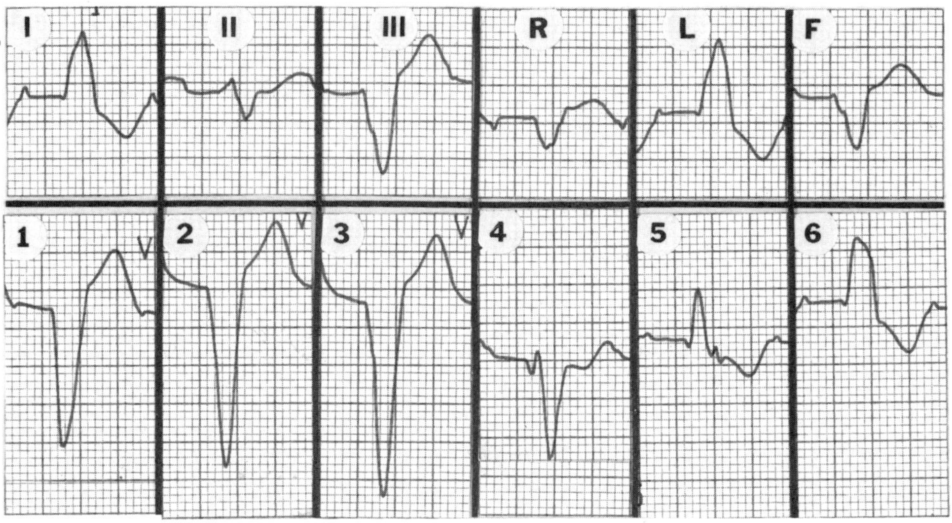

4-22.

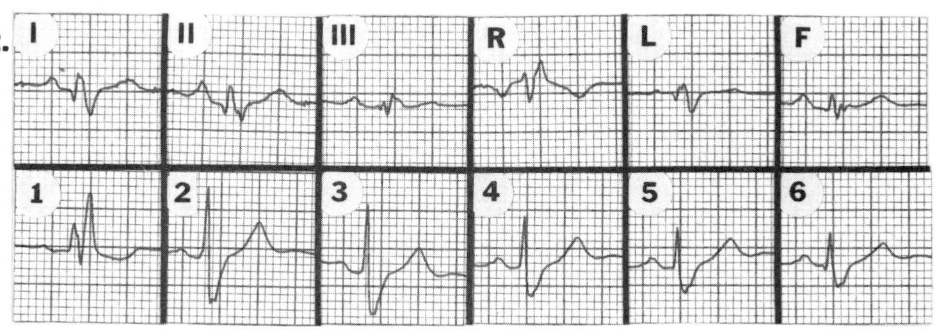

4-23.

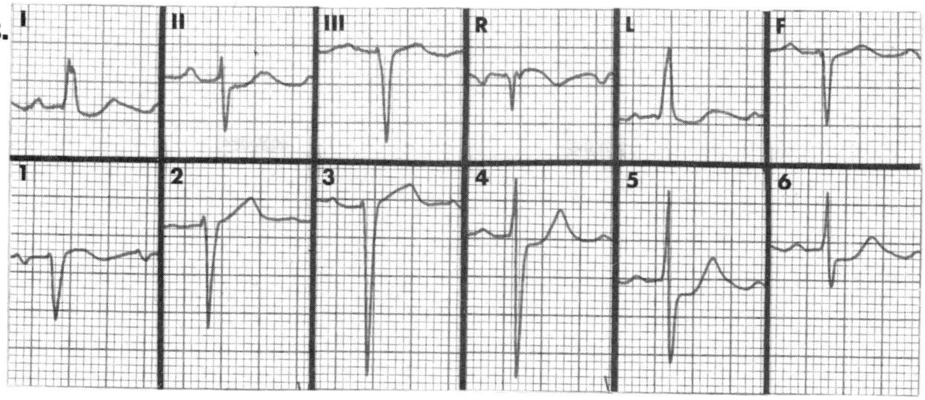

4-24.

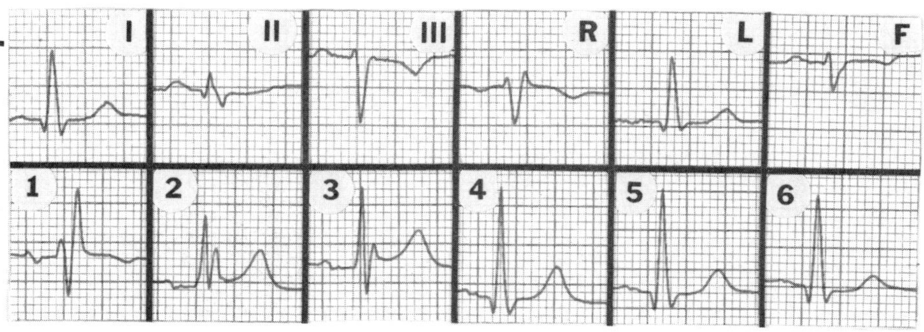

4-25.

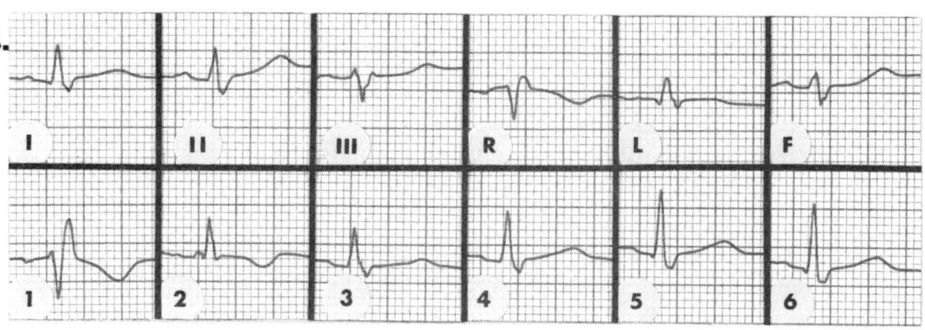

4-26.

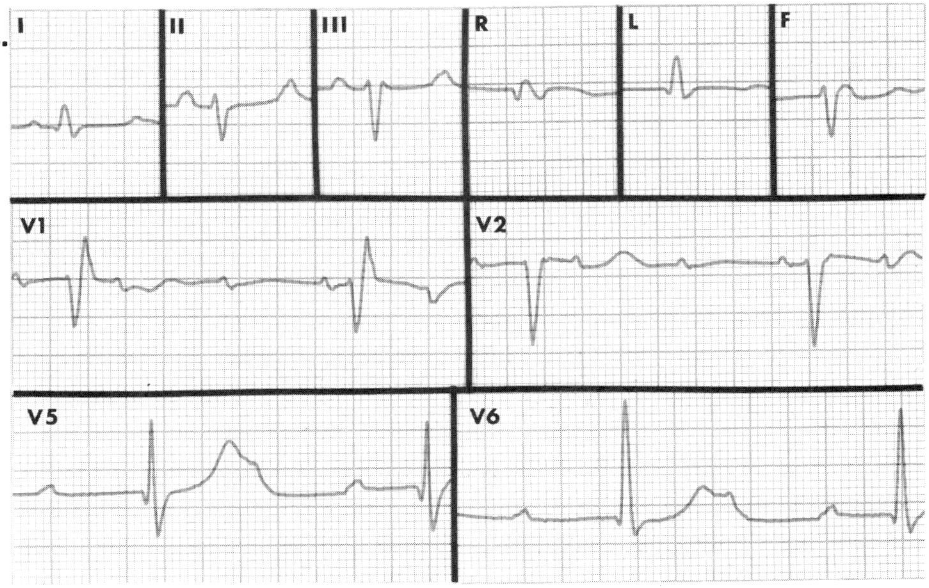

4-27.

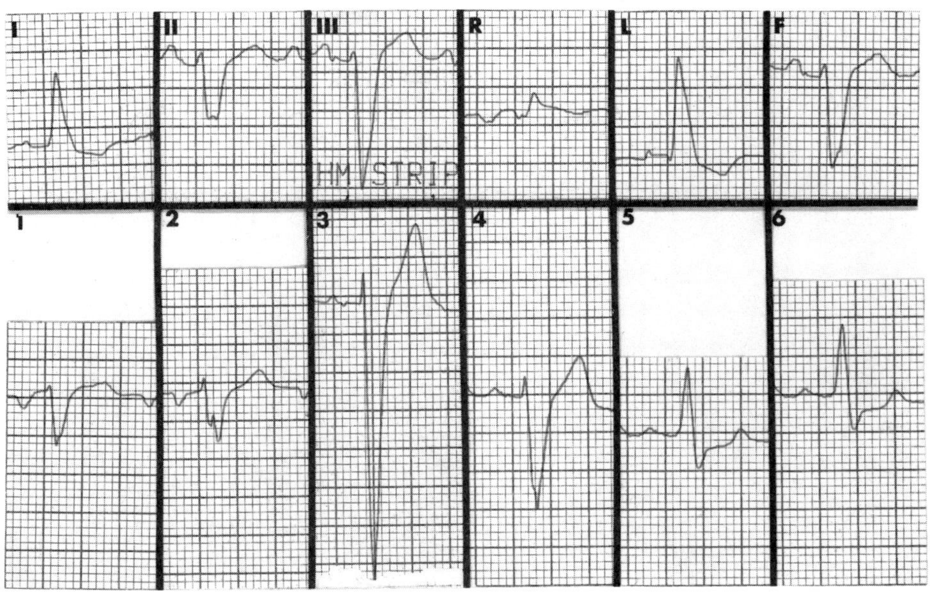

4-28.

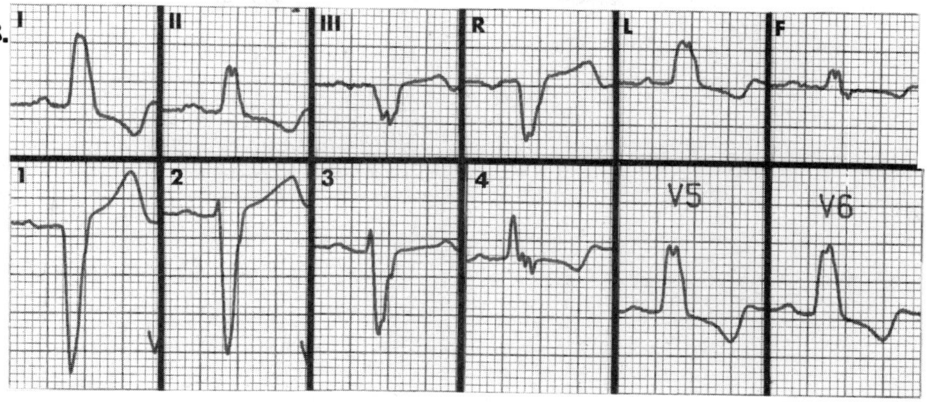

6/02

4-29.

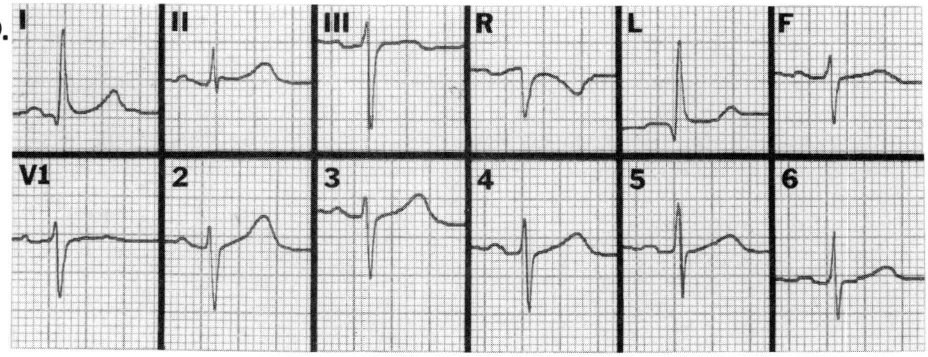

6/03

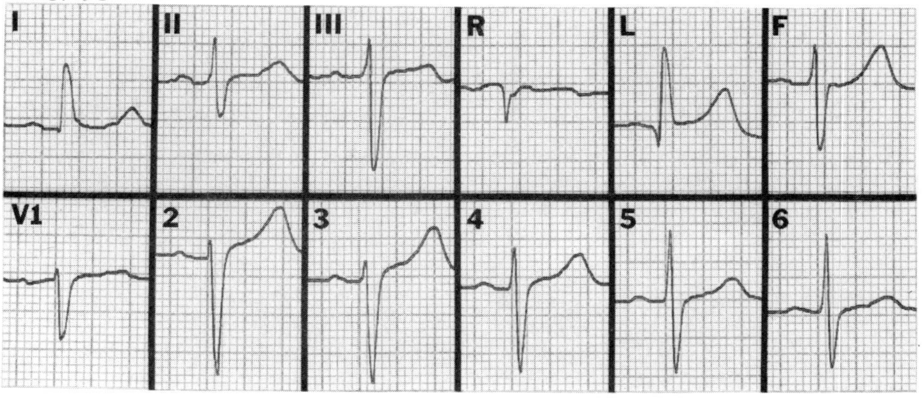

4-30.

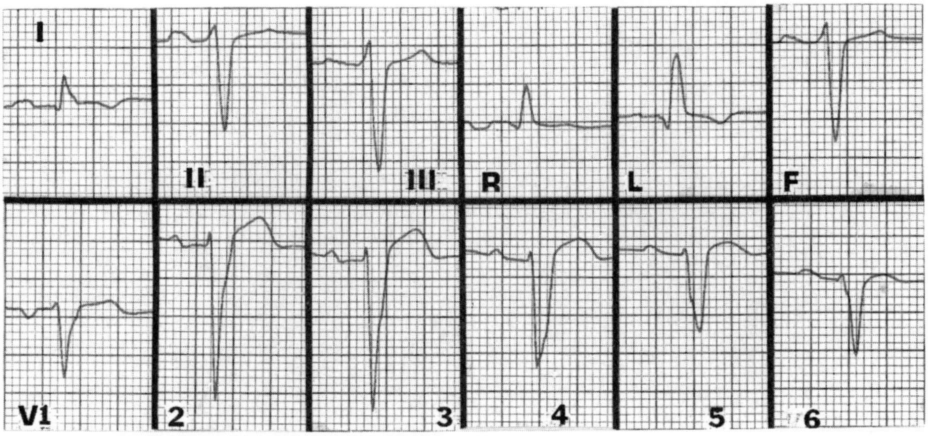

4-31.

1/11

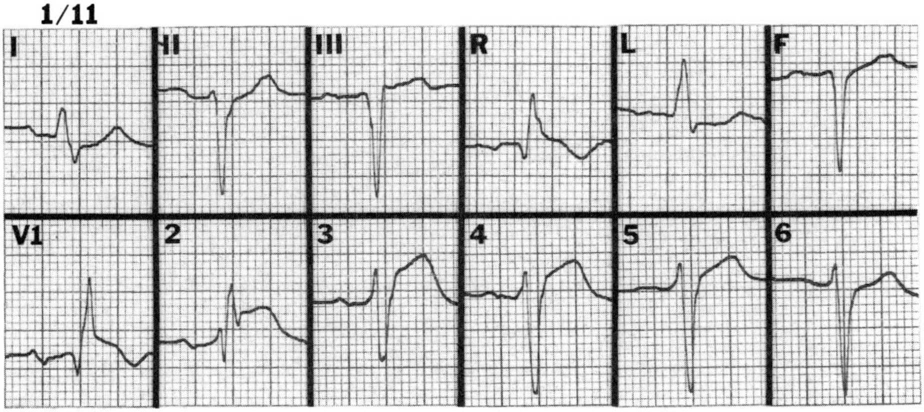

10/20

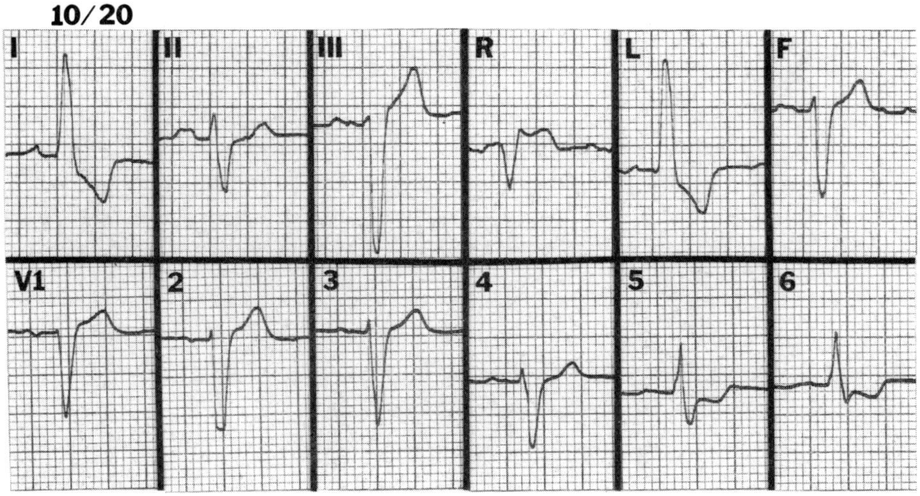

4-32.

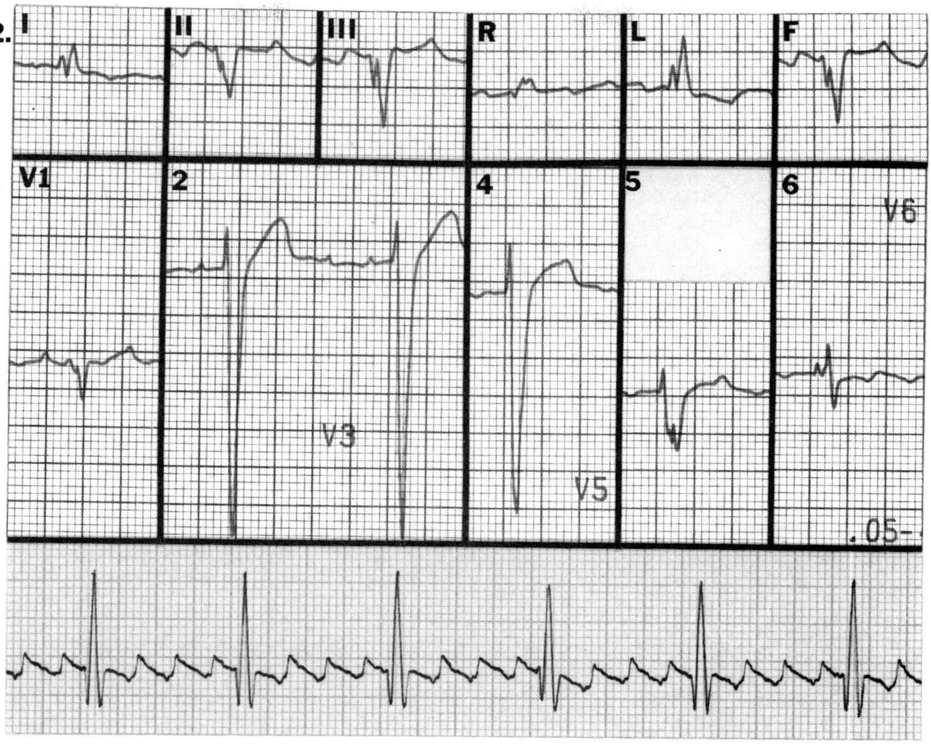

4-33.

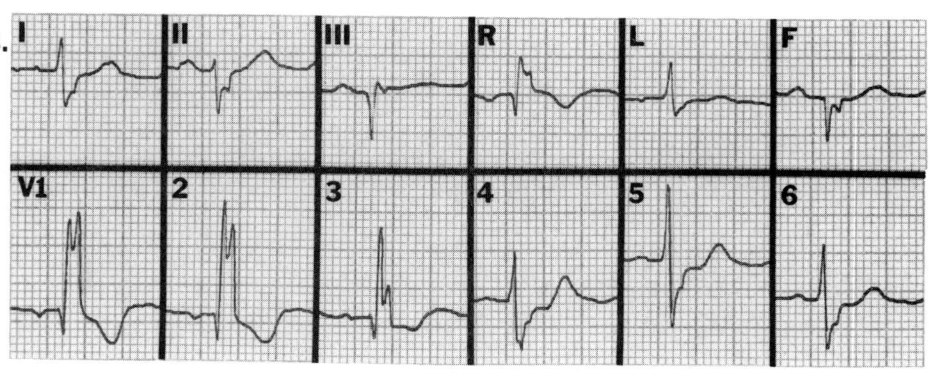

4-34.

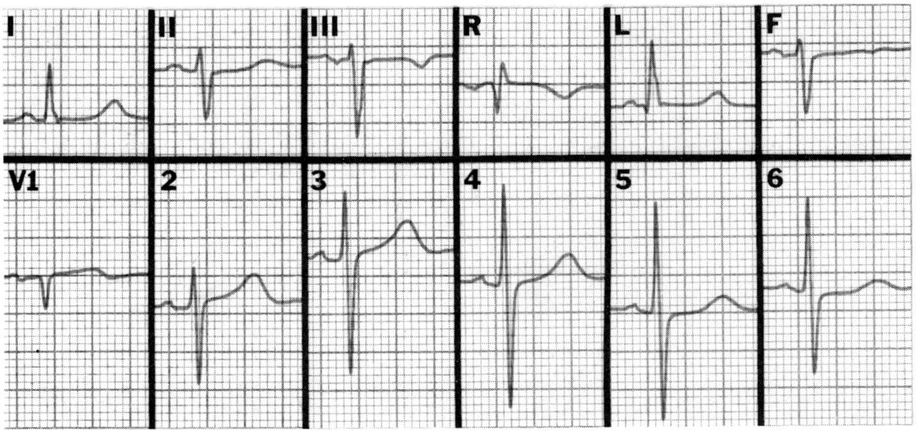

4-35.

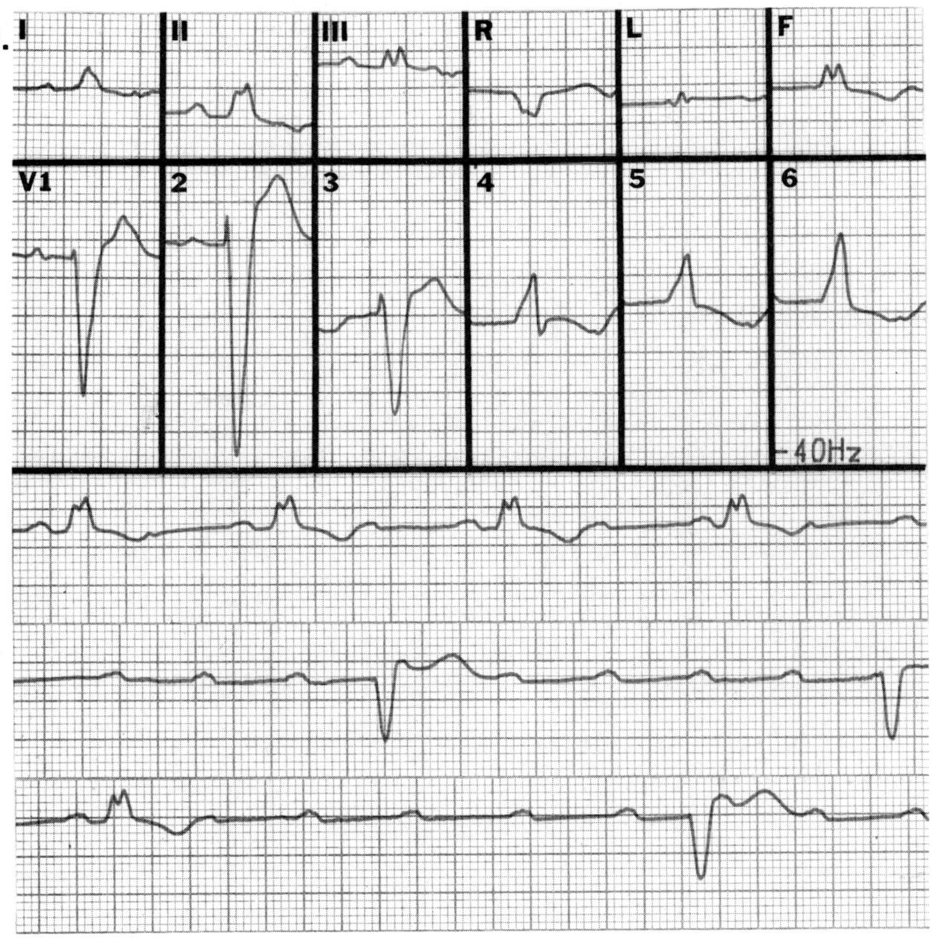

4-36.

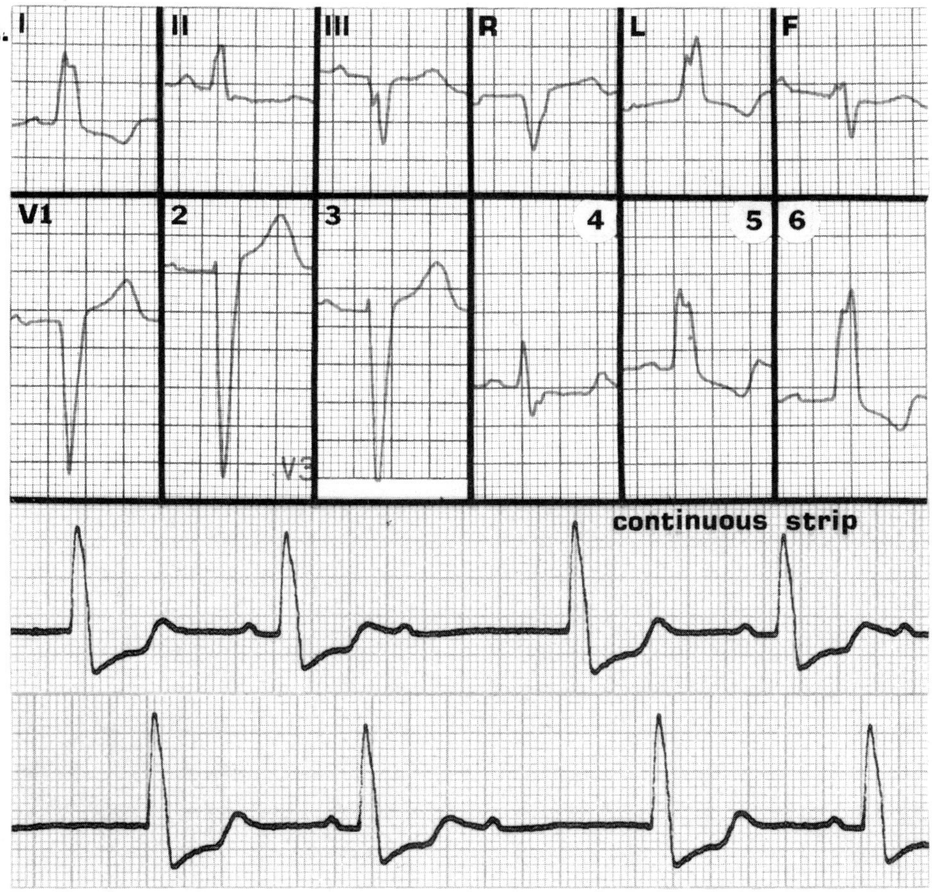

4-37.

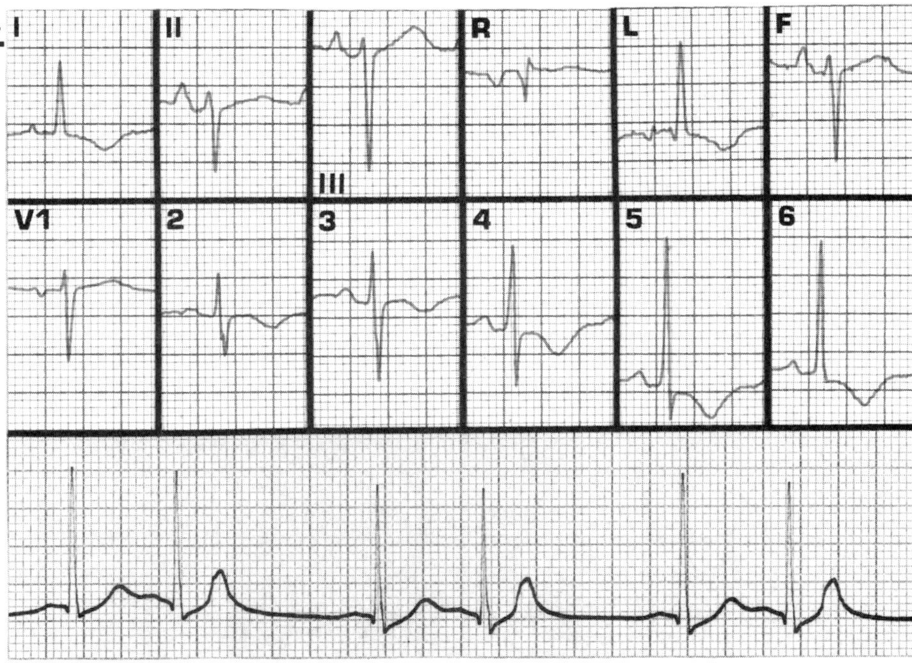

4-38.

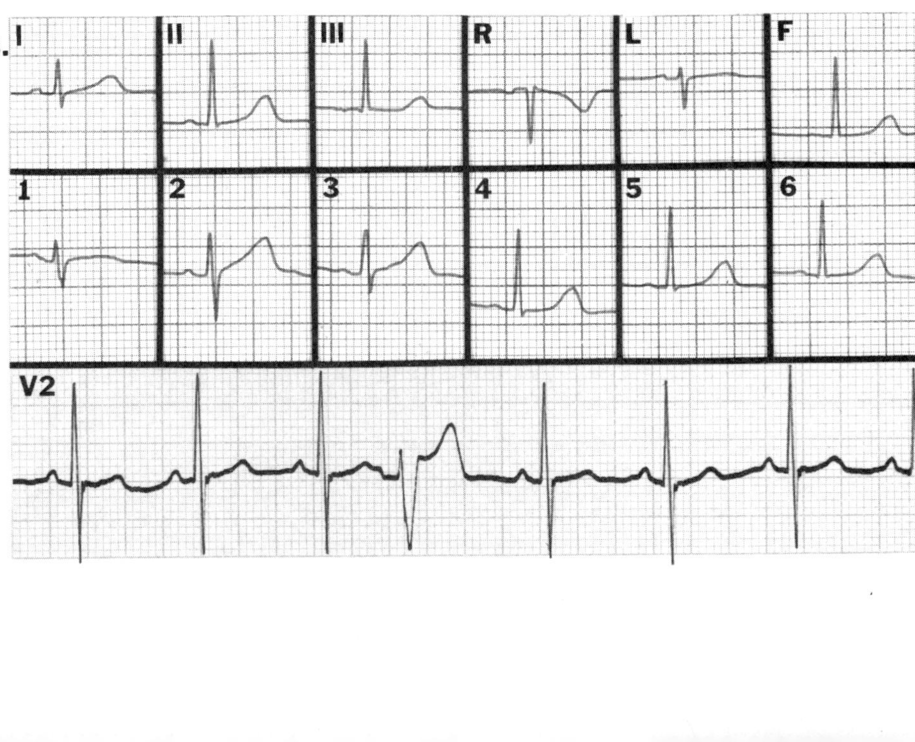

4-39.

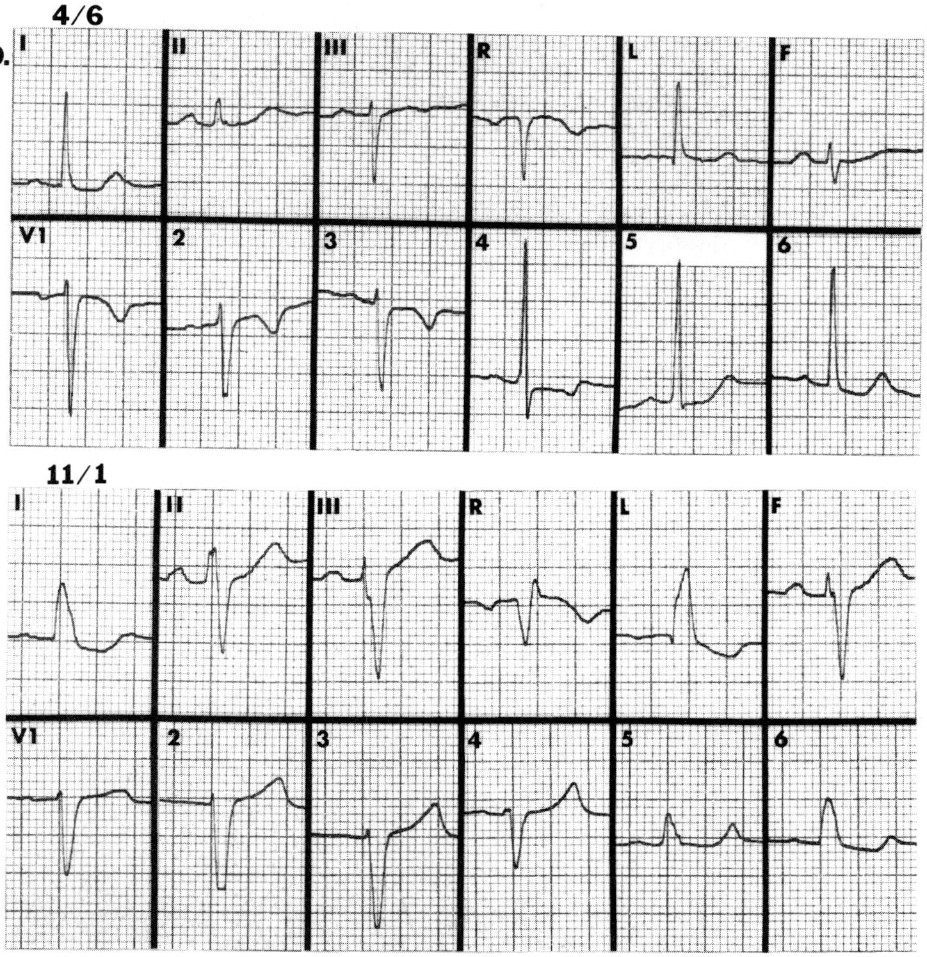

4-40.

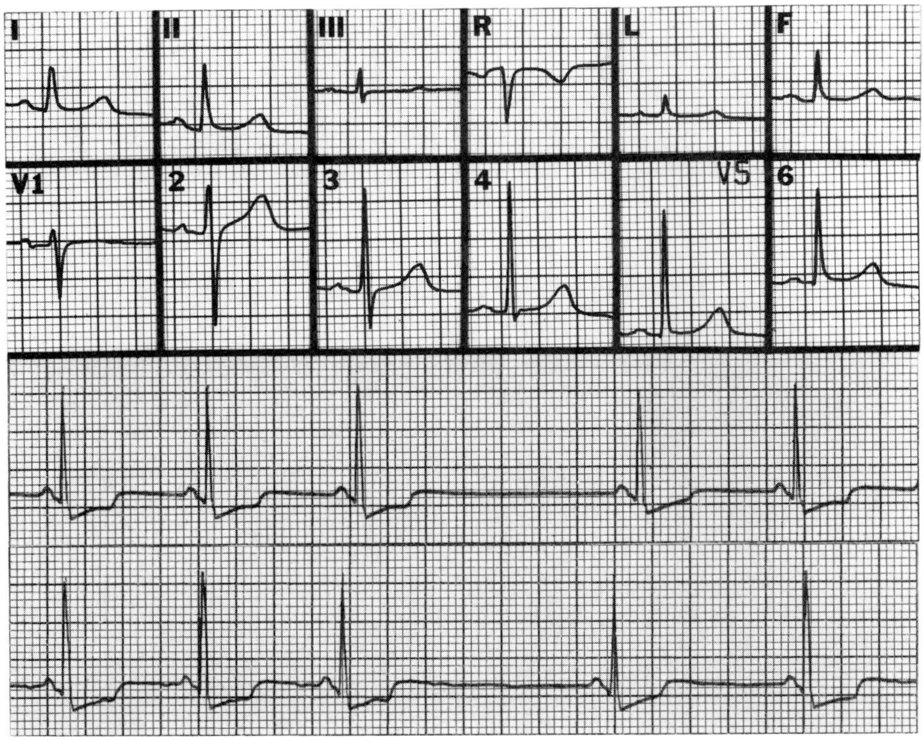

4-41.

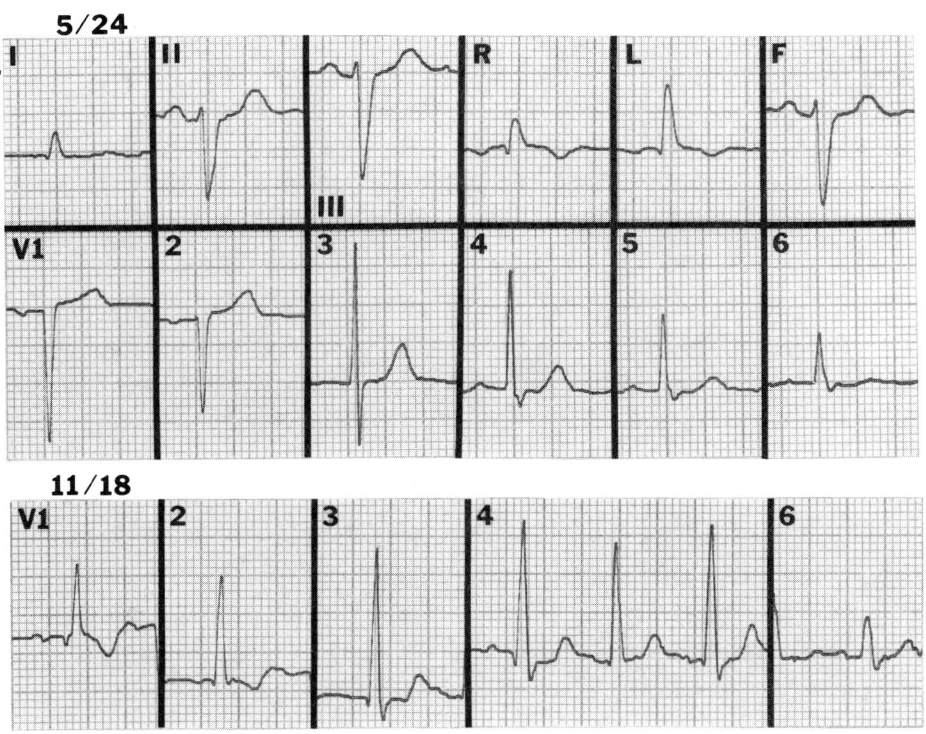

4-42.

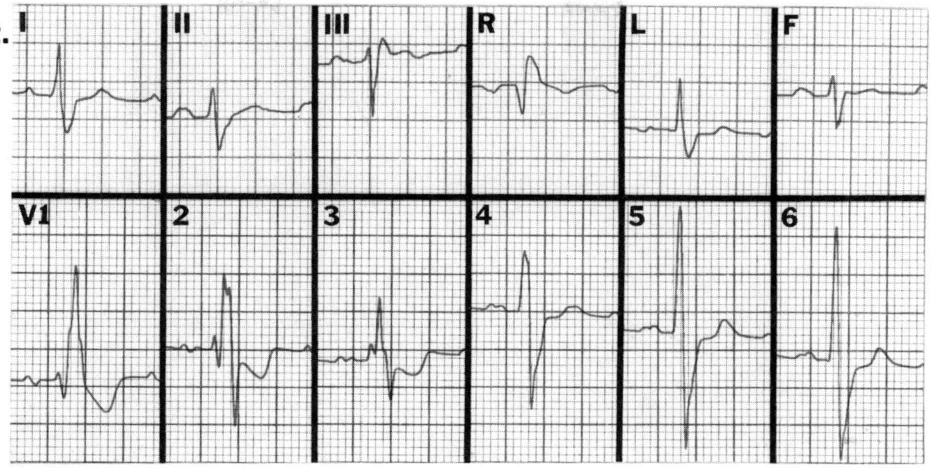

4-43.

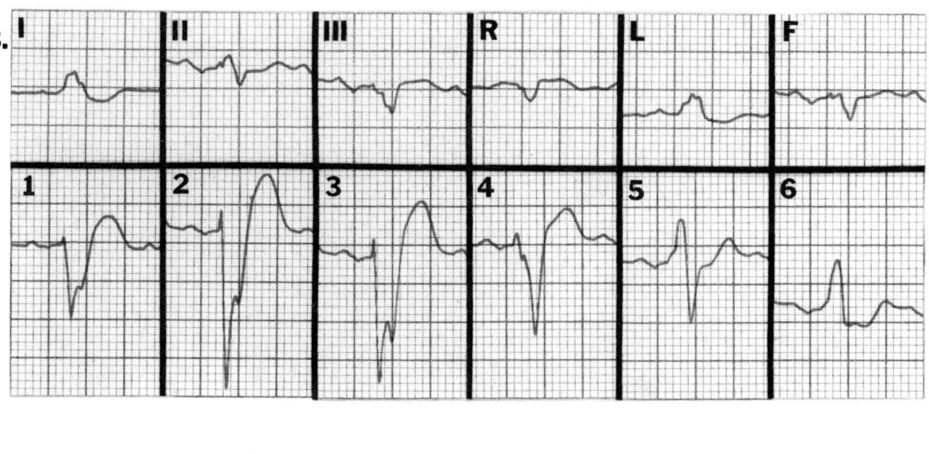

4-44.

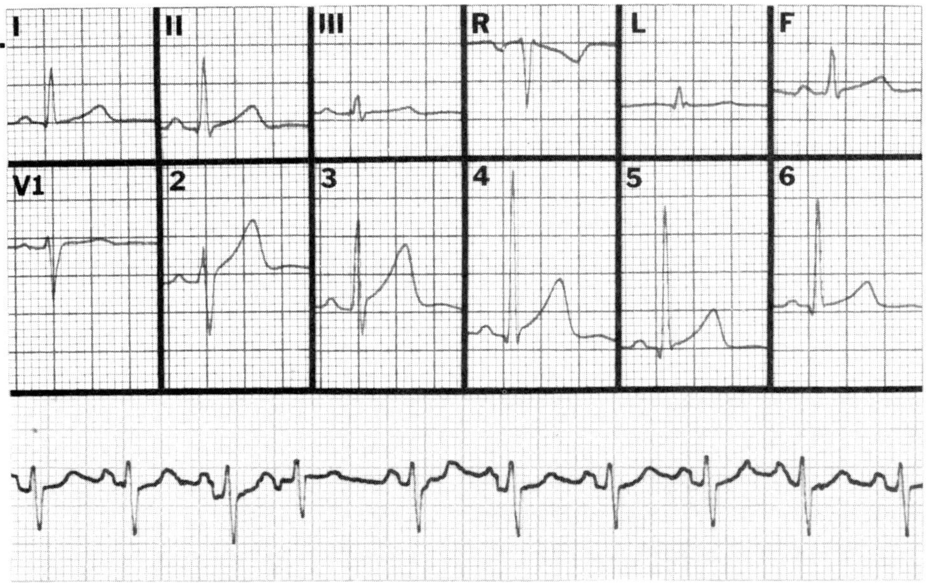

4-45.

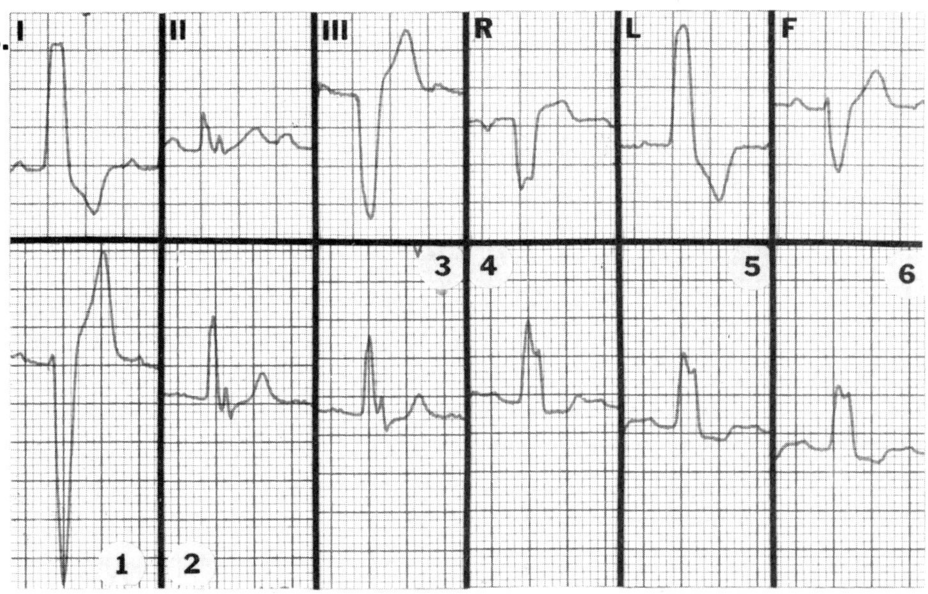

ANSWER KEY

Multiple Choice

1. c
2. d
3. a
4. b, a
5. a, d
6. a, c
7. d
8. c
9. b, d
10. c

Practice Strips

4–1. (ECG of 11/28)
Normal axis, +5 to +15 degrees.
Right bundle branch block.
(ECG of 11/29)
Normal axis, +5 to +15 degrees.
Early transition (V2).
Low voltage (13.5 mm).

4–2. Left axis deviation, −60 to −70 degrees.
LAFB.
RBBB.

4–3. Normal axis, +55 to +65 degrees.
Poor R wave progression.
LBBB.
1st degree AV block (PR 0.22).

4–4. Right axis deviation, +155 to +165 degrees.
Possible LPFB.
RBBB.
Sinus bradycardia, 54/minute, interpolated premature ventricular complex.

4–5. Normal axis, +25 to +35 degrees.
LBBB.

4–6. Left axis deviation, −50 to −60 degrees.
Poor R wave progression.
LBBB.
Ventricular tachycardia versus supraventricular tachycardia with LBBB.

4–7. Normal axis, +25 to +35 degrees.
Poor R wave progression.
LBBB.

4–8. (ECG of 5/03)
Left axis deviation, −10 to −20 degrees.
Poor R wave progression.
LBBB.
Sinus rhythm, 100/minute, block-acceleration dissociation, ventricular rate 62/minute.
(ECG of 5/04)
Left axis deviation, −40 to −50 degrees.
LAFB.
RBBB.
Atrial fibrillation.

4–9. Left axis deviation, −10 to −20 degrees.
Poor R wave progression.
LBBB.

4–10. (ECG of 9/29)
Left axis deviation, −5 to −15 degrees.
Atrial fibrillation.
(ECG of 9/30)
Left axis deviation, −10 to −20 degrees.
LBBB.
Atrial fibrillation with normalization of intraventricular conduction in the third complex of the upper strip.

4–11. Right axis deviation, +115 to +125 degrees.
LPFB.

4–12. Left axis deviation, −5 to −15 degrees.
Poor R wave progression.
LBBB.
Sinus rhythm, 88/minute with normalization of intraventricular conduction in the 4th beat of the upper strip and the third beat of the lower strip.

4–13. Left axis deviation, −55 to −65 degrees.
LAFB.
RBBB.

Junctional rhythm, 40/minute with reciprocation of the third junctional beat to produce a ventricular echo.

4–14. Normal axis, +55 to +65 degrees.
Early transition (V2).
Sinus tachycardia, 130/minute.

4–15. Right axis deviation, +115 to +125 degrees.
LPFB.
RBBB.
1st degree AV block (PR 0.22 second).

4–16. Left axis deviation, −55 to −65 degrees.
LAFB.
LBBB.
1st degree AV block (PR 0.22 second).

4–17. Normal axis, +5 to −5 degrees.
Poor R wave progression.
LBBB.

4–18. Right axis deviation, +115 to +125 degrees.
LPFB.
RBBB.

4–19. Normal axis, +5 to −5 degrees.
Poor R wave progression.
LBBB.
Sinus rhythm, 75/minute, second-degree AV block, type I (Wenckebach), complexes after the pauses produced by the blocked P waves exhibit incomplete left bundle branch block. The third complex in the fourth strip is an escape beat.

4–20. Left axis deviation, −55 to −65 degrees.
LAFB.
RBBB.

4–21. Left axis deviation, −10 to −20 degrees.
Poor R wave progression.
LBBB.
1st degree AV block (PR 0.28 second).

4–22. Right axis deviation, +160 to +170 degrees.
LPFB.
RBBB.

4–23. Left axis deviation, −55 to −65 degrees.
Poor R wave progression.
Late transition (V5).
LAFB.

4–24. Left axis deviation, −10 to −20 degrees.
RBBB.

4–25. Normal axis, +5 to +15 degrees.
RBBB.

4–26. Left axis deviation, −45 to −55 degrees.
Left anterior fascicular block.
RBBB.
Complete (third-degree) atrioventricular block.

4–27. Left axis deviation, −55 to −65 degrees.
LAFB.
LBBB.

4–28. Normal axis, +5 to −5 degrees.
LBBB.

4–29. (ECG of 6/02)
Left axis deviation, −10 to −20 degrees.
Late transition (V5).
(ECG of 6/03)
Left axis deviation, −40 to −50 degrees.
Late transition (V5).
LAFB.
NSIVCD versus LBBB.

4–30. Left axis deviation, −50 to −60 degrees.
Poor R wave progression.
Late transition (?).
LAFB.
NSIVCD.

4–31. (ECG of 1/11)
Left axis deviation, −80 to −90 degrees.
LAFB.
RBBB.
(ECG of 10/20)
Left axis deviation, −40 to −50 degrees.
Poor R wave progression.
Late transition (V5).

LAFB.
LBBB.

4–32. Left axis deviation, −70 to −80 degrees.
LAFB.
NSIVCD versus LBBB.
Atrial flutter, 4:1 conduction, ventricular rate 75/minute.

4–33. Extreme right axis deviation, +225 to +235 degrees.
LPFB.
RBBB.

4–34. Left axis deviation, −50 to −60 degrees.
Late transition (V6).
LAFB.

4–35. Normal axis, +50 to +60 degrees.
LBBB.
Second-degree block; 2:1 conduction with prolonged advanced block with escape beats.

4–36. Left axis deviation, −10 to −20 degrees.
Poor R wave progression.
LBBB.
Sinus rhythm, 73/minute. Second degree AV block. Capture beats preceded by P waves alternate with escape beats to establish an escape-capture bigeminy.

4–37. Left axis deviation, −55 to −65 degrees.
LAFB.
T wave inversion is noted in leads V2–V6.
Sinus tachycardia, 115/minute with pauses produced by nonconducted premature atrial beats (atrial trigeminy).

4–38. Normal axis, +55 to +65 degrees.
Normal ECG.
Sinus rhythm, 91/minute, premature atrial beat with left bundle branch block aberrant ventricular conduction.

4–39. (ECG of 4/6)
Left axis deviation, −5 to −15 degrees.
Poor R wave progression.
(ECG of 11/1)
Left axis deviation, −40 to −50 degrees.
Poor R wave progression.
LBBB.

4–40. Normal axis, +45 to +55 degrees.
Normal ECG.
Sinus rhythm, 75/minute. Probable sinoatrial block.

4–41. (ECG of 5/24)
Left axis deviation, −70 to −80 degrees.
LAFB.
(ECG of 11/18)
RBBB.

4–42. Right axis deviation, +210 to +220 degrees.
Probable LPFB.
RBBB.

4–43. Left axis deviation, −30 to −40 degrees.
Poor R wave progression.
LBBB.

4–44. Normal axis, +50 to +60 degrees.
Normal ECG.
Sinus tachycardia, 115/minute, premature atrial beat.

4–45. Left axis deviation, −5 to −15 degrees.
LBBB.

CHAPTER FIVE

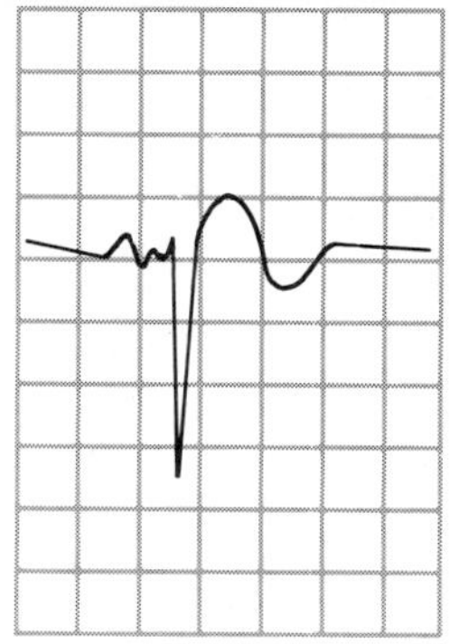

MYOCARDIAL ISCHEMIA AND INFARCTION

COGNITIVE GOALS

1. Identify the primary tool for diagnosing coronary artery disease.
2. Describe the principal branches of the left coronary artery and identify the myocardial segments supplied by each major branch.
3. Define the term **ramus intermedius.**
4. Describe the principal branches of the right coronary artery and identify the myocardial segment supplied by each major branch.
5. Describe the characteristics of a normal ST segment and T wave.
6. Describe the typical changes seen in the ST segment that are characteristic of Prinzmetal's angina.
7. Describe the typical changes seen in the ST segment that are characteristic of myocardial ischemia.
8. Identify the three classic ECG markers of acute myocardial infarction.
9. Name and identify the ECG characteristics of the stages of infarction.
10. Explain the importance of recognizing the hyperacute phase of infarction.
11. Define the terms **coving** and **cove-plane T wave.**
12. Identify the four principal myocardial segments.
13. Differentiate between **indicative** and **reciprocal** changes.
14. Identify the leads in which the indicative changes of anterior wall infarction are seen.
15. Identify the leads in which the indicative changes of inferior wall infarction are seen.
16. Identify the leads in which the indicative changes of lateral wall infarction occur.
17. Identify the leads in which the reciprocal changes of posterior wall infarction are seen.
18. Give the diagnostic criteria for posterior wall infarction.
19. List four recognized causes of ST segment depression in leads V1 to V4 during acute inferior wall infarction and explain the probable significance of this finding in the majority of patients.
20. Discuss why the term **non-Q infarction** is now preferred over the term **subendocardial infarction.**
21. Identify the significance of abnormal Q waves in ectopic ventricular beats.
22. Discuss the relationship between anterior wall infarction and right bundle branch block with or without axis deviation, and discuss the mortality rate in patients with this finding.

23. Identify the diagnostic criteria for the three degrees of atrioventricular block.
24. Differentiate between Mobitz type I and Mobitz type II block.
25. Discuss why it is impossible to reliably classify second-degree block with persistent 2:1 conduction ratio as to type.
26. Define the term **advanced** or **high-grade block.**

Coronary atherosclerosis, a progressive obliteration of the arterial lumen, continues to rank as the major health menace of the industrialized countries. Nearly one million Americans experience myocardial infarction (MI) or sudden cardiac death (SCD) each year, making coronary artery disease (CAD) the most common cause of death in men aged 35 to 44 and the most common cause of death in both sexes aged 45 to 54 (Vanden Belt et al, 1979). Around 600,000 new patients with CAD are diagnosed annually in the United States. Sudden cardiac death, defined as unexpected demise that occurs without prior diagnosed illness or as death within 2 hours of the onset of new symptoms, accounts for some 400,000 fatalitites per year, making it the leading cause of death among middle-aged men. In about 20 per cent of cases, SCD is the first manifestation of CAD (Sonnenblick and Lesch, 1981).

Many persons experiencing myocardial ischemia or infarction do not survive long enough to reach a hospital, often because the symptoms are misinterpreted or denied by the patient, or because ventricular fibrillation (VF) supervenes before the situation can be assessed and help summoned. Ischemia alone, without permanent occlusion of a coronary artery, can induce VF and SCD. For those who reach a facility alive, the in-hospital mortality rate for acute myocardial infarction (AMI) remains at 10 to 20 per cent despite the advent of coronary care units. Most of these deaths are due to mechanical, as opposed to arrhythmic, complications, notably cardiogenic shock resulting from pump failure.

Given the magnitude of this carnage, clinicians are intensely interested in identifying reliable diagnostic markers for CAD. Despite technologic advances, the **patient history** remains the primary diagnostic tool. The ECG is the most important secondary tool for detecting and localizing the site of ischemia or infarction and for diagnosing subsequent rhythm and conduction disturbances. The primary goals of this section include (1) a review of coronary artery anatomy, particularly as it relates to the conduction system, (2) identification of the ECG markers of ischemia and infarction, (3) discussion of the major myocardial segments and their blood supply, and (4) a brief review of the classification of atrioventricular (AV) block.

Coronary artery anatomy

The two coronary arteries, **left** and **right,** originate from the corresponding sinuses of Valsalva and are the first branches of the aorta. Their points of origin, as seen from within the aortic lumen, are called **ostia.**

The **left coronary artery,** also called the **left main coronary artery** (**1** in Fig. 5–1), begins in the left aortic sinus of Valsalva, passes behind the trunk of the pulmonary artery and emerges onto the anterior surface of the heart. Its distribution is illustrated in Figure 5–1. The left main coronary artery is a vessel of variable length, ranging from a very short trunk to a length of several centimeters. Upon reaching the anterior intraventricular sulcus, it divides into two constant branches, the left anterior descending artery, its more direct continuation, and the left circumflex artery.

The **left anterior descending artery** (**4** in Fig. 5–1) and its branches are the principal blood supply of the anterior myocardial segment, including the anterior left ventricular free wall and ventricular septum. Two important sets of secondary branches arise from the left anterior descending (LAD) artery, the **diagonal arteries** (**6** in Fig. 5–1) and the **septal perforating arteries (5).** The one to three diagonal branches supply the anterolateral wall of the left ventricle. The three to five septal perforating branches supply the anterior two thirds of the septum and the associated conduction structures, the right bundle branch, and the anterior radiations of the left bundle branch (Hurst et al, 1982; Rios et al, 1977).

The **left circumflex artery** (**3** in Fig. 5–1), the less direct continuation of the left main coronary artery, originates from it at an angle and curves inferiorly in the atrioventricular sulcus toward the inferior surface of the heart. It supplies the lateral wall of the left ventricle and the dorsal section of the left ventricular cone (compare Fig. 5–9). As many as three **obtuse marginal arteries** (**7** in Fig. 5–1) originate from the circumflex. In the majority of subjects the circumflex ends in a variable number of small muscular branches, but in 10 per cent the circumflex reaches the **crux** (the intersection of the atrioventricular and posterior interventricular sulci) and continues in the posterior interventricular sulcus as the **posterior descending artery** (PDA). When the PDA is supplied by the left circumflex artery, the subject is said to be "left coronary artery dominant."

At times the left coronary artery does not end in a true bifurcation but terminates in three or more branches. If a trifurcation is present, with three vessels originating from the terminus of the left main coronary artery, the most anterior is the left anterior descending (LAD) artery, the most posterior is the circumflex, and the remaining intermediate vessel is the **ramus intermedius** (**8** in Fig. 5–1).

The **right coronary artery** (**2** in Fig. 5–1) originates from the right aortic sinus of Valsalva, passes between the pulmonary artery and right atrial appendage, and turns downward in the atrioventricular sulcus toward the inferior surface of the right ventricle. In 55 per cent of the population, the sinoatrial node (**2** in Fig. 5–3) is supplied by a relatively large branch of the right coronary artery (**3** in Fig. 5–3), the **sinus node artery** (**1** in Fig. 5–3). As it circles the heart toward the inferior surface, the right coronary artery (RCA) supplies branches to the right atrium and ventricle (**2** in Fig. 5–3) and at the crux the important **atrioventricular nodal artery** branches from the RCA (**10** in Fig. 5–1, **7** in Fig. 5–3). At the crux the RCA turns sharply downward, forming the

1. **Left main**
2. **Right coronary**
3. **Circumflex**
4. **Left anterior descending**
5. **Septal perforators**
6. **Diagonals**
7. **Obtuse marginals**
8. **Ramus intermedius**
9. **Posterior descending**
10. **AV nodal**
11. **Septal perforators**

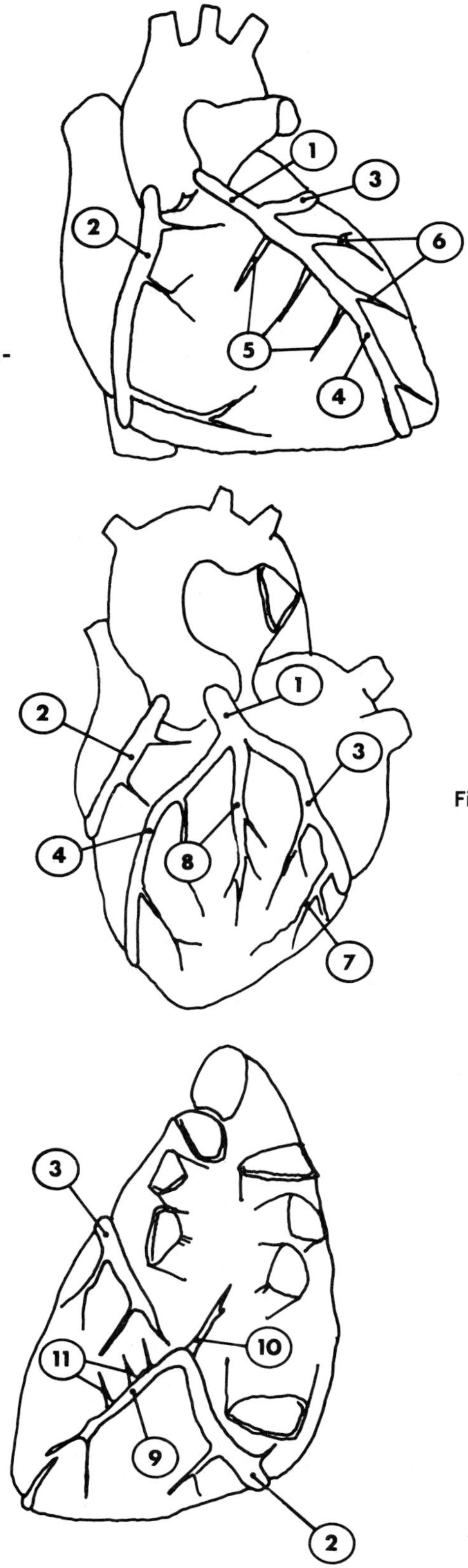

Figure 5–1. The coronary arteries.

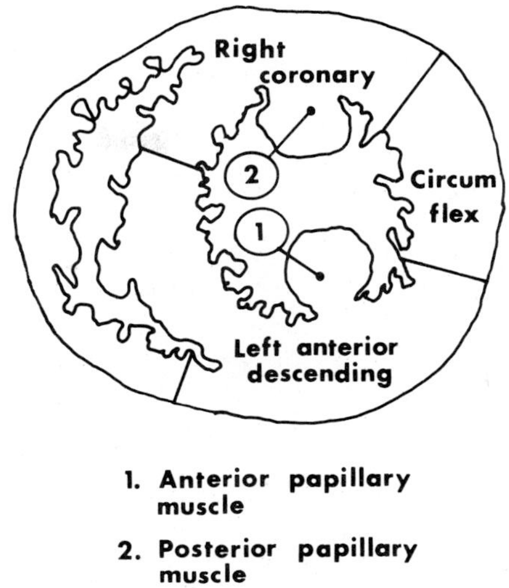

Figure 5–2. The segmental distribution of the coronary arteries.

"shepherd's crook," to continue as the **posterior descending artery** (**9** in Fig. 5–1; **10** in Fig. 5–3). The posterior descending artery is the parallel counterpart of the left anterior descending artery (**5** in Fig. 5–3) and, like the LAD, supplies **septal perforating branches** (**11** in Fig. 5–1) to the posterior one third of the septum and associated conduction structures, the posterior and septal radiations (**6** and **9** in Fig. 5–3) of the left bundle branch. The septal perforating branches of the right and left coronary arteries form anastomoses, establishing an important source of collateral circulation. When the posterior descending artery is supplied by the right coronary artery, as in the majority of cases, the subject is said to be "right coronary artery dominant."

Myocardial ischemia

It cannot be overemphasized that the primary tool for diagnosing myocardial ischemia is the patient history. Evidence of angina or anginal equivalent, such as shortness of breath, must be carefully sought, bearing in mind that many patients have a strong sense of denial. The occurrence of "chest pain" is often flatly denied, while questions about chest tightness, pressure, and squeezing elicit positive responses. Some deny any discomfort related to the chest but describe referred sensations in the hands, arms, jaws, or teeth. The discomfort may be perceived as numbness, aching, tingling, or burning, or as sensation so poorly characterized that no term for it is volunteered. Angina is often dismissed as heartburn, upset stomach, gallbladder pain, or musculoskeletal discomfort. These misidentifications may become more attractive if the anginal attack is accompanied by nausea; vomiting; cool, clammy skin; or other manifestations of sickness such as increased salivation.

The ECG findings that imply myocardial ischemia may be totally absent from a tracing taken at rest. In fact, it may be flatly stated that **a normal ECG**

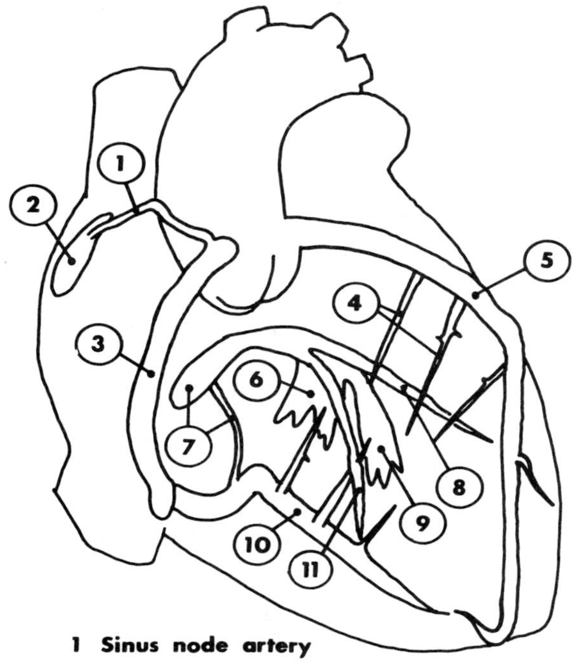

1 Sinus node artery
2. Sinus node
3. Right coronary artery
4. Septal perforators
5. Left anterior descending artery
6. Left posterior fascicle
7. AV node & artery
8. Left anterior fascicle
9. Left septal fascicle
10. Posterior descending artery
11. Right bundle branch

Figure 5–3. The segmental circulation to the conduction system.

taken while a person is comfortable and at rest is meaningless as far as detection of ischemia is concerned.

Some of the ECG findings suggestive of ischemia are illustrated in Figure 5–4. These markers all involve changes in the **ST segment** and **T wave.** The first panel shows a normal QRS-T complex. Note that the upslope of the T wave is gradual (**1** in Fig. 5–4) and that the ST segment merges imperceptibly with the proximal limb of the T wave without any abrupt angles or changes in polarity. A normal ST segment displays a gentle upward slope, that is, **it is not flat.** Further, the ST segment initially lies in the same plane as the isoelectric line, that is, **it is not elevated or depressed.**

Ischemia often causes **ST segment depression** with a sharp angle at the junction of the ST segment and T wave (**2** and **3** in Fig. 5–4). **Flattening** of the ST segment, with or without ST segment depression, is a suspicious finding. Another commonly observed indication of ischemia is **T wave inversion** (**4** in Fig. 5–4). Typically inverted (negative) T waves are relatively narrow and

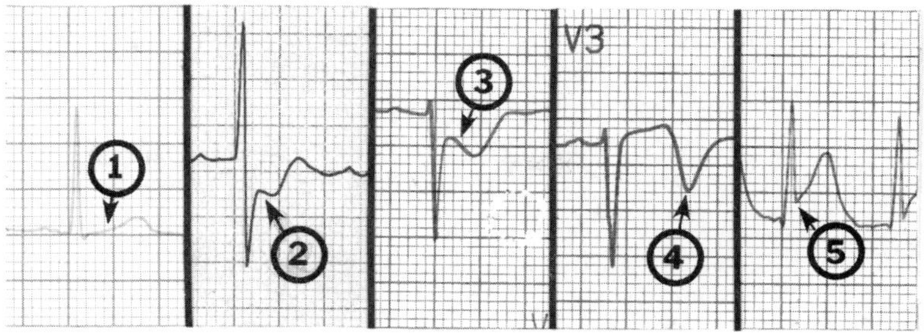

Figure 5–4. The electrocardiographic signs of ischemia.

symmetrical. They are known by several names including **coronary T waves, Pardee T waves** (after a describer), and **arrowhead T waves.** Non-Q infarctions, fully evolved cases of pericarditis, and left ventricular hypertrophy are other common causes of T wave inversion. Further T wave changes are described in the discussion of myocardial infarction.

The classic pattern of ST segment depression that usually indicates myocardial ischemia is in sharp contrast to the behavior of the ST segment that occurs during **variant** or **Prinzmetal's angina.** During Prinzmetal's angina attacks, which are usually due to transient coronary artery spasm, the ECG reveals ST segment **elevation** (**5** in Fig. 5–4), which returns to the baseline after the episode of vascular spasm is over.

Myocardial infarction

According to classic ECG theory, three markers are used for the diagnosis of acute myocardial infarction: (1) **inverted T waves,** (2) **elevated ST segments,** and (3) **abnormal Q waves.** In the classic paradigm, inverted T waves are thought to represent myocardial ischemia in a zone surrounding the infarcted area, ST segment elevation to represent myocardial injury, and pathologic Q waves to indicate the presence of necrosis. Pathologic Q waves are 0.04 second or more wide and appear in the leads facing the infarcted area. Classically, ischemic changes (inverted T waves) and injury (ST segment elevation) are regarded as a reversible finding, but infarction (abnormal Q waves) is regarded as irreversible.

A significant number of cases of infarction do not present in the classic manner and result in ECG findings that cause even experienced electrocardiographers to miss the presence of or underestimate the extent of an infarction using ECG criteria alone. In addition, other conditions, including the cardiomyopathies, left ventricular hypertrophy, and the Wolff-Parkinson-White syndrome, can produce spurious infarct patterns. These caveats are mentioned to emphasize the importance of integrating the ECG into the total patient data. The ECG is an imperfect assessment tool, not a magic wand, even in the hands of the most experienced and erudite. Fortunately, the majority of myocardial infarctions can be readily diagnosed or at the very least strongly suspected by ECG during their acute and most dangerous phase.

The ECG pattern of infarction typically **evolves in stages.** The **hyperacute,** or very earliest stage, represents the first ECG manifestations of infarction, but disappears rapidly. The **acute** phase is observed in the first day to a week after infarction begins. The **recent** phase reflects an infarction less than 1 month old, and the term **old** infarction is reserved for healing infarctions that are generally more than 3 months old. A fifth category, **age undetermined,** is often encountered when the stage of an infarction cannot be estimated with any certainty (Surawicz et al, 1978).

The hallmarks of various stages are shown in Figure 5–5. Panel **A** illustrates a normal QRS-T complex. Note that the junction of the QRS complex and the ST segment, the **J point,** is at the isoelectric line and that the ST segment exhibits a gradual upward slope as it merges imperceptibly with the ascending limb of the T wave (**1** in panel **A**).

The earliest stage of infarction, the **hyperacute phase,** is characterized by abnormally tall, symmetrical T waves (**1** in panel **B**) with or without associated ST segment elevation. Hyperacute change represents the first ECG evidence of an "infarction in progress" and its prompt recognition assumes increasing importance with the current emphasis on timely restoration of circulation to infarcting segments of myocardium (Kennedy, 1987). Unless hyperacute changes are recognized for what they are, the first opportunity to diagnose an acute infarction will, unfortunately, be missed.

As the infarction progresses to the **acute phase,** ST segment elevation occurs in those leads facing the infarcted area (**1** in panel **C**) and persists as a feature of later stages (**1** in panels **D** and **E**). Early in the evolution of the infarct pattern, the T waves begin to invert (**2** in panels **D, F,** and **G**). Finally, abnormal Q waves, the classic sine qua non of infarction, appear in the leads facing the infarcted area (**2** in panel **C, 3** in panels **D, F,** and **G**). Elevation of the ST segment and T wave inversion in leads facing the necrotic area often combine

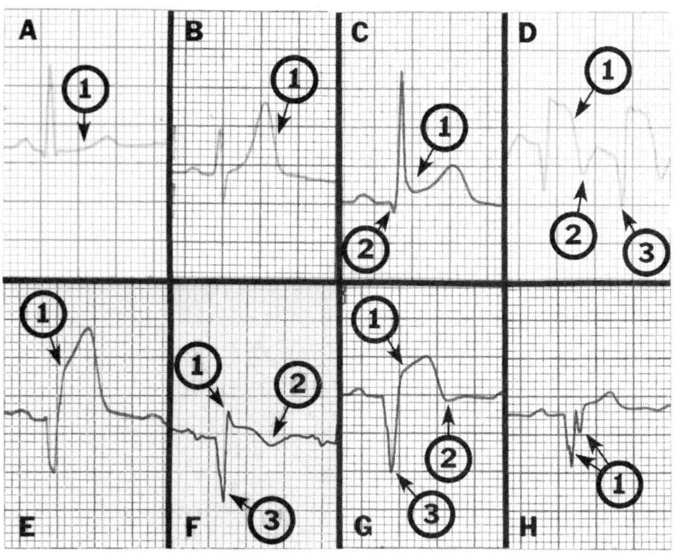

Figure 5–5. The electrocardiographic signs of infarction.

to produce a gracefully arched ST-T complex, which is said to exhibit **coving.** The distal limb of the inverted T wave straightens (or "planes") so that the resulting ST segment and T wave have acquired the name **cove-plane T wave** (**1** and **2** in panel **D** illustrate this effect). In many cases, ST segment elevation raises the J point (**1** in panel **E**). An abnormal Q wave may consist of two successive negative waves written below the baseline so that a **QS complex** results (**1** in panel **H**).

As the infarction progresses through the **recent** to the **old** phase, ST segment elevation subsides and the T waves regain their normal positive polarity, as shown in panel **H.** In upwards of 10 per cent of cases that initially show abnormal Q waves, the Q waves eventually disappear and the ECG becomes nondiagnostic for infarction (Silverman and Silverman 1979). The reliability of the Q wave as an indicator of necrosis is thrown further into doubt by the finding that transient Q waves appear during episodes of ischemia and disappear after the ischemia resolves (Bashour, 1983; Bateman et al, 1983).

Basically, four major myocardial segments are distinguished electrocardiographically: (1) **anterior,** (2) **inferior,** (3) **lateral,** and (4) **posterior.** A task force on terminology recognized these and certain subsegmental infarctions, which are listed in Table 5–1 (Surawicz et al, 1978).

Anterior wall myocardial infarction (AWMI) is diagnosed when T wave inversion, ST segment elevation, and Q waves are seen in the precordial leads. The infarction may be localized to the septal area (V1, V2), or may involve all or part of the left ventricular free wall (V3 to V6). An evolving anteroseptal infarction is shown in Figure 5–6, in which coving of the ST segments, T wave inversion, and abnormal Q waves are noted in leads V1 to V4. The low amplitude of the QRS complexes in V5 and V6 probably represents loss of voltage owing to necrosis of the myocardium underlying those leads. AWMI is associated with serious atrioventricular conduction defects preceded by right or left bundle branch block, a higher incidence of cardiogenic shock, and a higher average mortality than is typical of infarctions of other segments. *Initially* a hyperdynamic cardiovascular response characterized by tachycardia and hypertension predominates. The occluded artery is almost always the left anterior descending, the "artery of sudden death" or "the widowmaker" in the jargon of pathologists and cardiologists.

Inferior wall infarction is diagnosed by ST segment elevation, T wave inversion, and Q waves in the inferior leads (II, III, aVF). Figure 5–7 illustrates the hyperacute phase of an inferior wall infarction (IWMI). The leads facing

Table 5–1. SEGMENTAL AND SUBSEGMENTAL INFARCTIONS

Segment	Q Waves
Anterior	V3, V4
Septal	V1, V2
Anteroseptal	V1–V4
Lateral	I, aVL, V5, V6
Anterolateral	I, aVL, V3–V6
Inferior	II, III, aVF
Posterior	Wide R waves V1, V2

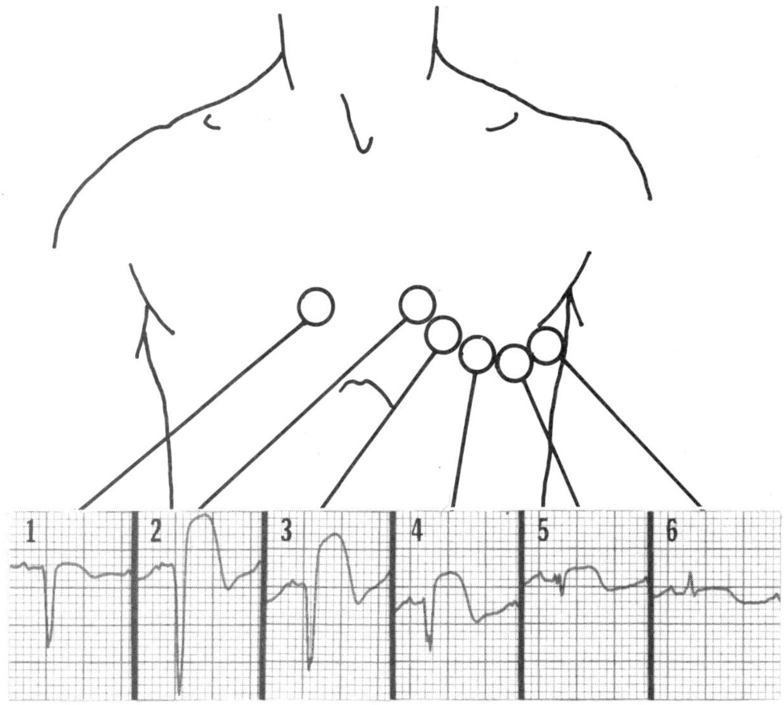

Figure 5–6. Anterior wall myocardial infarction.

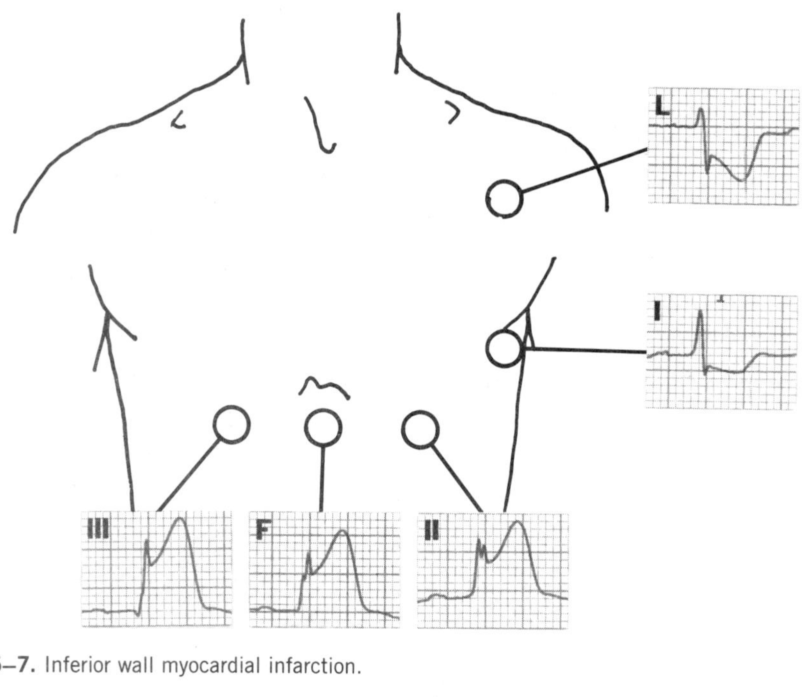

Figure 5–7. Inferior wall myocardial infarction.

the area of infarction record the expected ECG changes, which at this stage consist of marked ST segment elevation, upward displacement of the J point, and pointed, symmetrical T waves. ECG changes in the leads *facing* the infarcted area are collectively called **indicative changes.** Leads *facing away from* the infarcting segment, in this case leads I and aVL, record a mirror image consisting of depressed ST segments and J point depression. Changes in leads remote from the infarcting segment are collectively known as **reciprocal changes.** Inferior wall infarctions are *initially* characterized by hypodynamic circulatory responses such as bradyarrhythmias, particularly sinus bradycardia and accelerated idioventricular rhythm (AIVR), and hypotension. Occasionally patients exhibit other signs of increased vagal tone such as wheezing, increased salivation, and high-grade AV block precipitated by Valsalva maneuvers such as straining. Inferior wall infarction is usually due to obstruction of the right coronary artery.

Diagnosis of a remote IWMI, particularly after the ST segment and T wave changes have normalized, is often difficult. A wide Q wave is a normal feature in lead III in 4 per cent of the population, and Q waves are also commonly seen in lead III as a result of cor pulmonale, right bundle branch block, and left ventricular hypertrophy (Silverman and Silverman, 1979). About 10 per cent of subjects with IWMI exhibit an **rS** pattern in leads III and aVF owing to concomitant left anterior fascicular block. In a study of 48 patients with confirmed IWMI, Shettigar and associates found that only 15 per cent with healed infarctions retained Q waves in all three inferior leads and that 29 per cent did not retain Q waves in any of the inferior leads (Shettigar et al, 1974).

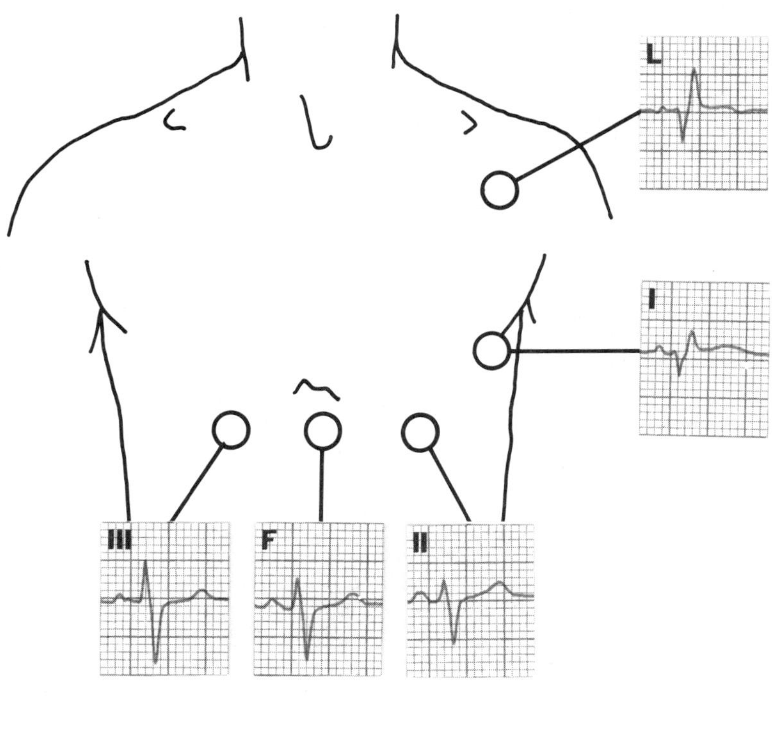

Figure 5–8. Lateral wall myocardial infarction.

Lateral wall infarction (LWMI) is diagnosed by ST-T wave changes and Q waves in the lateral leads I, aVL, V5, and V6 (Fig. 5–8). LWMI generally results from occlusion of the circumflex artery or one of its major branches. Conduction deficits of any kind rarely appear. The case shown in Figure 5–8 demonstrates that ST segment elevation and T wave inversion resolve as an infarction heals and the event becomes more remote in time. Although traditional teaching has maintained that Q waves in the lateral leads are specific for infarctions of the lateral wall, recent studies have cast a shadow of doubt on the specificity of these findings (Movahed and Becker, 1984; Warner et al, 1986).

Although **posterior wall infarction (PWMI)** is not an uncommon event, it goes virtually unmentioned in many critical care courses and rates only passing reference in many ECG texts. PWMI can occur as an isolated event or in conjunction with infarctions of the inferior or lateral walls. The posterior segment is located dorsally, at the base of the left ventricular "cone," and is oriented toward the vertebral column. It is usually supplied by the distal branches of the circumflex artery or the right coronary artery or both. The area and blood supply of the posterior segment are shown in Figure 5–9.

In an older terminology the inferior myocardial segment, represented by leads II, III, and aVF, was called the "posterior" wall and the anatomically posterior segment per se was not known to have electrocardiographic representation. Not until relatively recently was posterior infarction recognized as a separate ECG entity. The authors who described PWMI and established the ECG criteria for its diagnosis used the terms "strictly posterior" or "true posterior" in an attempt to avoid confusion (Perloff, 1964). Diagnosis of PWMI poses a problem because none of the conventional leads face that segment and also because the distance of the posterior segment from the surface leads tends to diminish the sensitivity of those leads to changes that take place during

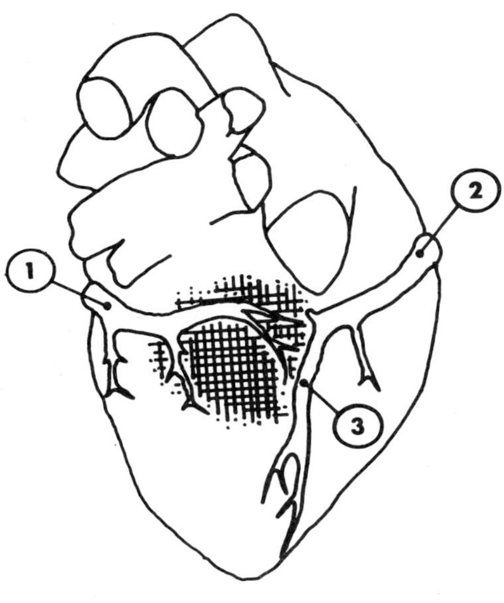

Figure 5–9. The posterior myocardial segment and its blood supply. *1*, Circumflex artery; *2*, right coronary artery; *3*, posterior descending artery.

infarction of the posterior wall. In the cases of PWMI, diagnosis is made entirely on the basis of indirect or reciprocal changes that appear in the leads opposite the posterior segment, leads V1 to V3. Unfortunately, the absence of diagnostic changes in those leads does not exclude the possibility of posterior infarction (Eisenstein et al, 1985).

The characteristic triad of (1) **tall R waves,** (2) **depressed ST segments,** and (3) **tall, symmetrical T waves** in leads V1 or V2 or both is a mirror image of the usual triad of deep Q waves, elevated ST segments, and inverted, symmetrical T waves recorded by leads facing infarctions in other segments. The ECG criteria for acute PWMI include:

1. An increase in the duration and amplitude of the R wave in leads V1 to V3
2. Tall, wide, symmetrical T waves in leads V1 to V3
3. Depression of the ST segments in leads V1 to V3
4. Evidence of coexisting infarction in the inferior (II, III, aVF) or lateral (I, aVL, V5, V6) leads
5. **Voltage dropoff,** a marked loss of R wave amplitude, in the left precordial leads (V5, V6)

Increased amplitude (height) and duration (width) of the R waves in V1 to V2 or V3 are the most reliable of the criteria for PWMI. Increased amplitude of the R waves results in an R:S ratio equal to or greater than 1 in those leads. In the normal right ventricular complex, an **rS** complex, the R:S ratio is usually less than 1. The width of the R wave follows the same criterion used to identify abnormal Q waves (0.04 second or more). Complete descriptions of the ECG findings and examples of tracings have been published in the nursing and medical literature (Perloff, 1964; Schamroth, 1984; Conner, 1985). A recent study indicates that PWMI by ECG correlates quite well with circumflex artery lesions that result in damage to the basal and lateral left ventricular wall. When found in combination with IWMI, as is often the case, the additional finding of PWMI identifies patients with severe disease of both the circumflex and the right coronary arteries (Bough and Korr, 1986).

The typical findings of PWMI are shown in Figure 5–10. Tall R waves are observed in leads V1 to V3, as are tall, symmetrical T waves. Voltage dropoff (low R wave amplitude) is noted in leads V5 and V6. In this particular case, a distal obstruction of the circumflex artery was demonstrated angiographically.

Inferior wall infarction with precordial ST segment depression

Depression of the ST segments in leads V1 to V4 is a common finding in cases of acute IWMI. The significance of such ST segment depression in the right precordial leads is currently a subject of much research and debate among electrocardiographers. At least four mechanisms have been invoked to account for this constellation of findings: (1) **reciprocal change,** (2) **remote ischemia,**

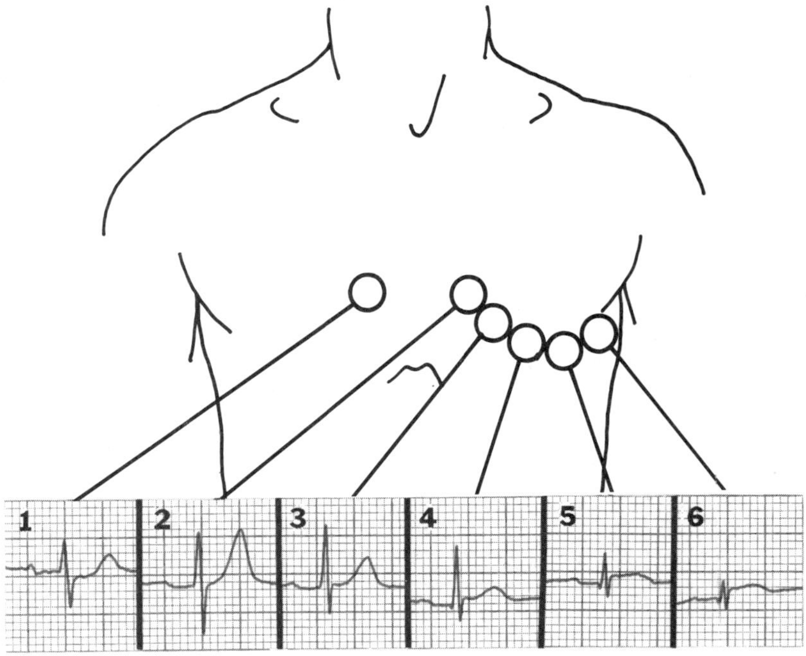

Figure 5–10. Posterior wall myocardial infarction.

(3) **more extensive necrosis,** and (4) **the hyperacute phase of posterior wall infarction.**

Investigators who propose the reciprocal change theory believe that precordial ST segment depression accompanying IWMI represents an essentially benign electrical phenomenon that does not add significantly to morbidity or mortality (Goldberger, 1975; Croft et al, 1982; Wasserman et al, 1983). However, based on the same ECG criteria, a number of studies have identified a subset of patients with more extensive infarctions, increased morbidity and mortality, and poorer long-term prognosis with an increased propensity for recurrent infarction. In a study of 162 patients, Hlatky and coworkers noted a 13 per cent in-hospital mortality rate for those exhibiting ST segment depression in leads V1 to V4 during the acute stage of IWMI versus a 4 per cent mortality rate for patients with acute IWMI but no right precordial changes (Hlatky et al, 1985). A recent study in Sweden, based on 229 subjects, concluded that acute IWMI combined with ST segment depression in the anterior chest leads predicted larger infarctions, an increased incidence of congestive heart failure and significant hypotension, and a higher 5-year mortality rate (Herlitz and Hjalmarson, 1987). Other studies have documented evidence of larger infarct size as determined by serum enzyme levels, echocardiographic evidence of more pronounced wall motion abnormalities, and a greater decrease in ejection fraction among subjects with precordial ST segment depression and IWMI (Shah et al, 1980; Goldberg et al, 1981; Gibson et al, 1982; Gelman and Saltups, 1982; Nasmith et al, 1982; Ong et al, 1983; Boden et al, 1984; Dewhurst and Muir,

1985; Berland et al, 1986; Lembo et al, 1986; Ruddy et al, 1986). Remote ischemia due to coexisting obstructions in the left anterior descending artery has been advanced as another cause of precordial ST depression (Dunn et al, 1979; Schuster and Bulkley, 1981; Salcedo et al, 1981; Tendera and Campbell, 1983), and the hyperacute phase of simultaneous posterior wall infarction is another documented cause (Schamroth, 1984). The weight of current evidence indicates that precordial ST segment depression present during the acute phase of inferior infarction is not an innocent finding in the majority of cases but rather is a marker of more extensive infarction, either posterior, inferobasal, or inferoapical (Pierard et al, 1986); more serious congestive failure; and higher probability of future cardiac disease or death.

Figure 5–11 illustrates serial ECGs obtained from a 35-year-old male. The tracing of August 30 shows indicative hyperacute changes in the inferior leads (II, III, aVF), consisting of ST segment elevation (**1** in Fig. 5–11) and an expected reciprocal change in lead aVL that consists of ST segment depression **(2).** In addition, marked ST segment depression **(3)** is noted in the right precordial leads (V1 to V4). The tracing of September 3 shows pathologic Q waves in the inferior leads **(4)** with QS complexes in leads III and aVF. In the second tracing, the zone of transition has moved rightward, and tall R waves **(5)** and pointed,

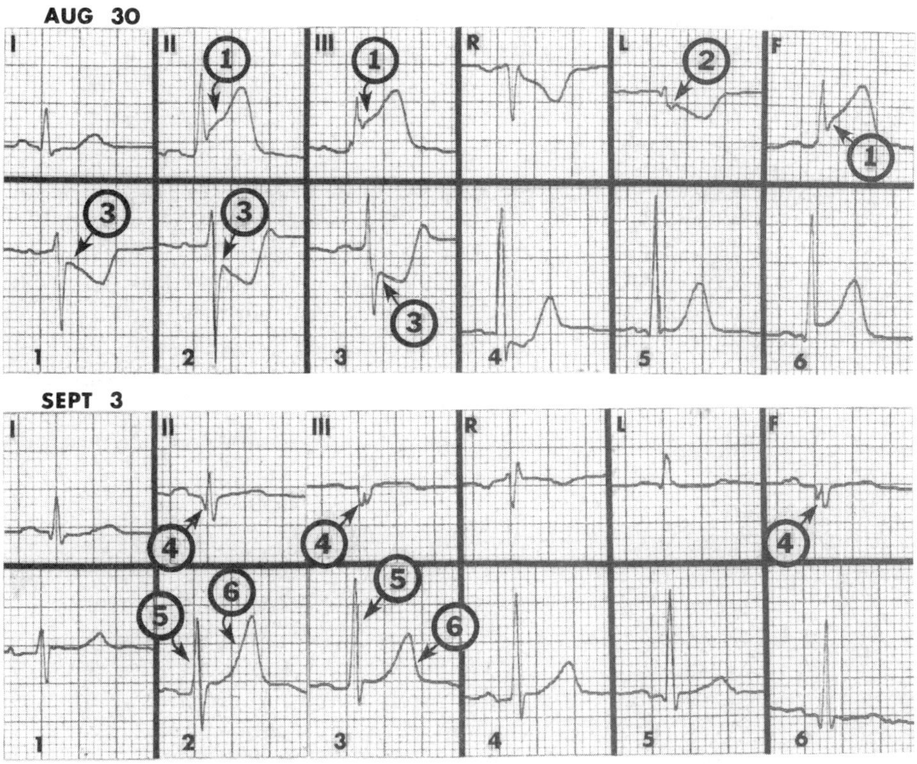

Figure 5–11. Precordial ST segment depression (V1–V3) representing hyperacute phase of posterior wall infarction.

symmetrical T waves **(6)** are now present in leads V2 and V3. These findings suggest the diagnosis of PWMI in addition to IWMI.

Non-Q infarctions

Traditional teaching has regarded the Q wave as the essential marker of a transmural (or full-thickness) infarction of the myocardium. Infarctions not involving the entire thickness of the myocardium (or "subendocardial infarctions") were thought to produce only ST segment and T wave changes without the appearance of abnormal Q waves. Many recent studies have shown this distinction to be untenable: infarctions that involve less than the complete thickness of the ventricular wall are known to produce Q waves. On the other hand, infarctions of the complete thickness of the myocardium occasionally do *not* produce diagnostic Q waves. Rarely an infarction may not produce any diagnostic changes on the ECG. Infarctions that do not produce Q waves are still frequently called "subendocardial infarctions" on the false assumption that only full-thickness, transmural, infarctions produce Q waves. The term "subendocardial" is lacking in specificity and is being replaced in the literature by the term **non-Q infarction,** a more accurate appelative that leaves open the question of the thickness of the infarction and the completeness of the infarction process (Phibbs, 1983; Spodick, 1983).

Although absolute consensus among studies is lacking, it appears that as a rule infarctions that exhibit Q waves carry a higher *initial* mortality rate and that patients with Q infarctions tend to have more evidence of left ventricular damage as measured by such parameters as end-diastolic pressure and ejection fraction (Zema, 1985). Non-Q infarctions appear more likely to represent *partial* infarction, which is prone to extend itself later to encompass the full thickness of the myocardial wall. Such infarctions are said to "complete." Extension or completion of a non-Q infarction at a later date, sometimes within days or weeks, carries a significant risk to the patient (Goldberger, 1984; Chou, 1986). Non-Q infarctions often display marked T-wave inversion in both the limb and precordial leads. The negative T waves are usually symmetrical and their depth may equal or surpass the height of the associated QRS complexes.

Q waves in ectopic ventricular beats

Resolution of Q waves is of such frequent occurrence that it is estimated that only 85 per cent of tracings will still have diagnostic Q waves a year after infarction (Rios et al, 1977). However, the asynchronous depolarization of the myocardium that results from premature ventricular beats can unmask Q waves that do not still appear in normally conducted beats. With the exception of leads aVR and V1, a QR or QRS noted in a premature ventricular beat warrants strong suspicion of a previous infarction even if the complexes of normal beats do not show Q waves. To be diagnostically significant, the QRS complex of

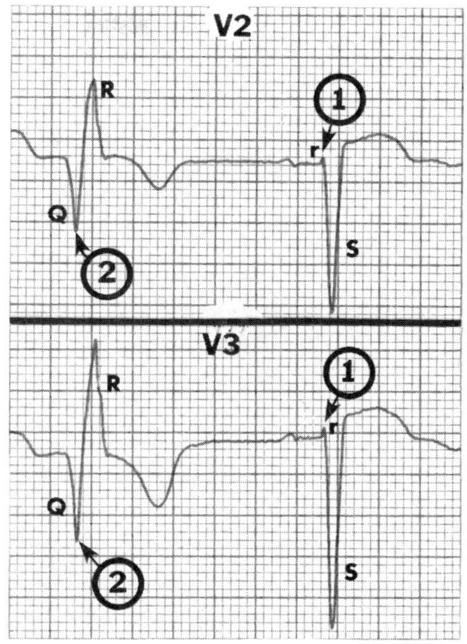

Figure 5–12. Diagnostic Q waves in ventricular ectopic beats.

the ventricular premature beat **must have a strong, positive component.** Completely negative complexes (QS) are fairly common in ectopic ventricular beats and are *not* diagnostically significant (Goldberger, 1984; Schamroth, 1984).

An example of diagnostic Q waves in ventricular premature beats is given in Figure 5–12. Leads V2 and V3 are shown. The normal complexes begin with small **r waves (1)** followed by deep **S waves,** whereas the ventricular complexes begin with wide **Q waves (2)** followed in each case by a strong positive component (R wave). The remainder of the tracing showed diagnostic Q waves in the normal beats in leads I, aVL, and V6. The Q waves in the ectopic beats likely indicate the existence of a more extensive previous infarction than is obvious from an examination of the normal beats.

Conduction deficits

Bundle branch and fascicular block are frequent complications of anterior wall infarction. The in-hospital mortality accompanying bundle branch block, with and without associated fascicular block, is shown in Table 5–2. It is

Table 5–2. CONDUCTION DEFECTS AND ASSOCIATED MORTALITY

Block	Mortality	Pump Failure
LAFB	27%	64%
LPFB	47%	69%
RBBB	40%	70%
RBBB + LAFB	42%	66%
RBBB + LPFB	59%	75%

From Saksena and Sung, 1980.

immediately obvious from an examination of the statistics in this table that the majority of patients with intraventricular conduction deficits die from mechanical, not electrical, causes; that is, pump failure and resulting cardiogenic shock account for many more deaths than does ventricular asystole due to bilateral bundle branch block.

An estimated 20 per cent of cases in which right bundle branch block is a complication of acute infarction will progress to complete loss of atrioventricular conduction. The majority of these subjects will also have fascicular block. In most instances this form of conduction loss represents bilateral bundle branch block, which is usually temporary but which is associated with a very high mortality rate in spite of pacing. Conduction loss in a bundle branch nearly always signifies extensive destruction of ventricular muscle. Atrioventricular block in the setting of anterior wall infarction is usually sudden in onset, is preceded by bundle branch block, and is accompanied by high mortality. AV block associated with inferior wall infarction, although more common, does not appear to add a significant increase to the mortality rate even if it progresses to complete AV block, provided it is treated promptly (Brown et al, 1969; Norris et al, 1972; Hindman et al, 1978).

Classification of atrioventricular block

First-degree AV block is a prolongation of the PR interval to more than 0.20 second in adults or to more than 0.18 second in children under age 14. Various forms of AV block are illustrated diagrammatically in Figure 5–13.

Second-degree AV block is defined as intermittent failure of some sinus impulses to reach the ventricles. It is divided into two subtypes: Mobitz type I or Wenckebach and Mobitz type II. **Wenckebach** or **Mobitz type I** second-degree block (Fig. 5–13) is characterized by progressive increases in conduction delay culminating in complete failure of impulse transmission. Block of the last sinus impulse in each cycle results in a momentary pause in the ventricular rhythm, which is usually less than twice the basic sinus cycle length. The first PR interval after each pause is shorter than the last PR interval before the pause. The conduction ratio of a Wenckebach cycle is determined by the number of P waves to the number of QRS complexes (P:QRS). Atypical Wenckebach cycles are very common and are of clinical interest because they can be (and have been) confused with Mobitz type II block (El-Sherif et al, 1978; Denes et al, 1975; Conner, 1987).

Mobitz type II second-degree block is diagnosed when all *consecutive* PR intervals, both before and *after* the blocked P wave, remain the same length. Mobitz type II is a manifestation of bilateral bundle branch block in most cases and is rare.

Second-degree block with persistent 2:1 or 3:1 ratios of conduction poses a diagnostic dilemma because the most helpful diagnostic feature for distinguishing between Mobitz type I and type II, the behavior of *consecutive* PR intervals, is absent. Almost all cases of 2:1 AV block are simply variants of the

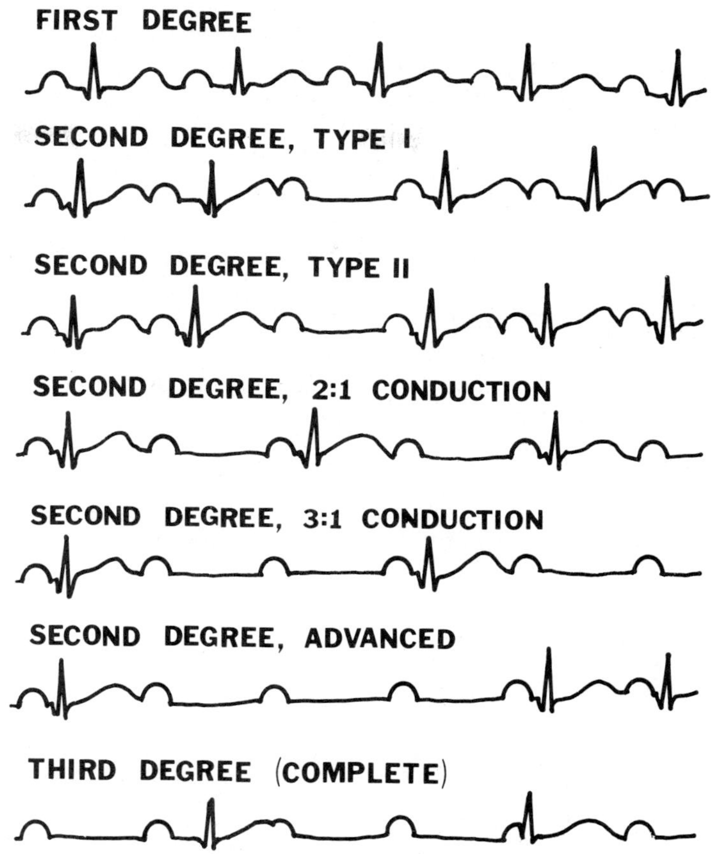

Figure 5–13. A simplified classification of atrioventricular block.

Mobitz type I (Wenckebach) variety. Most cases of persistent 3:1 AV conduction are probably type I variants also. Some authors customarily classify all 2:1 block as Mobitz type II because all the PR intervals are the same length. However, unless *two or more consecutive* PR intervals are available for inspection in some part of the record, no attempt should be made to classify persistent 2:1 or 3:1 blocks as to type (Narula, 1979; Pick and Langendorf, 1979; Marriott, 1983).

Advanced or **high-grade AV block** is a form of second-degree block diagnosed when *two or more consecutive* sinus impulses are blocked at atrial rates less than 150 per minute (Fig. 5–13). This form of second-degree AV block is more common in the setting of anterior wall infarction and represents a variant of Mobitz type II block in those cases. Its onset is often abrupt and is preceded by right bundle branch block in most cases. Advanced AV block is also frequently observed as an agonal arrhythmia.

Third-degree or **complete AV block** refers to *prolonged, total* loss of atrioventricular conduction, which results in asynchronous, independent atrial and ventricular activity (atrioventricular dissociation). A confident diagnosis of complete heart block cannot be made unless the ventricular rate is *less than 40 per minute.* In the setting of anterior wall infarction, complete AV block may result in ventricular asystole. In inferior wall infarction, ventricular asystole is rarely seen as a result of third-degree AV block.

Atrioventricular block complicating AWMI and IWMI almost invariably progresses in definite *stages*, but the progression of events differs markedly. Atrioventricular block in the setting of AWMI is infranodal, representing transient or persistent bilateral bundle branch block, and progresses in stages from fascicular block to bundle branch block to complete AV block. In nearly all cases, AV block complicating IWMI is nodal and progresses in stages from first-degree block to second-degree block (generally Mobitz type I, or 2:1) to advanced or third-degree block.

Relatively minor degrees of block can combine with relatively fast escape rhythms to produce prolonged independent atrial and ventricular activity, atrioventricular dissociation, that closely mimics third-stage block in appearance. An undefined degree of block, often only first-degree, combined with interference from a subsidiary junctional or ventricular escape rhythm, can cause prolonged dissociation, a state of affairs for which Marriott has coined the useful term **block-acceleration dissociation** (Marriott, 1983).

References

Bashour, TT. **Am Heart J** 106:780–783, 1983.
Bateman, TM, et al. **Am Heart J** 106:1421–1426, 1983.
Berland, J, et al. **Am Heart J** 111:481–488, 1986.
Boden, WE, et al. **Am J Cardiol** 54:1216–1223, 1984.
Bough, EW, and Korr, KS. **J Am Coll Cardiol** 7:990–996, 1986.
Brown RW, et al. **Am Heart J** 78:460–466, 1969.
Chou, T-C. **Electrocardiography in Clinical Practice,** 2nd ed. Grune & Stratton, New York, 1986, pp 161–162.
Conner, RP. **Crit Care Nurse** 5:20–24, 1985.
Conner, RP. **Heart Lung** 16:506–518, 1987.
Croft, CW, et al. **Am J Cardiol** 50:428–436, 1982.
Denes, P, et al. **Am Heart J** 89:26–31, 1975.
Dewhurst, NG, and Muir, AL. **Am J Med** 78:765–770, 1985.
Dunn, RF, et al. **Circulation** 60:451–457, 1979.
Eisenstein, I, et al. **Chest** 88:409–416, 1985.
El-Sherif, N, et al. **Br Heart J** 40:1376–1383, 1978.
Gelman, JS, and Saltups, A. **Br Heart J** 48:560–565, 1982.
Gibson, RS, et al. **Circulation** 66:732–741, 1982.
Goldberg, HL, et al. **Am J Cardiol** 48:1009–1015, 1981.
Goldberger, AL. **Myocardial Infarction, Electrocardiographic Differential Diagnosis,** 2nd ed. CV Mosby, 1979, p 20.
Herlitz, J and Hjalmarson, A. **Clin Cardiol** 10:529–534, 1987.
Hindman, MC, et al. **Circulation** 58:689–699, 1978.
Hlatky, MA, et al. **Am J Cardiol** 55:325–329, 1985.
Hurst et al, **The Heart**, 5th Ed. McGraw-Hill, New York, 1982, p 1126.
Kennedy, JW. **Heart Lung** 16:740–745, 1987.
Lembo, NJ, et al. **Circulation** 74:57–63, 1986.
Marriott, HJL. **Practical Electrocardiography,** 7th ed. Williams & Wilkins, Baltimore, 1983, pp 347–348.
Movahed, A, and Becker, LC. **J Am Coll Cardiol** 4:660–666, 1984.
Narula, OS. **Cardiac Arrhythmias, Electrophysiology, Diagnosis and Management.** Williams & Wilkins, Baltimore, 1979, p 92.
Nasmith, J., et al. **Ann Intern Med** 96:22–26, 1982.

Norris, RM, et al. **Am Heart J** 84:560–566, 1972.
Ong, L, et al. **Am J Cardiol** 51:734–739, 1983.
Perloff, JK. **Circulation** 30:706–718, 1964.
Phibbs, B. **J Am Coll Cardiol** 1:561–564, 1983.
Pick, A, and Langendorf, R. **Interpretation of Complex Arrhythmias.** Lea & Febiger, Philadelphia, 1979, p 219.
Pierard, LA, et al. **Am J Cardiol** 57:82–85, 1986.
Rios, JC, et al. **Clinical Electrocardiographic Correlations.** FA Davis, Philadelphia, 1977, pp 65–67.
Ruddy, T, et al. **Am Heart J** 112:1210–1216, 1986.
Saksena, S, and Sung RJ. **Pract Cardiol** 6:99–122, 1980.
Salcedo, JR, et al. **Am J Cardiol** 48:1003–1008, 1981.
Schamroth, L. **The Electrocardiography of Coronary Artery Disease.** 2nd ed. Blackwell Scientific, Oxford, 1984, pp 58–59, 129–131.
Schuster, EH, and Bulkley, BH. **N Engl J Med** 305:1101–1105, 1981.
Shah, PK, et al. **Am J Cardiol** 46:915–921, 1980.
Shettigar et al, **Am Heart J** 88:170–175, 1974.
Silverman, ME, and Silverman, BD. **The Heart, Update I.** McGraw-Hill, New York, 1979, pp 13–45.
Sonnenblick, EH, and Lesch, M. **Sudden Cardiac Death.** Grune & Stratton, New York, 1981, pp 1–4.
Spodick, DH. **Am J Cardiol** 51:913–915, 1983.
Surawicz, B, et al. **Am J Cardiol** 41:130–138, 1978.
Tendera, M, and Campbell, WB. **Am J Cardiol** 54:994–996, 1984.
Vanden Belt, RJ, et al. **Cardiology: A Clinical Approach.** Year Book Medical Publishers, Chicago, 1979, pp 224–225.
Warner, RA, et al. **Am J Cardiol** 58:431–435, 1986.
Wasserman, AG, et al. **Am Heart J** 106:516–520, 1983.
Zema, MJ. **Am J Med** 78:391–398, 1985.

SELF-ASSESSMENT

Multiple Choice

1. The normal ST segment:

   a. is flat.
   b. contains an angle, the J point, marking its junction with the T wave.
   c. displays a gradual upward slope and merges imperceptibly with the T wave.
   d. may be either elevated or depressed but is not flat.

2. Variant or Prinzmetal's angina is associated with:

   a. widespread ST segment depression and T wave inversion.
   b. abnormal Q waves that disappear after the angina subsides.
   c. transient ST segment elevation that persists during the bout of angina.
   d. no diagnostically significant ST segment or T wave changes.

3. The hyperacute phase of myocardial infarction:

   a. is the earliest phase and because it is transient is often missed.
   b. is characterized by abnormally tall, symmetrical T waves or by ST segment elevation without T wave inversion.
   c. is marked by ST segment elevation and Q waves.
   d. choices *a* and *b*.

4. The indicative changes of anterior infarction are seen in leads:

   a. II, III, aVF
   b. aVR, aVL, aVF
   c. I, aVL
   d. V3, V4

5. The leads in which the reciprocal changes of posterior infarction are seen are:

   a. V1–V3
   b. I, aVL, V5, V6
   c. II, III, aVF
   d. V1–V6

6. The term **non-Q infarction** refers to:

   a. a nontransmural infarction.
   b. an infarction characterized electrocardiographically by ST segment and T wave changes only.
   c. a subendocardial infarction.
   d. an infarction in which only reciprocal changes register on the ECG.

The following multiple choice questions are based on the 12-lead ECGs and rhythm strips in cases 5–1 to 5–50.

7. Inferior wall infarctions (IWMI) are diagnosed from ST-T changes and/or Q waves in (cases 5–1, 5–7, 5–9, 5–11, 5–12, 5–24, 5–34, 5–40, 5–45, and 5–50):

   a. I, II, III.
   b. II, III, aVF.
   c. V1–V6.
   d. I, aVL.

8. In the setting of acute inferior wall infarction, ST segment depression in the precordial leads V1–V4 correlates with (cases 5–7, 5–12, 5–29, and 5–42):

   a. more extensive infarction (inferobasal or inferoapical).
   b. the hyperacute phase of posterior wall infarction.
   c. remote ischemia due to coexisting obstruction of the left anterior descending artery.
   d. all of the above.

9. In the setting of anterior wall infarction (AWMI), ventricular asystole due to atrioventricular block is preceded by (cases 5–23, 5–33, and 5–43):

   a. left axis deviation.
   b. right axis deviation.
   c. right bundle branch block and axis deviation.
   d. Mobitz type I second-degree block.

10. Atrioventricular block with a 2:1 or even 3:1 conduction ratio is often observed in the setting of (cases 5–9, 5–17, 5–18, and 5–35):

    a. anterior wall infarction.
    b. inferior wall infarction.
    c. posterior wall infarction.
    d. lateral wall infarction.

11. Sudden pauses in ventricular rhythm during infarction may be due to (cases 5–1, 5–4, 5–10, 5–12, 5–13, 5–19, 5–23, 5–35, 5–45, and 5–50):

    a. premature atrial beats or premature junctional beats.
    b. nonconducted atrial premature beats or premature ventricular beats.
    c. sinoatrial block or atrioventricular block.
    d. all of the above.

12. The hyperacute phase of infarction is diagnosed primarily by the observation of (cases 5–8, 5–12, 5–24, 5–29, 5–32, 5–41, and 5–43):

    a. diagnostic Q waves in leads facing the infarcted area.
    b. tall, symmetrical T waves with or without ST segment elevation.
    c. reciprocal changes in the leads facing away from the infarcted area.
    d. marked T wave inversion in the leads facing the infarcted segment.

13. Anterior wall infarctions (AWMI) are diagnosed from ST-T changes or Q waves or both in (cases, 5–3, 5–4, 5–5, 5–8, 5–10, 5–14, 5–15, 5–23, 5–26, 5–32, 5–33, 5–36, 5–38, and 5–43):

    a. V1–V6.
    b. I, aVL.
    c. II, III, aVF.
    d. reciprocal changes in V1–V3.

14. Posterior wall infarctions (PWMI) are diagnosed by tall R waves and tall, symmetrical T waves in (cases 5–2, 5–25, 5–29, 5–30, and 5–37):

    a. II, III, aVF.
    b. I, aVL.
    c. V1–V3.
    d. I, aVL, V5, V6.

Practice Strips

In the ECGs that follow, determine the (1) axis, (2) zone of transition, (3) presence of low voltage, (4) presence of poor R wave progression, (5) fascicular block, (6) bundle branch block or nonspecific intraventricular conduction delay, (7) ischemia or infarction by the involved segment, (8) diagnosis of arrhythmias.

Many ECGs in this and the following sections are serial tracings taken hours to days apart. The times or dates or both are indicated on the tracings.

5-1.

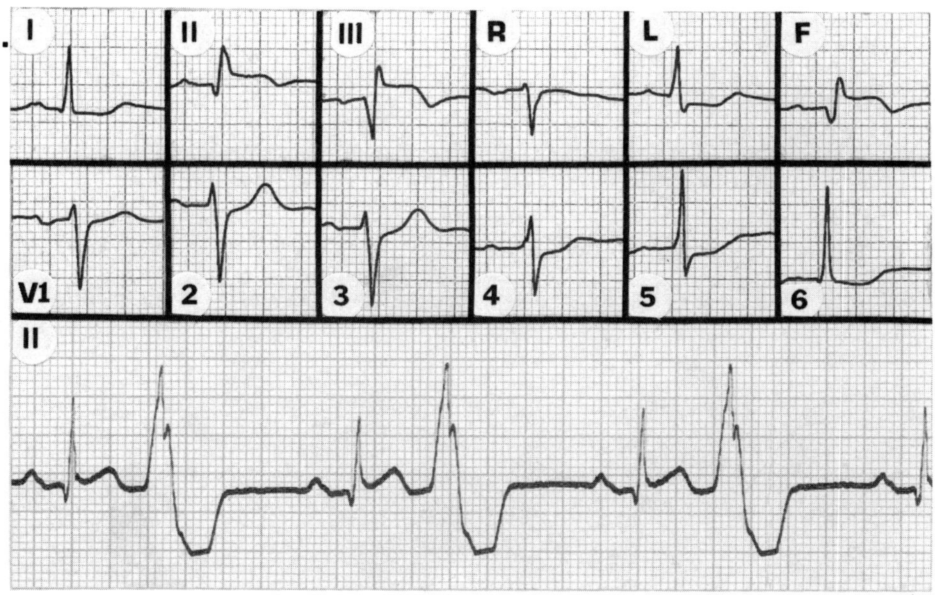

5-2.

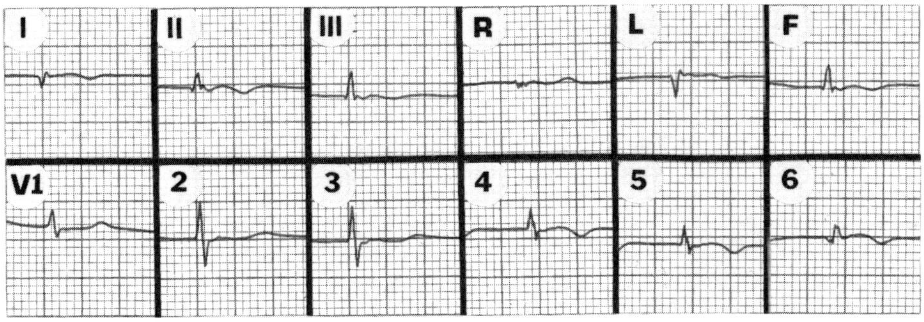

5-3.

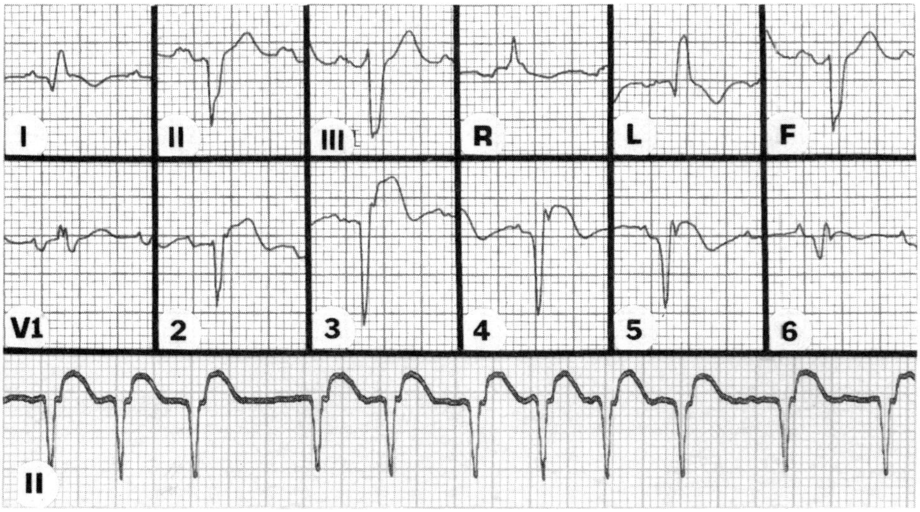

5-4.

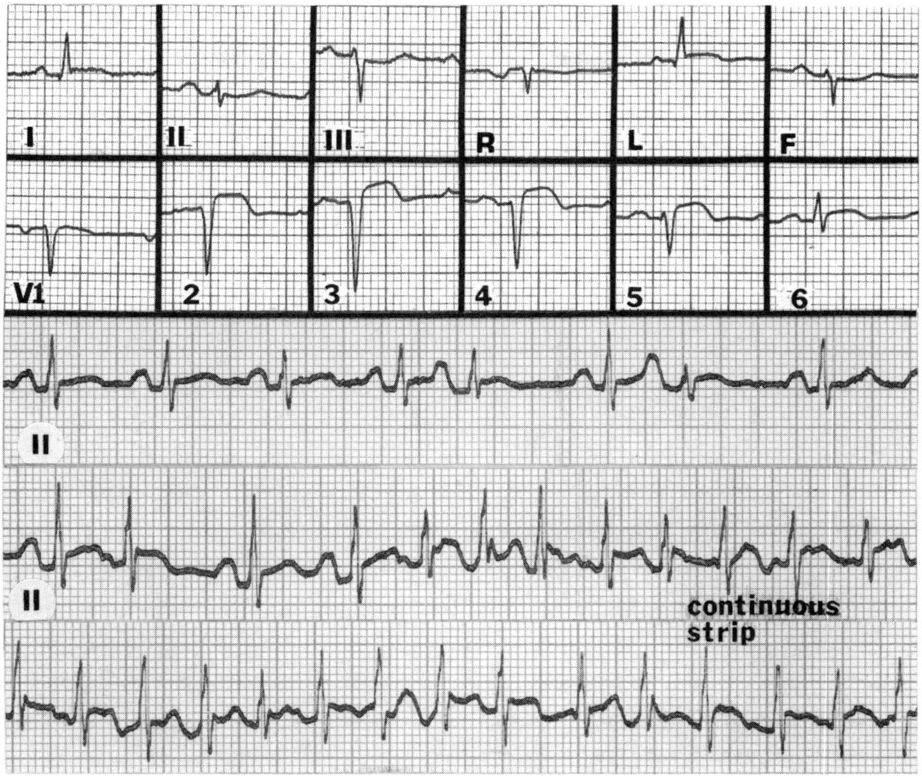
I
II
III
R
L
F
V1
2
3
4
5
6
II
II
continuous
strip

5-5.

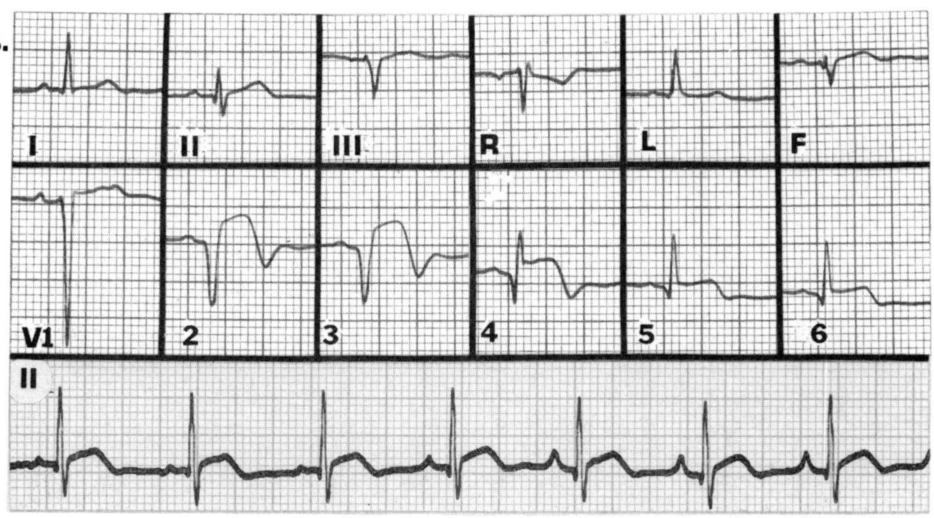
I
II
III
R
L
F
V1
2
3
4
5
6
II

5-6.

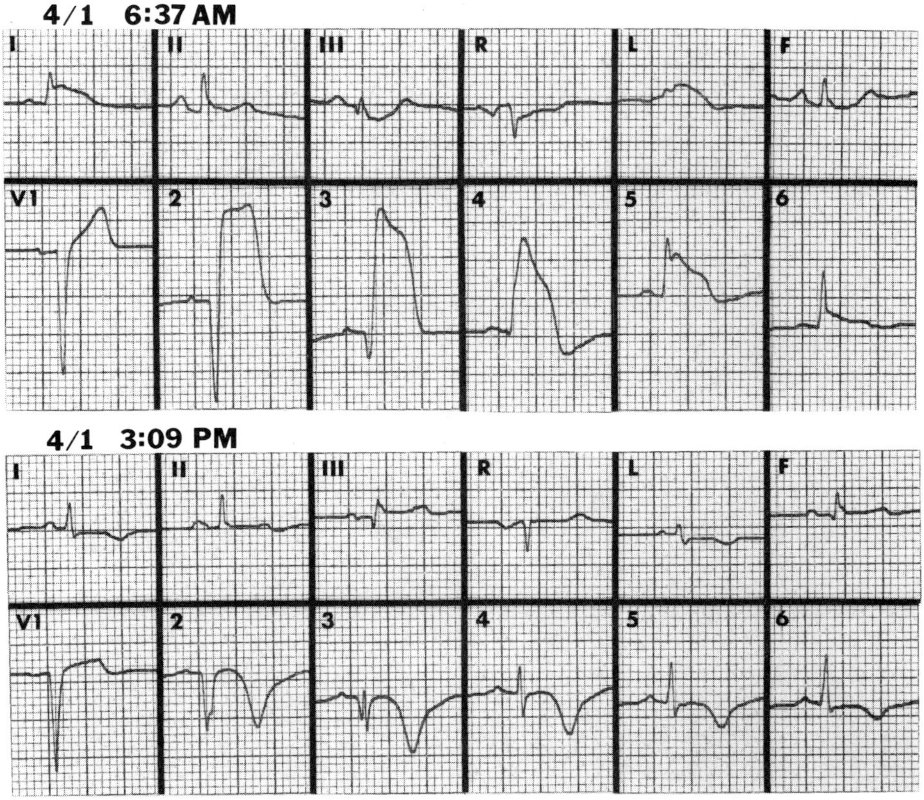
4/1 6:37 AM
I
II
III
R
L
F
V1
2
3
4
5
6
4/1 3:09 PM
I
II
III
R
L
F
V1
2
3
4
5
6

5-7.

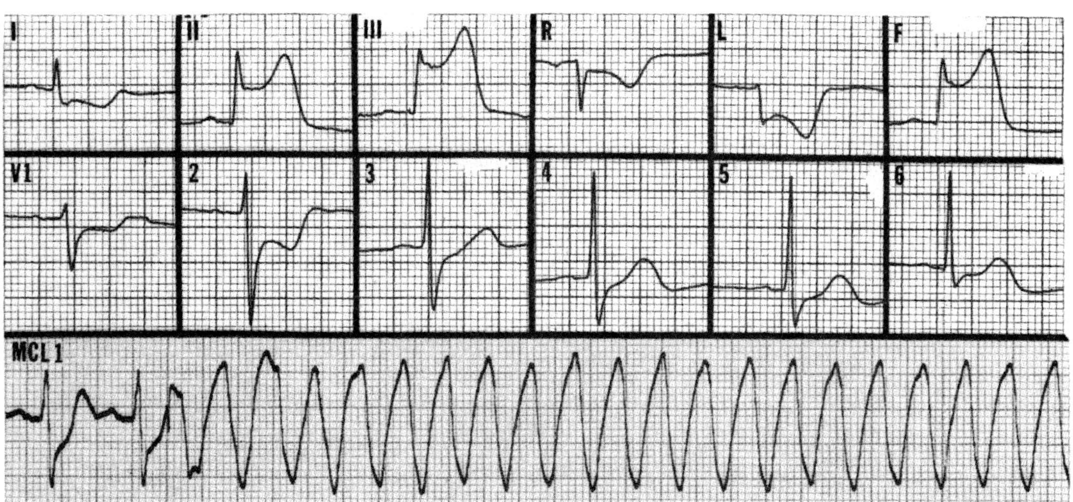
I
II
III
R
L
F
V1
2
3
4
5
6
MCL 1

5-8.

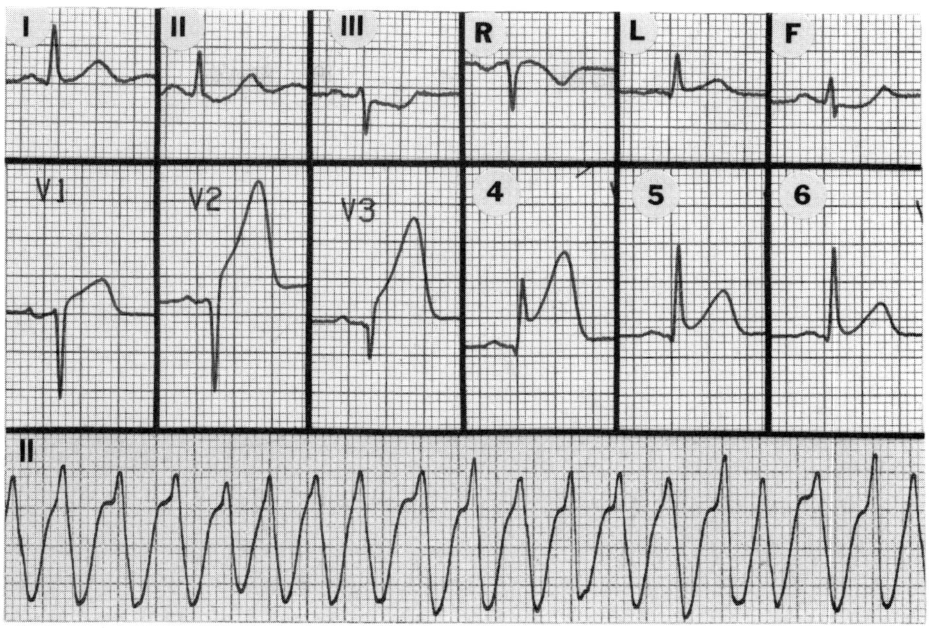

5-9.

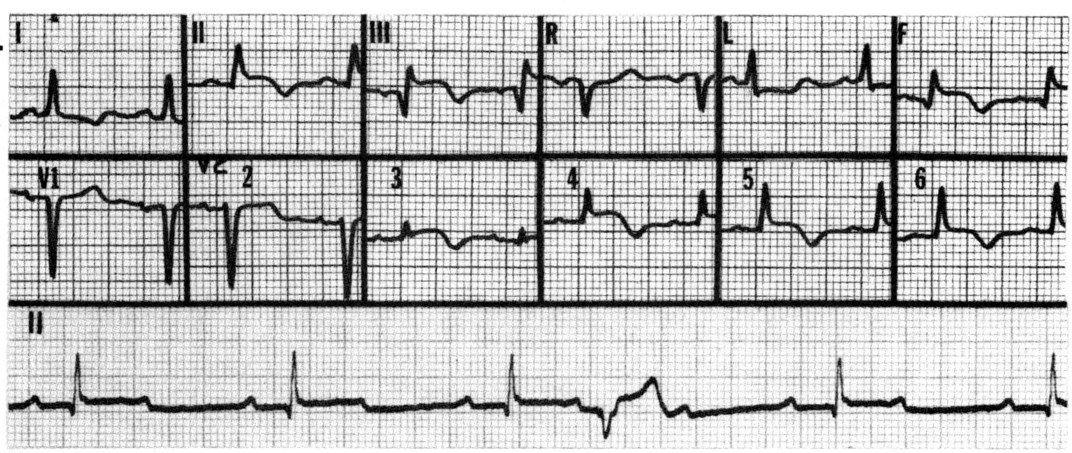

5-10.

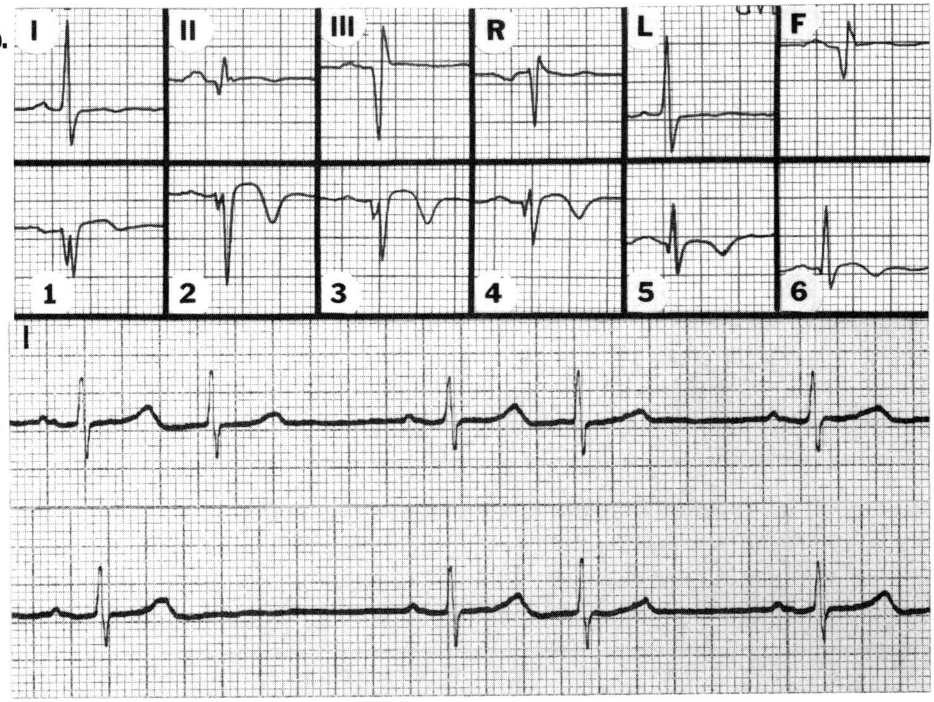

5-11.

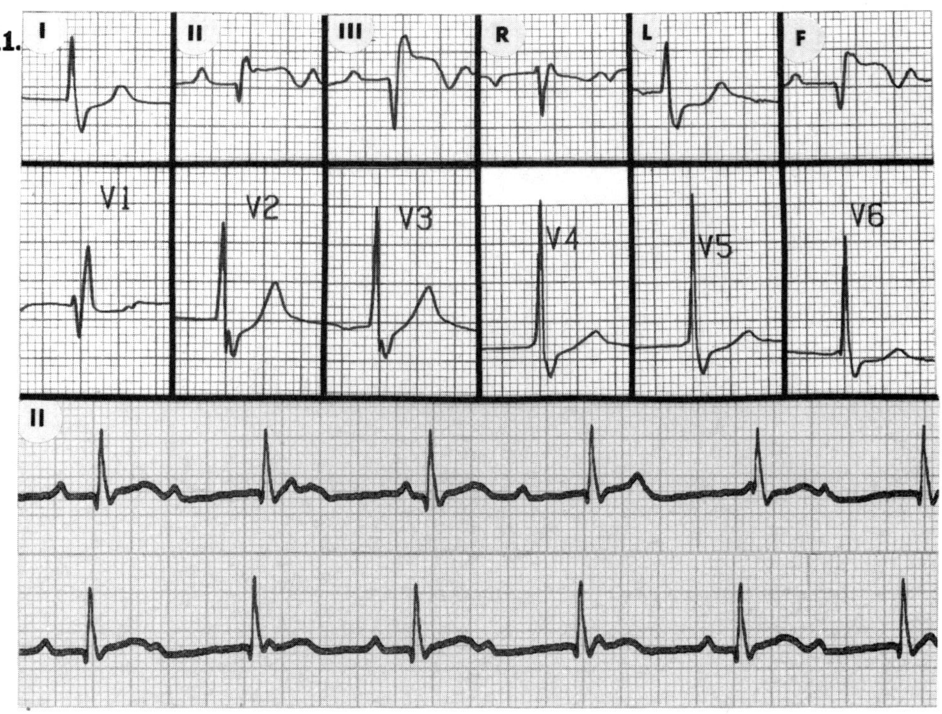

5-12.

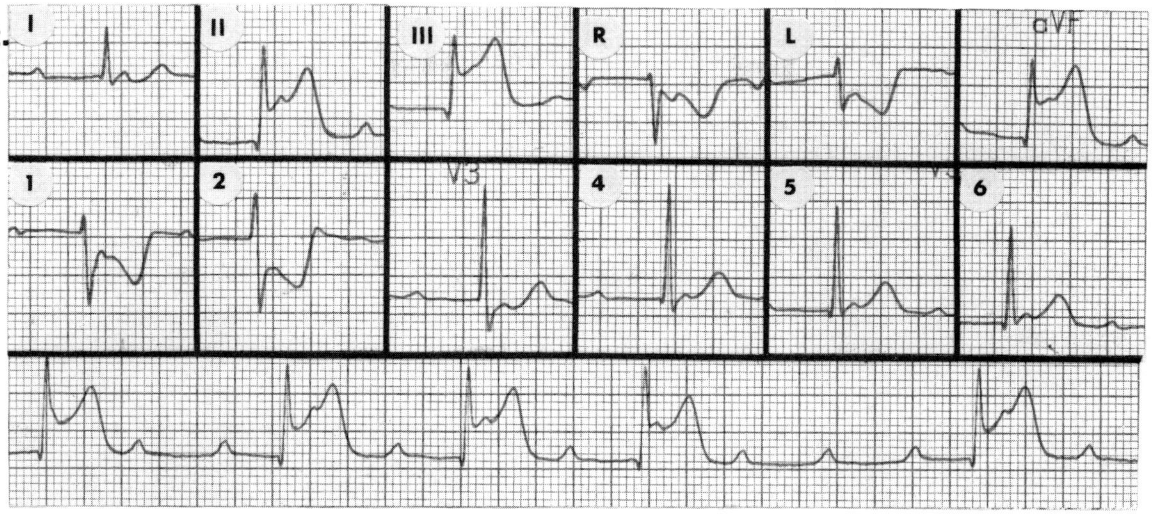

5-13

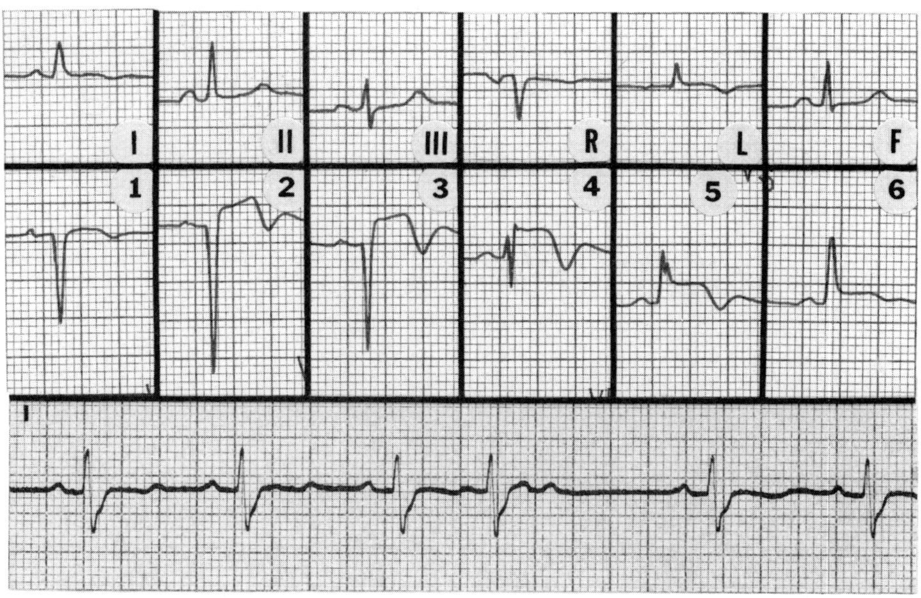

5-14.

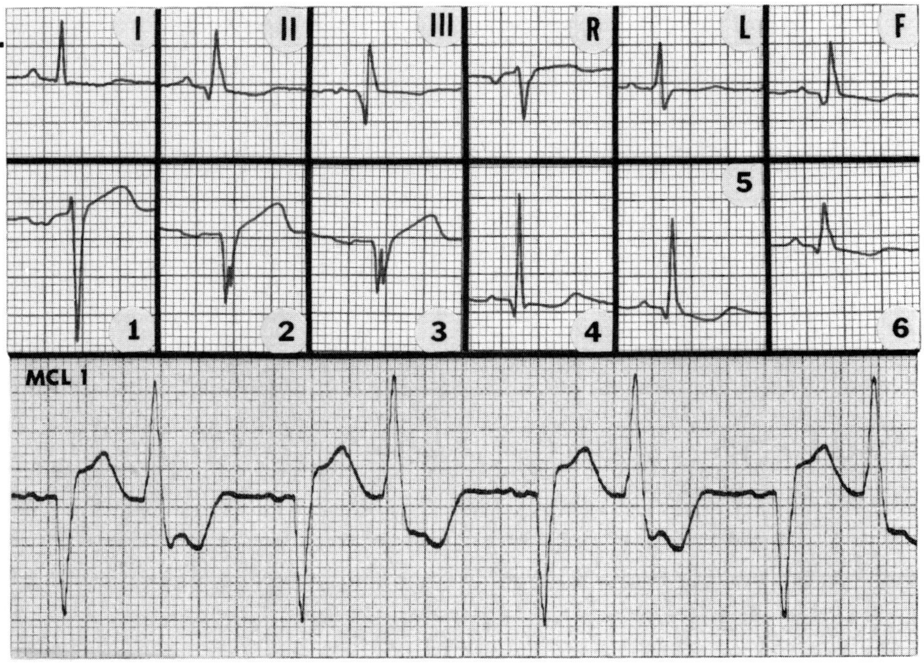

5-15.

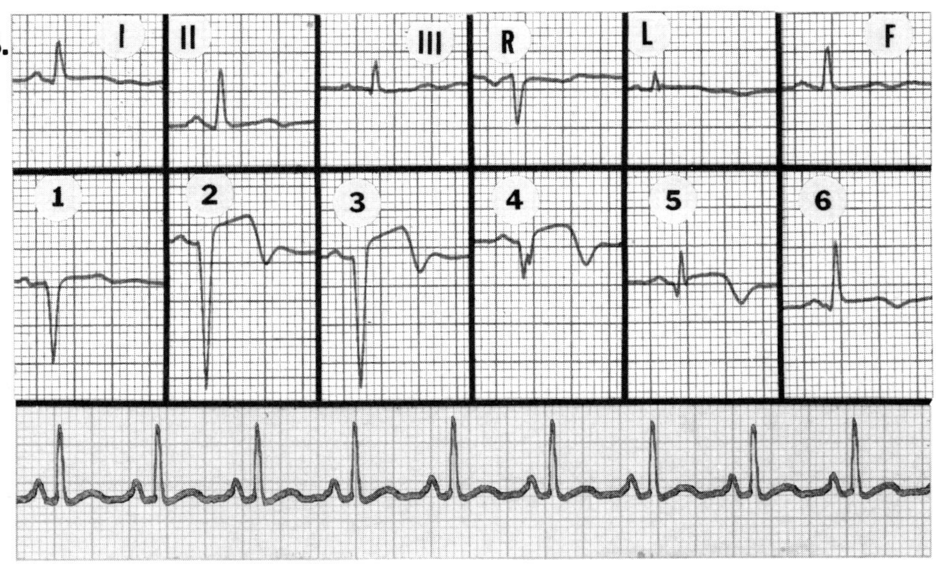

5-16.

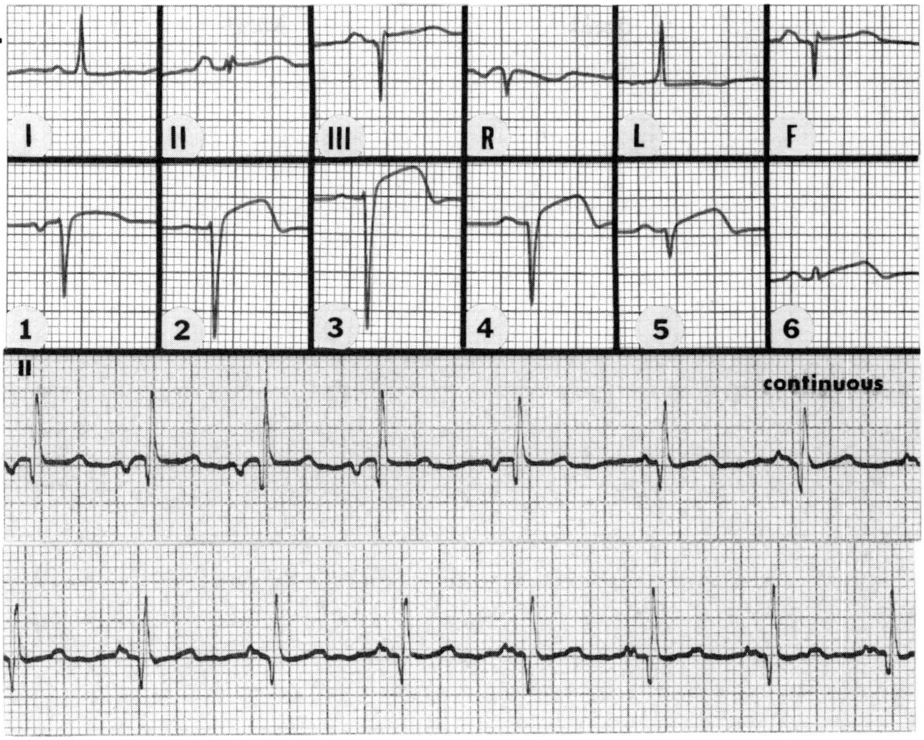

5-17.

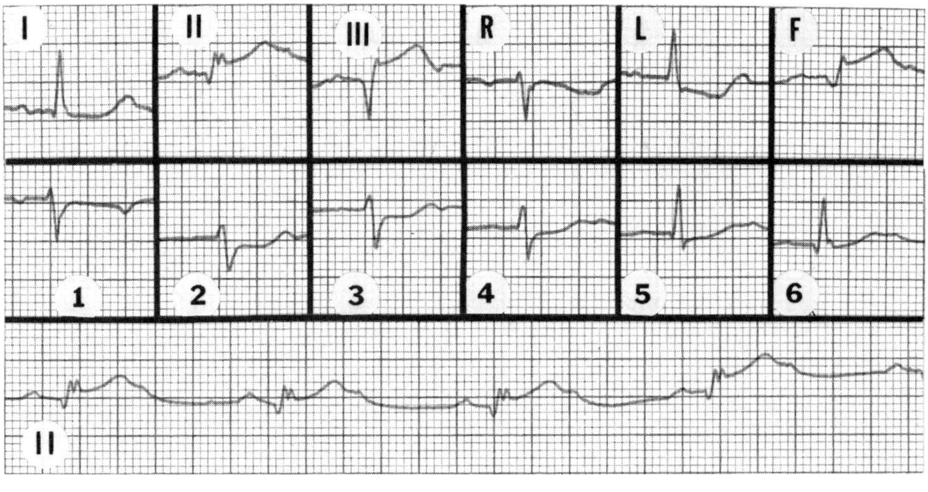

5-18.

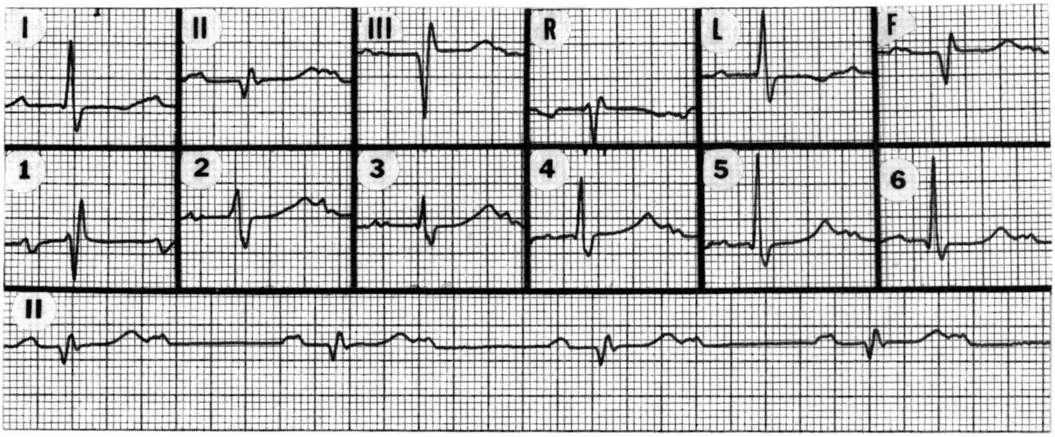

5-19.

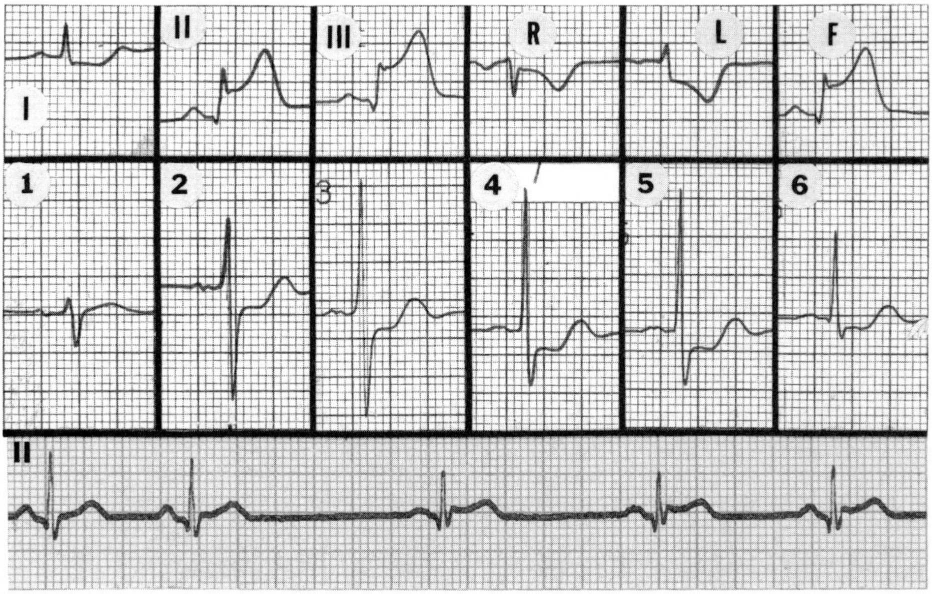

5-20.

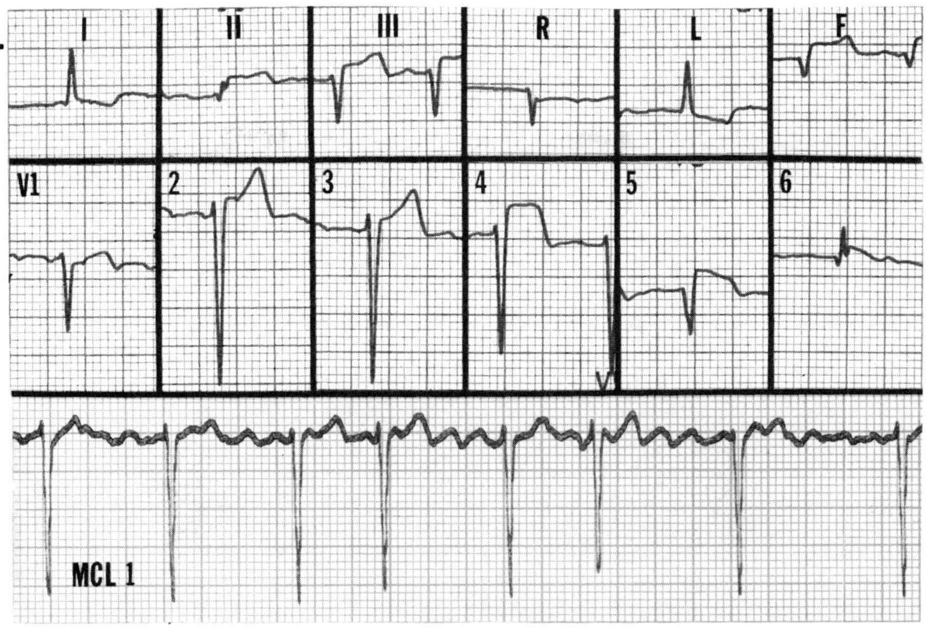

5-21.

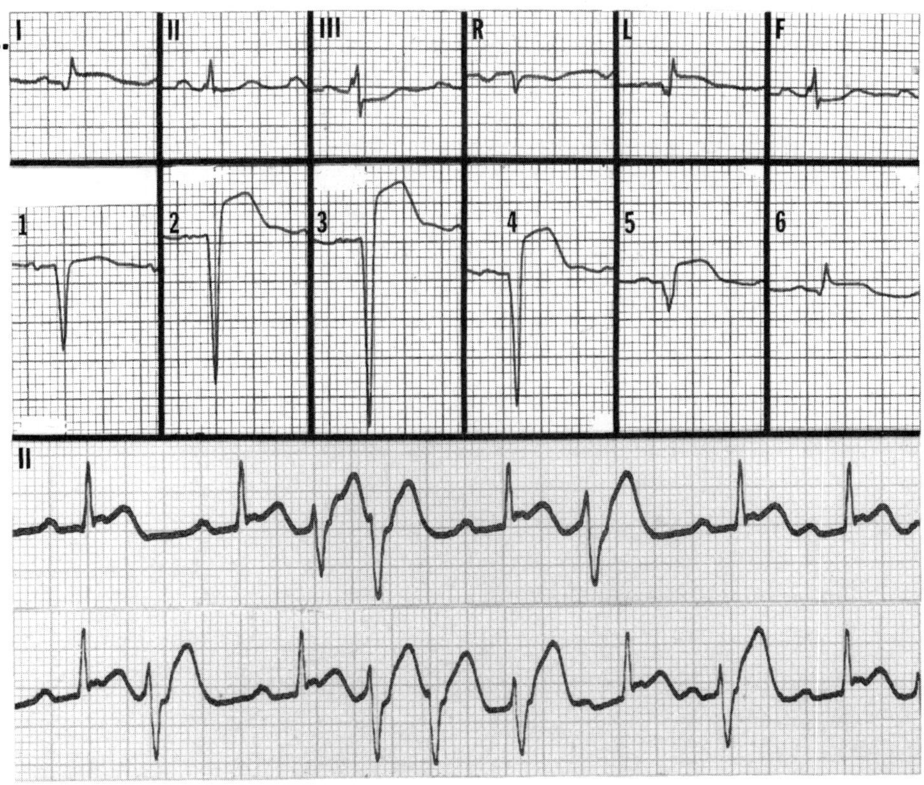

5-22.

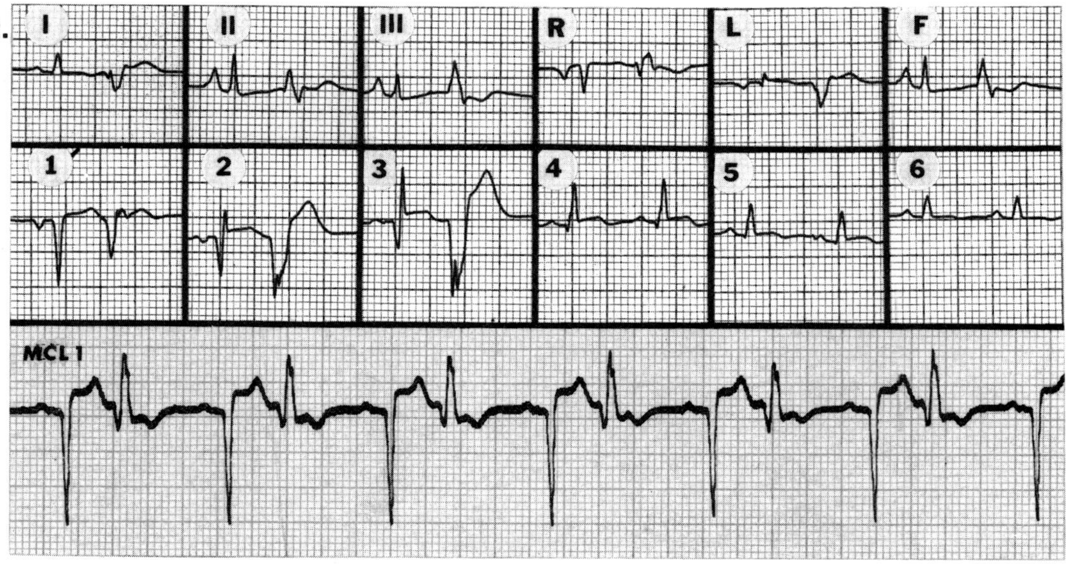

5-23.

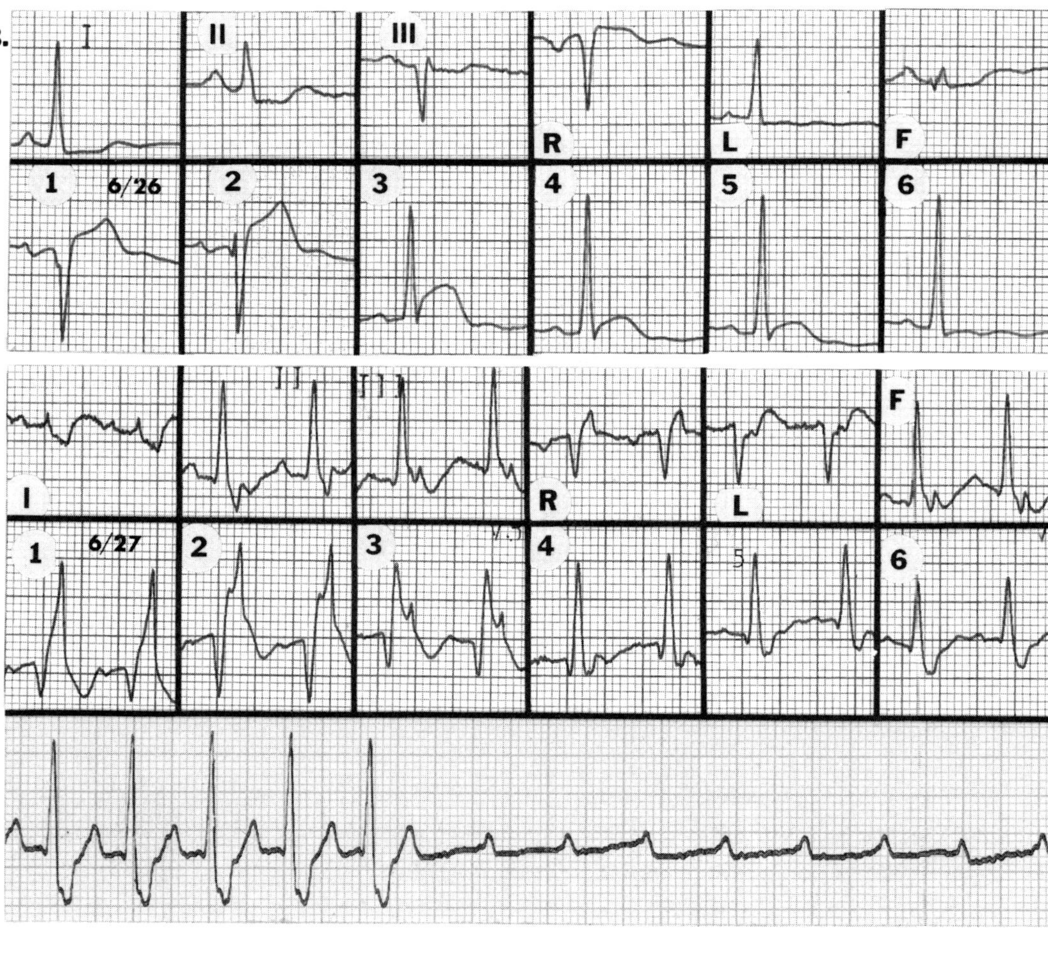

5-24.

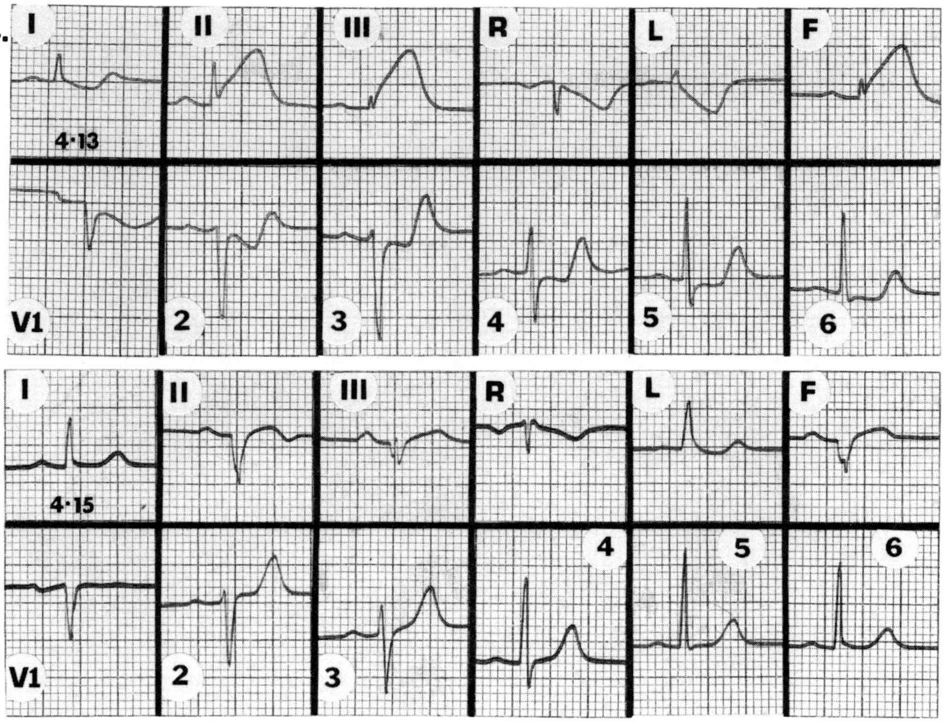
I
II
III
R
L
F
4·13
V1
2
3
4
5
6
I
II
III
R
L
F
4·15
4
5
6
V1
2
3

5-25.

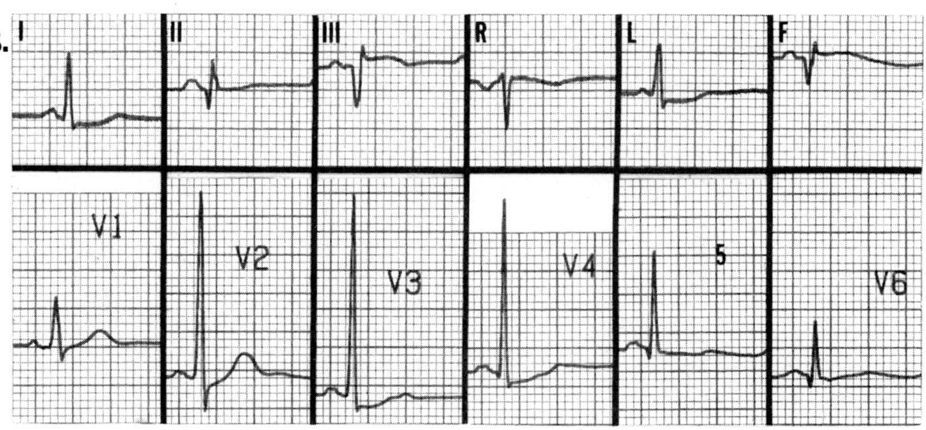
I
II
III
R
L
F
V1
V2
V3
V4
5
V6

5-26.

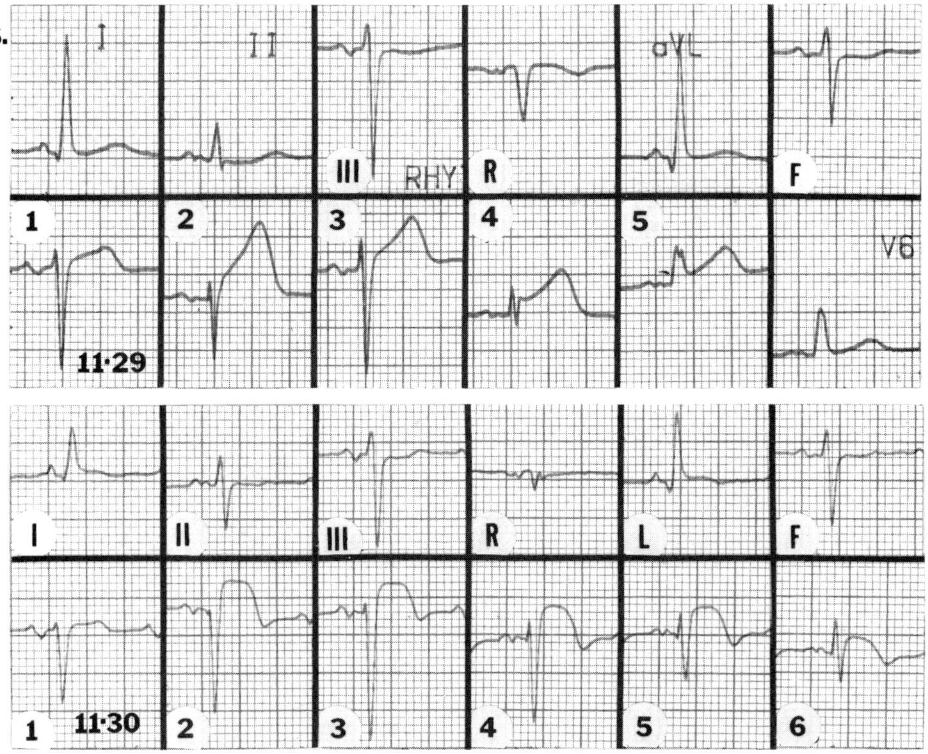
I
II
III
RHY
R
aVL
F
1
2
3
4
5
V6
11·29
I
II
III
R
L
F
1
11·30
2
3
4
5
6

5-27.

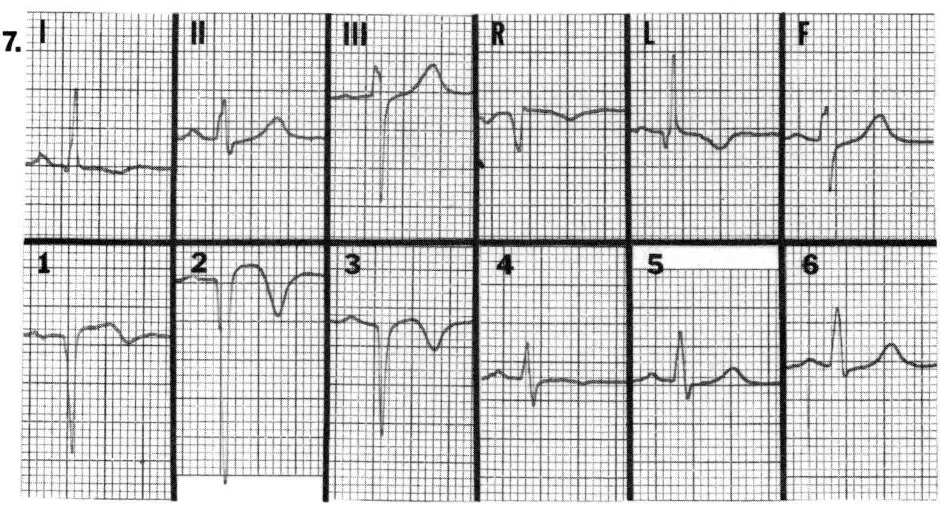
I
II
III
R
L
F
1
2
3
4
5
6

5-28.

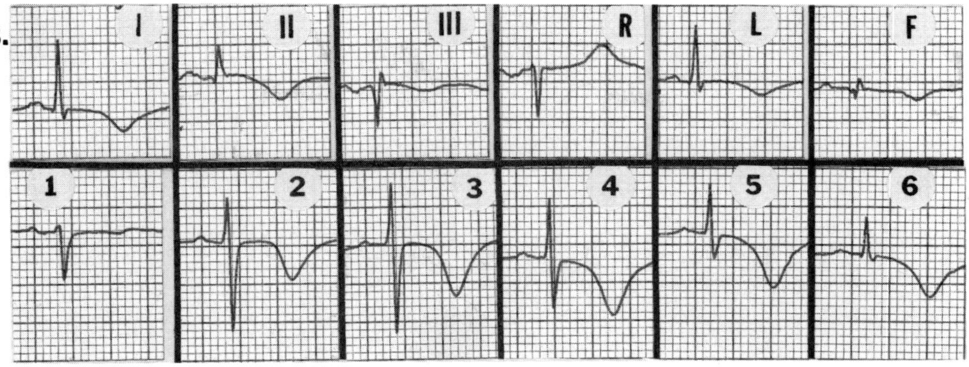
I
II
III
R
L
F
1
2
3
4
5
6

5-29.

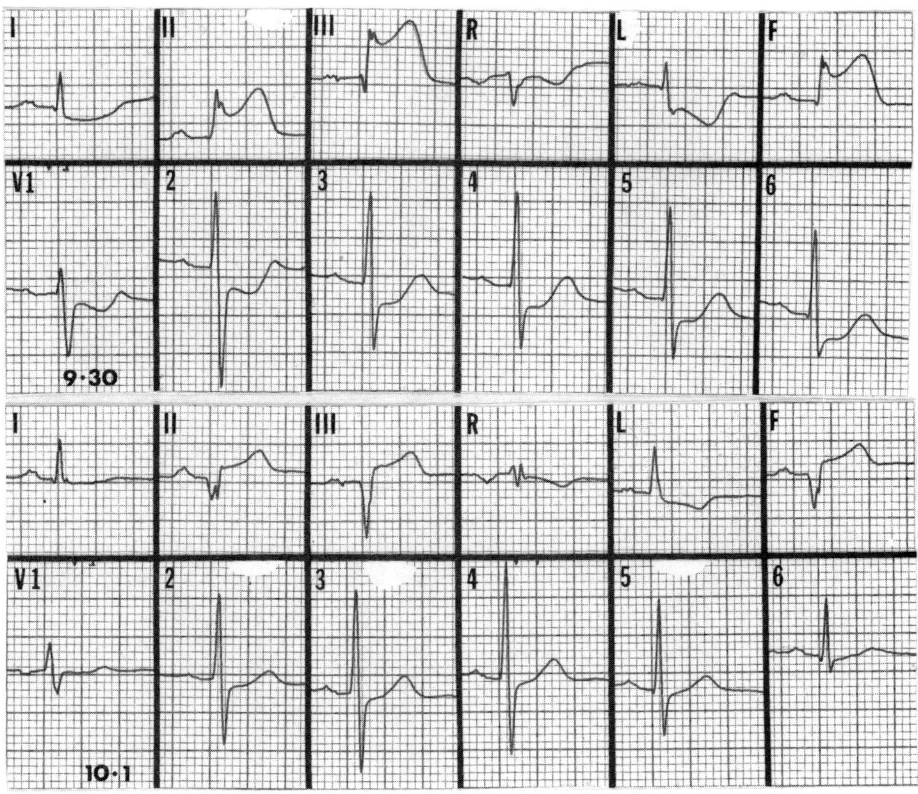
I
II
III
R
L
F
V1
2
3
4
5
6
9·30
I
II
III
R
L
F
V1
2
3
4
5
6
10·1

5-30.

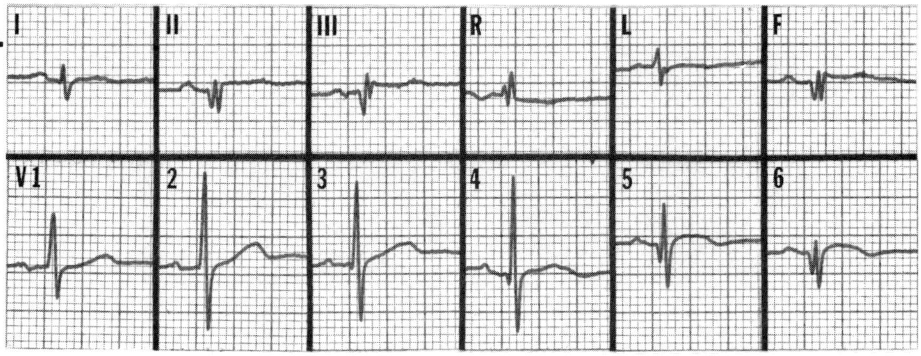
I
II
III
R
L
F
V1
2
3
4
5
6

5-31.

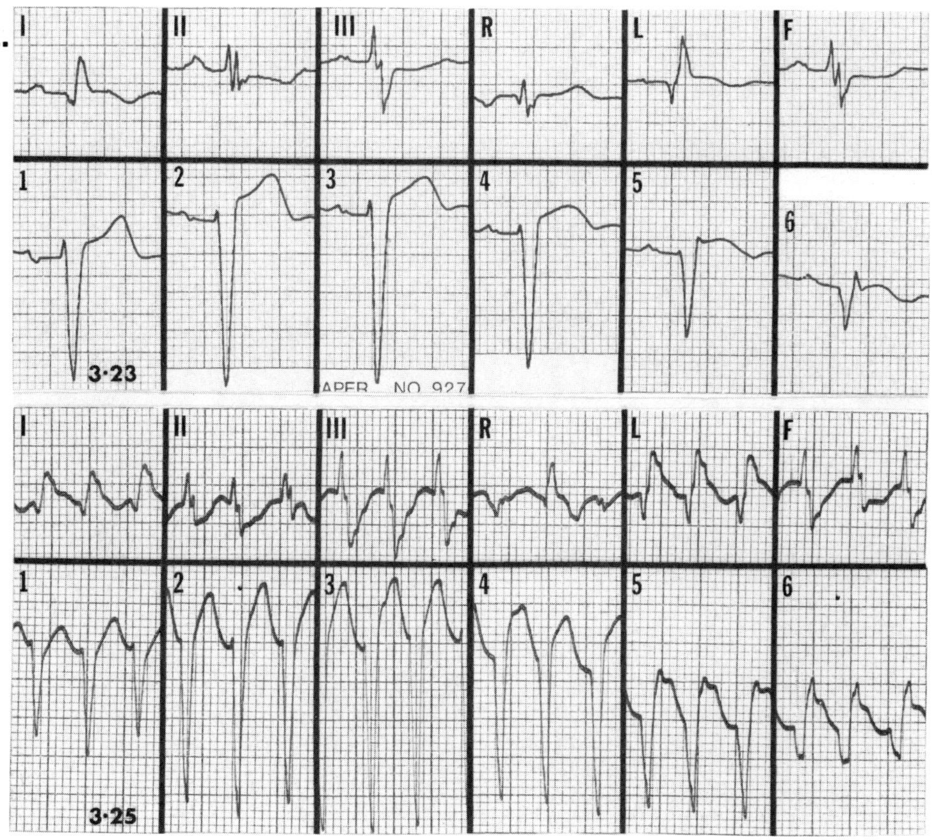
I
II
III
R
L
F
1
2
3
4
5
6
3·23
I
II
III
R
L
F
1
2
3
4
5
6
3·25

5-32.

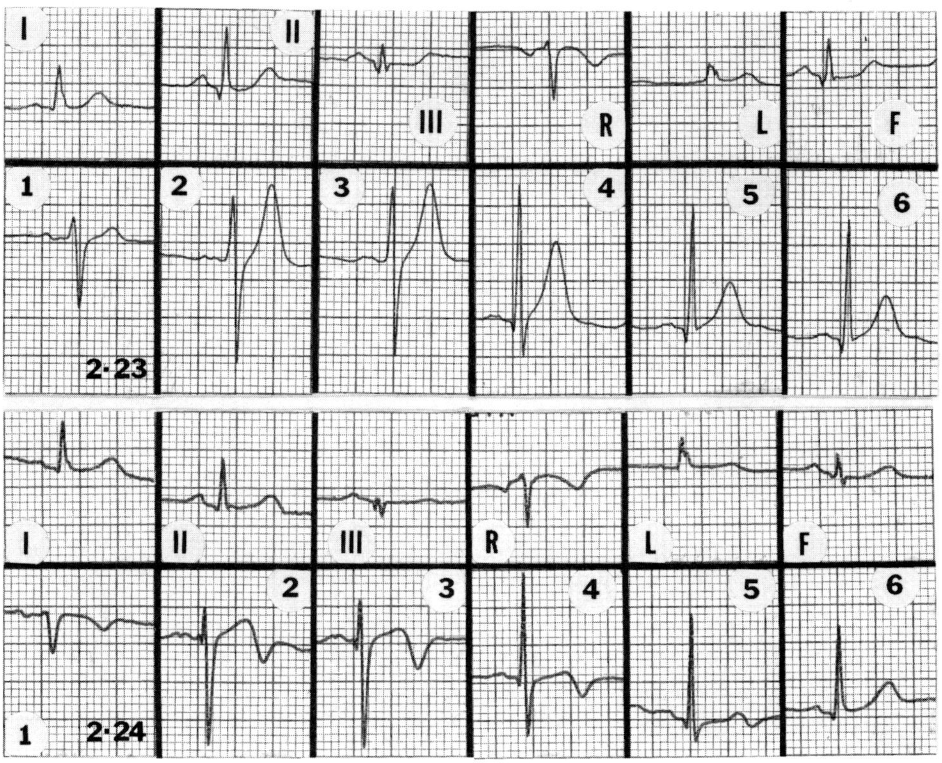

5-33.

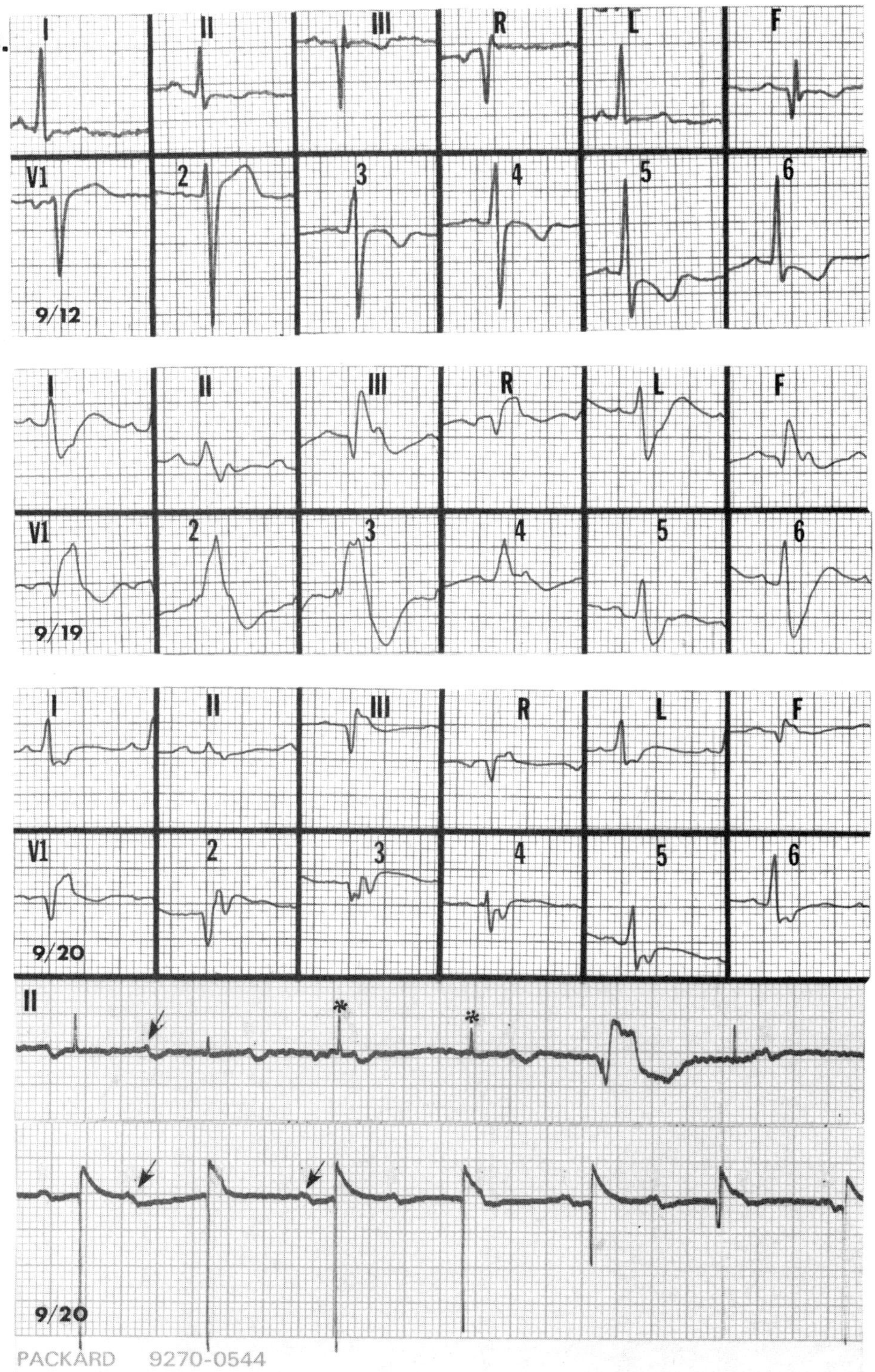
I
II
III
R
L
F
V1
2
3
4
5
6
9/12
I
II
III
R
L
F
V1
2
3
4
5
6
9/19
I
II
III
R
L
F
V1
2
3
4
5
6
9/20
II
*
*
9/20
PACKARD 9270-0544

5-34.

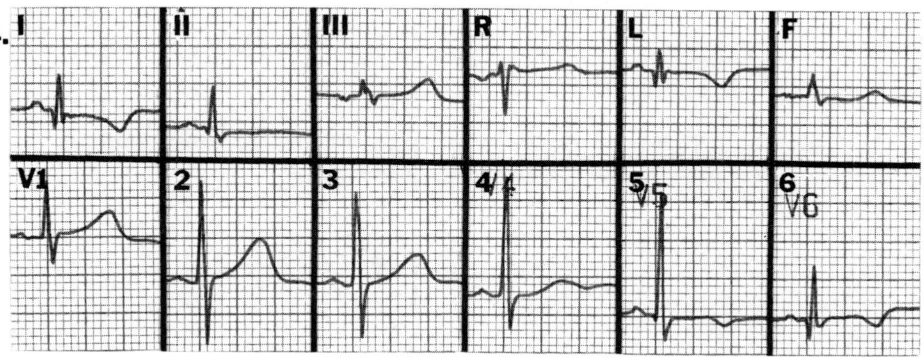

5-35.

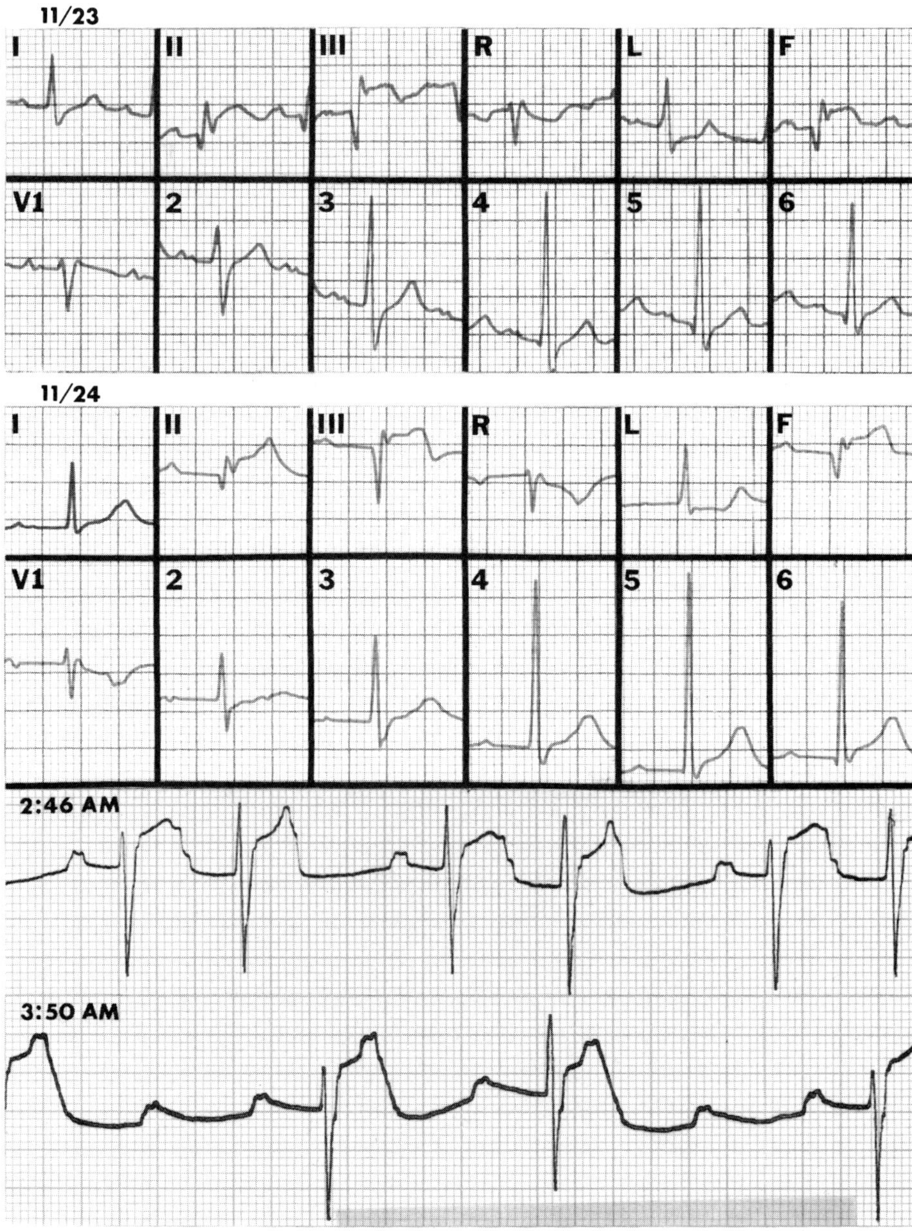
11/23
I
II
III
R
L
F
V1
2
3
4
5
6
11/24
I
II
III
R
L
F
V1
2
3
4
5
6
2:46 AM
3:50 AM

5-36.

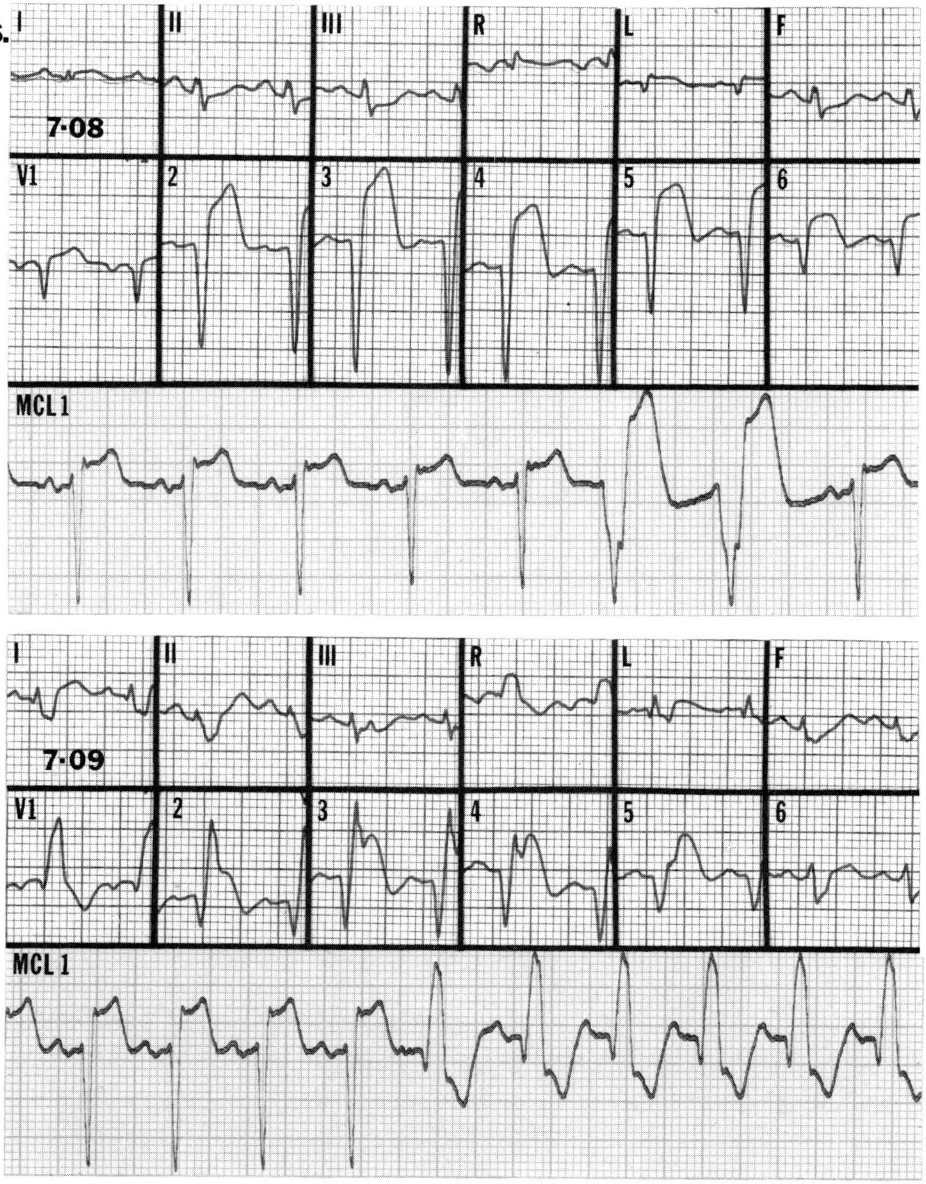

5-37.

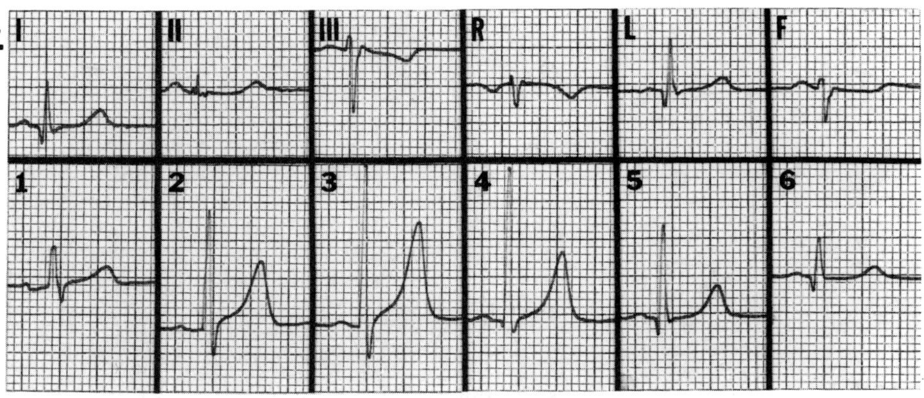

5-38.

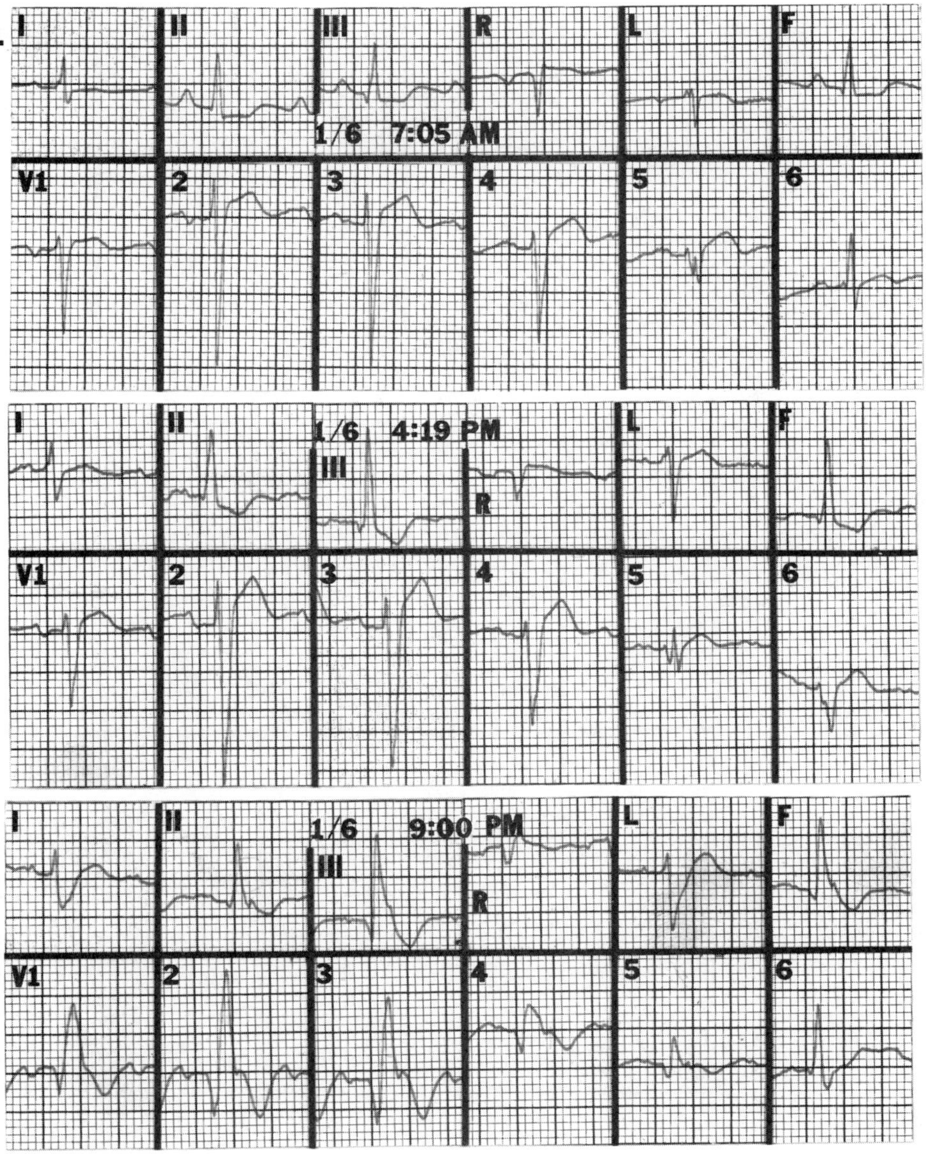

5-39.

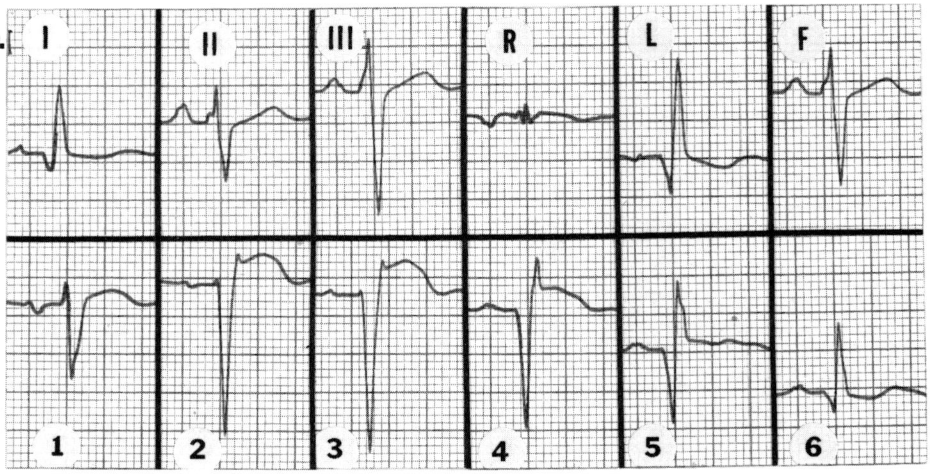
I
II
III
R
L
F
1
2
3
4
5
6

5-40.

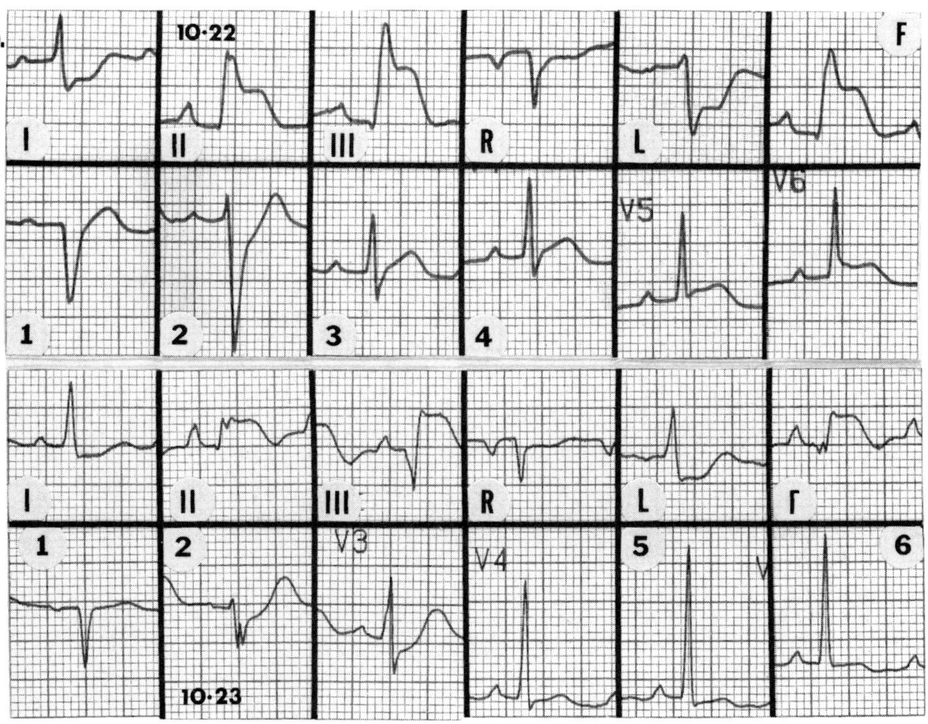
10·22
F
I
II
III
R
L
V5
V6
1
2
3
4
I
II
III
R
L
1
2
V3
V4
5
6
10·23

5-41.

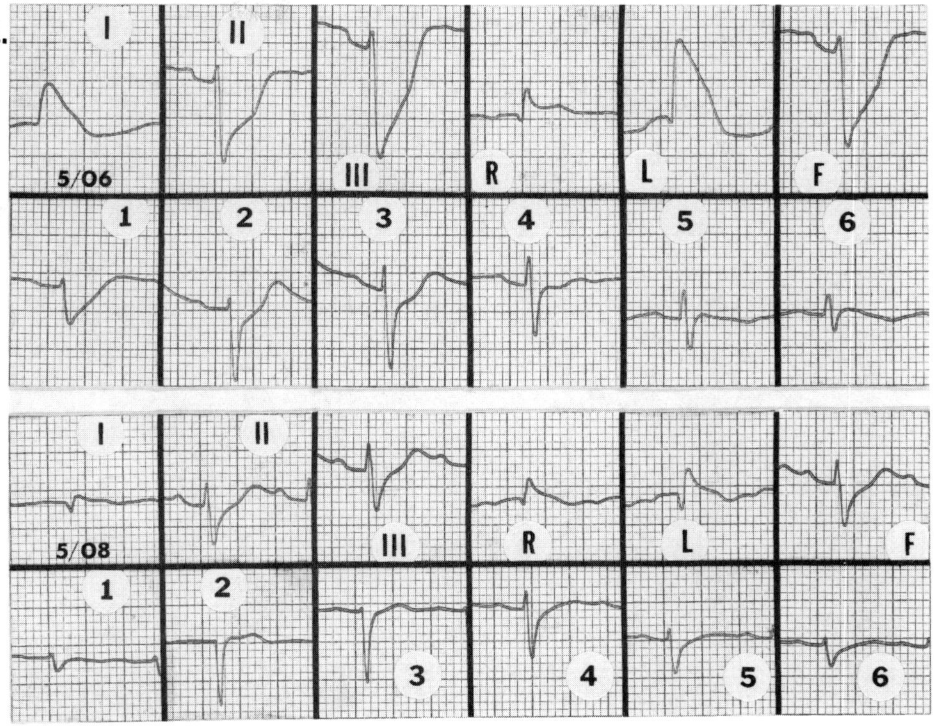
I
II
III
R
L
F
5/06
1
2
3
4
5
6
I
II
III
R
L
F
5/08
1
2
3
4
5
6

5-42.

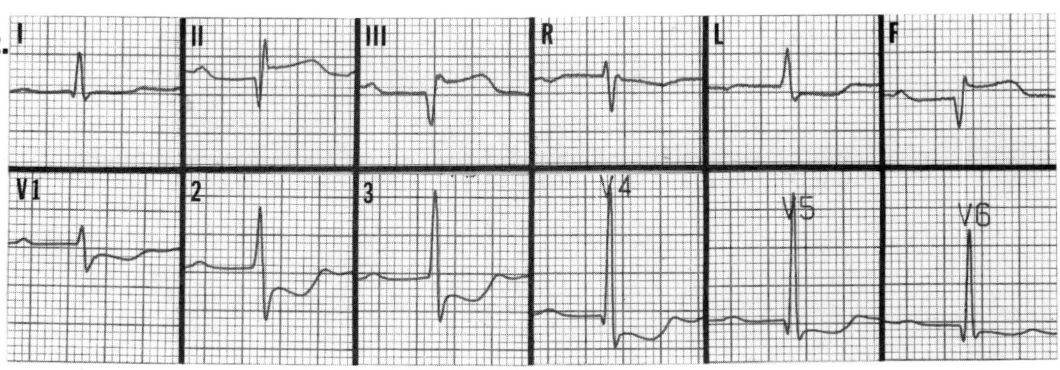
I
II
III
R
L
F
V1
2
3
V4
V5
V6

5-43.

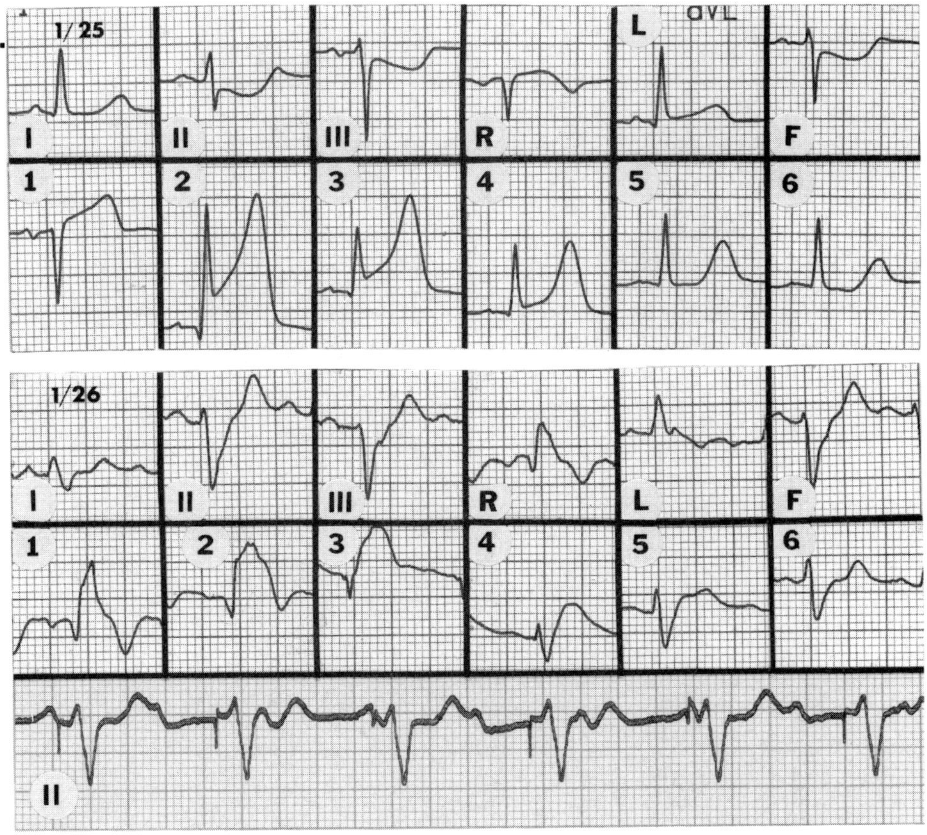
1/25
aVL
I
II
III
R
L
F
1
2
3
4
5
6
1/26
I
II
III
R
L
F
1
2
3
4
5
6
II

5-44.

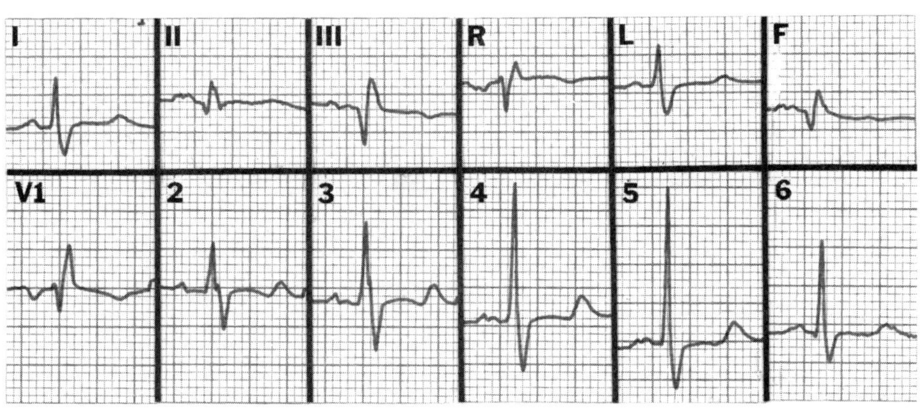
I
II
III
R
L
F
V1
2
3
4
5
6

5-45.

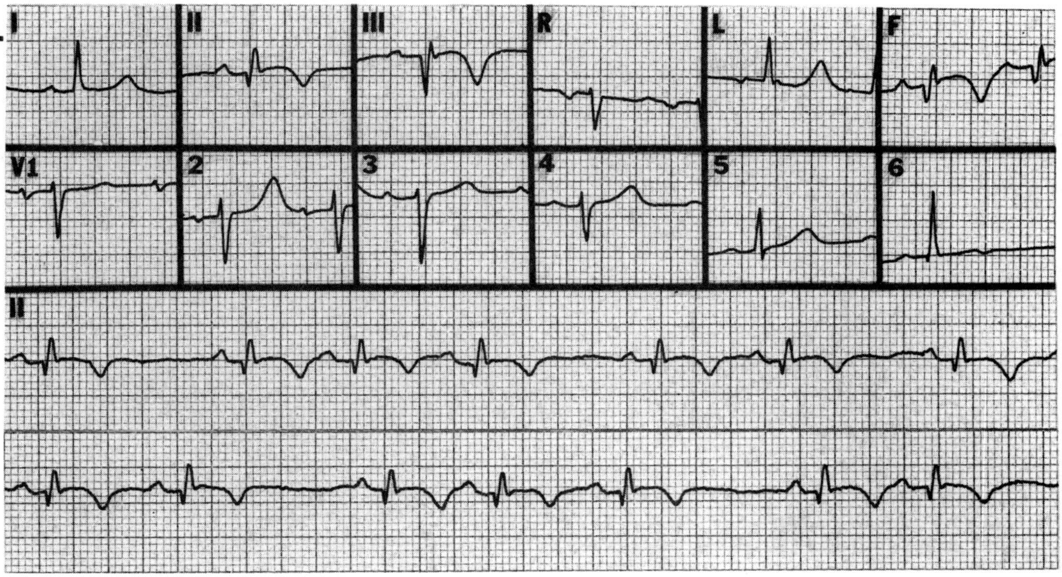

5-46.

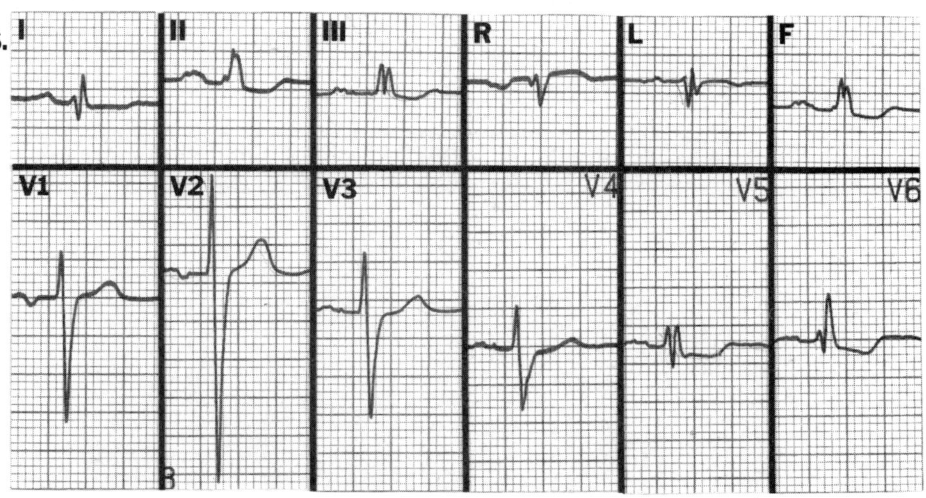

5-47.

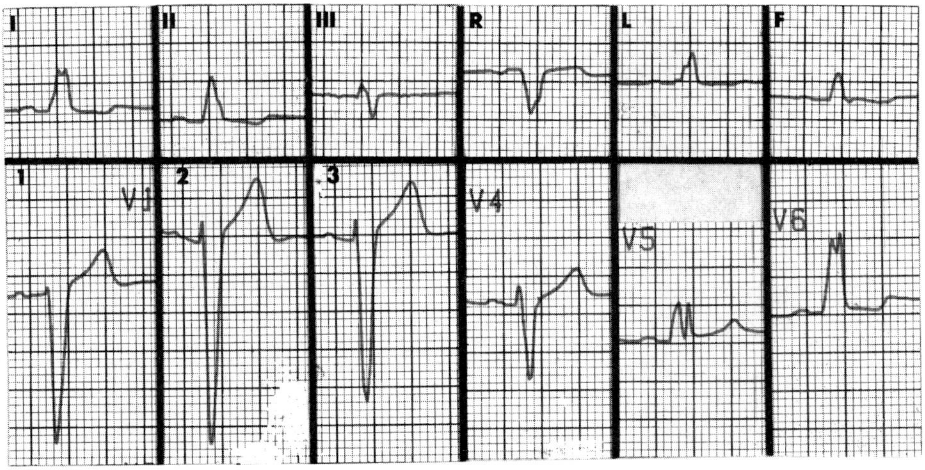

5-48.

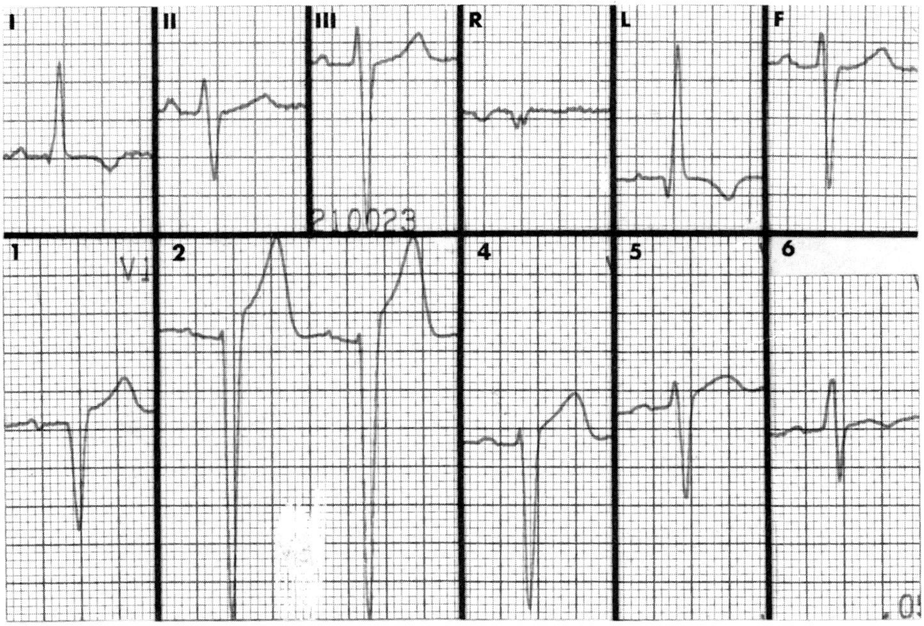

5-49.

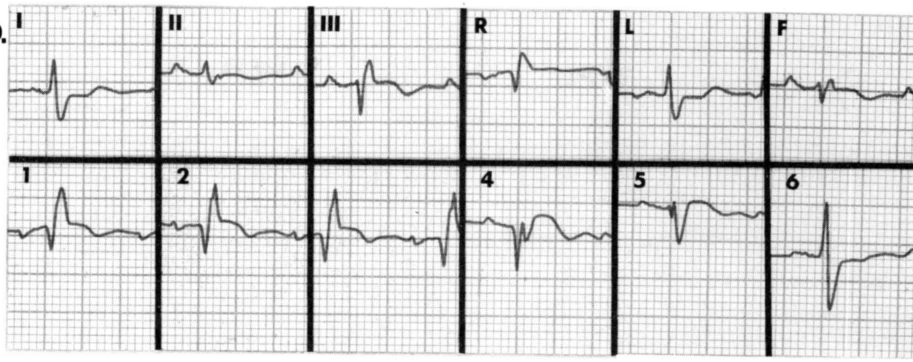

5-50.

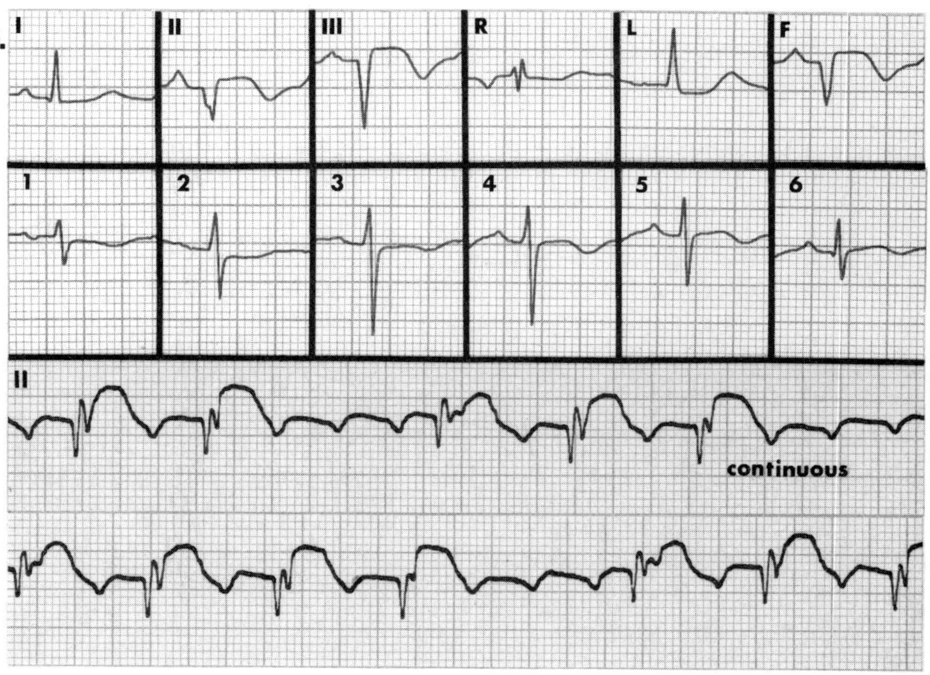

5-51.

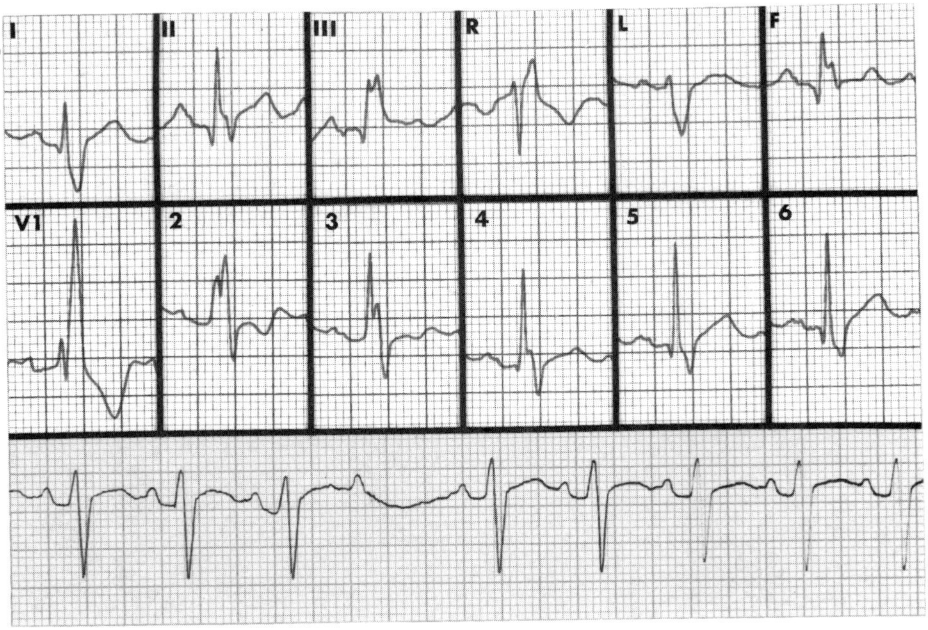

9/10

5-52.

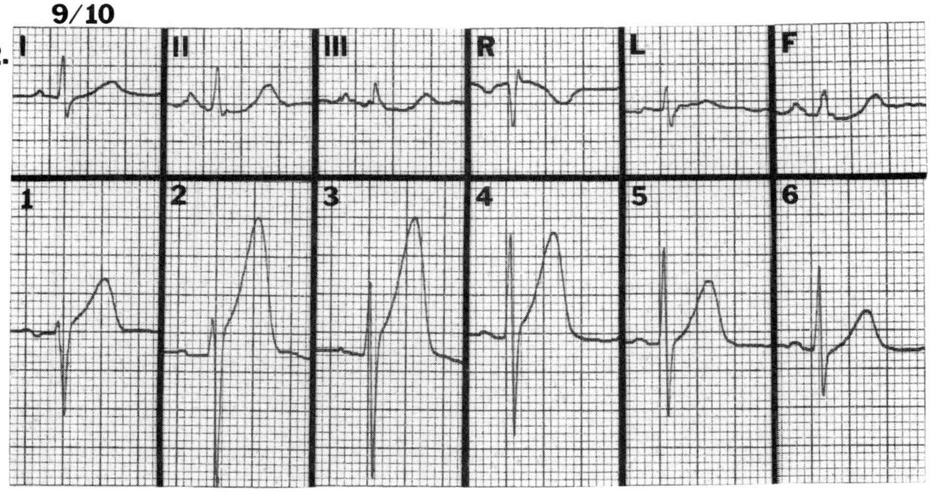

9/11

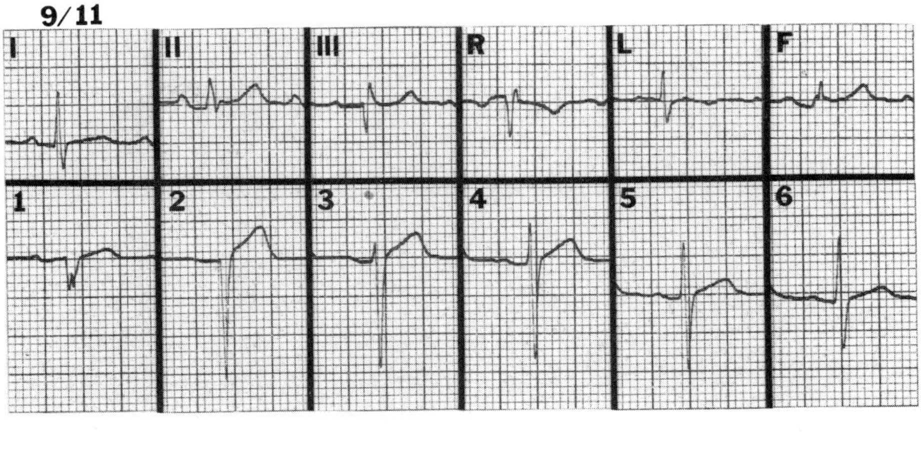

5-53.

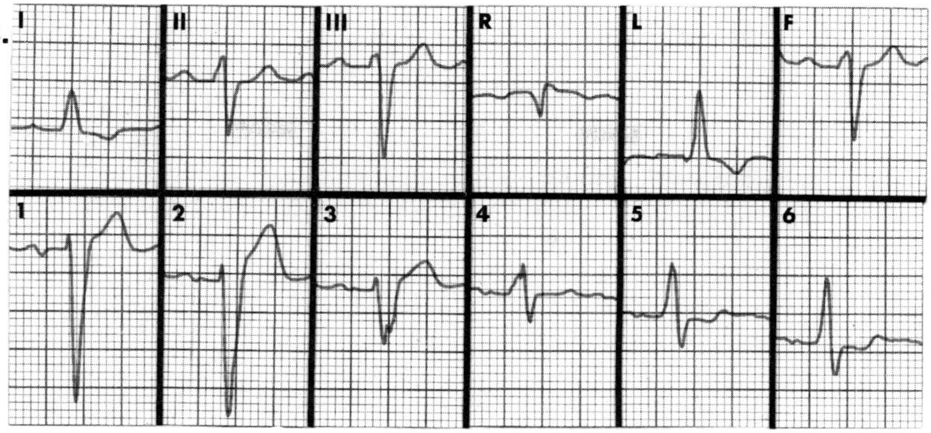

5-54.

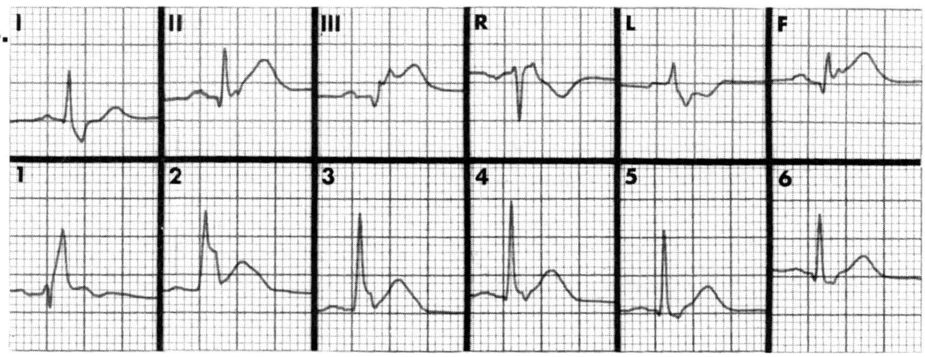

5-55.

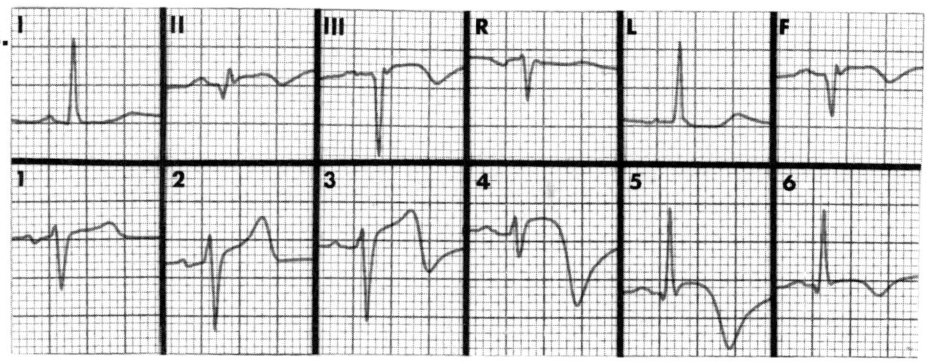

ANSWER KEY

Multiple Choice

1. c
2. c
3. d
4. d
5. a
6. b
7. b
8. d
9. c
10. b
11. d
12. b
13. a
14. c

5–1. Normal axis +5 to −5 degrees.
Late transition, V4–V5.
Normal voltage, poor R wave progression.
IWMI (II, III, aVF).
Ventricular bigeminy.

5–2. Right axis deviation, +115 to +125 degrees.
Early transition, V1.
Low voltage, (8.0 mm).
LWMI (I, aVL, V6).
PWMI (V1–V3).

5–3. Left axis deviation, −65 to −75 degrees.
Late transition, (?).
Normal voltage, poor R wave progression.
A-LWMI (I, aVL, V3–V6).
LAFB.
Atrial fibrillation.

5–4. Left axis deviation, −40 to −50 degrees.
Late transition, V6.
Normal voltage, poor R wave progression.
A-SWMI.
LAFB.
Sinus rhythm, 75/minute, premature atrial beats precipitating atrial fibrillation.

5–5. Normal axis, 0 to −10 degrees.
Normal transition, V4.
Normal voltage, poor R wave progression.

A-SWMI (V2–V4).
Possible old IWMI.
Wandering atrial pacemaker.

5–6. (ECG of 4/1, 6:37 A.M.)
Normal axis, +40 to +50 degrees.
AWMI, acute phase (V2–V6).
(ECG of 4/1, 3:09 P.M.)
Normal axis, +55 to +65 degrees.
AWMI, acute phase, evolving (V2–V6).

5–7. Normal axis, +55 to +65 degrees.
Normal transition, V3.
Normal voltage
IWMI, hyperacute phase (II, III, aVF with reciprocal changes in I, aVL, V1–V6).
Two beats of normal sinus rhythm followed by ventricular tachycardia triggered by a pacemaker spike.

5–8. Normal axis, +15 to +25 degrees.
Normal transition, V3–V4.
Normal voltage, poor R wave progression.
A-SWMI, acute phase (V1–V5).
Ventricular tachycardia.

5–9. Normal axis, +25 to +35 degrees.
Normal transition, V3–V4.
Normal voltage.
IWMI (II, III, aVF).
Anterior and lateral wall ischemia (I, aVL, V3–V6).
Second-degree AV block, 2:1 conduction, premature ventricular beat.

5–10. Left axis deviation, −5 to −15 degrees.
Late transition, V4–V5.
Normal voltage, poor R wave progression.
IWMI, old (II, III, aVF).
A-SWMI, acute (V1–V4).
Sinus rhythm with conducted and nonconducted atrial premature beats.

5–11. Right axis deviation, +110 to +120 degrees.
IWMI (II, III, aVF).
RBBB.
Atrioventricular dissociation (probable block-acceleration dissociation).

5–12. Normal axis, +55 to +65 degrees.
Normal transition, V2–V3.

Normal voltage.
IWMI, hyperacute phase (II, III, aVF with reciprocal changes in aVL, V1–V3).
Second-degree AV block, 2:1 conduction; advanced AV block with 4:1 conduction.

5–13. Normal axis, +55 to +65 degrees.
Late transition, V4–V5.
Normal voltage, poor R wave progression.
A-SWMI, acute phase (V1–V4).
Sinus rhythm, 73/min, premature junctional beat.

5–14. Normal axis, +40 to +50 degrees.
Normal transition, V3–V4.
Normal voltage, poor R wave progression.
IWMI, old (II, III, aVF).
A-SWMI, acute (V1–V4).
Ventricular bigeminy.

5–15. Normal axis, +55 to +65 degrees.
Late transition, V5.
Normal voltage, poor R wave progression.
A-SWMI, acute (V2–V4).
Sinus tachycardia, 120/minute.

5–16. Left axis deviation, −10 to −20 degrees.
Late transition, V6.
Normal voltage, poor R wave progression.
IWMI, old (III, aVF).
A-LWMI, acute (V2–V6).
Wandering atrial pacemaker.

5–17. Normal axis, +5 to +15 degrees.
Normal transition, V4.
Normal voltage, poor R wave progression.
IWMI, acute phase (II, III, aVF with reciprocal changes in aVL, V2–V4).
Second-degree AV block, 2:1 conduction.

5–18. Left axis deviation, −15 to −25 degrees.
Normal voltage.
IWMI, old (II, III, aVF).
RBBB.
Second-degree AV block, 2:1 conduction.

5–19. Normal axis, +50 to +60 degrees.
Normal transition, V3.
Normal voltage.

IWMI, hyperacute phase (II, III, aVF with reciprocal changes in I, aVL, V2–V6).
Sinus arrhythmia.

5–20. Left axis deviation, −10 to −20 degrees.
Late transition, V5–V6.
Normal voltage, poor R wave progression.
IWMI, age indeterminate (II, III, aVF).
A-LWMI, acute (V3–V6).
Atrial fibrillation.

5–21. Normal axis, +55 to +65 degrees.
Low voltage (13.0 mm), poor R wave progression.
Late transition, V6.
LWMI (I, aVL, V5, V6).
A-SWMI (V2–V4).
Sinus rhythm, 79/minute, first-degree AV block (PR 0.24), frequent premature ventricular complexes, some in couplets and triplets.

5–22. Normal axis, +55 to +65 degrees.
Low voltage (11.0 mm).
A-SWMI, age indeterminate (V2–V4).
Ventricular bigeminy. Note right axis deviation of premature ventricular complexes.

5–23. (ECG of 6/26).
Normal axis, +5 to −5 degrees.
Normal transition, V2–V3.
Normal voltage.
A-SWMI, hyperacute phase (V1–V5).
(ECG of 6/27)
Right axis deviation, +110 to +120 degrees.
A-SWMI, acute (V1–V5).
LPFB.
RBBB.
Second-degree AV block, high-grade, ventricular asystole.

5–24. (ECG of 4/13)
Normal axis, +50 to +60 degrees.
Normal transition, V3–V4.
Low voltage (10.0 mm) and poor R wave progression.
IWMI, hyperacute phase (II, III, aVF, reciprocal changes in I, aVL, V1–V6).
(ECG of 4/15)
Left axis deviation, −10 to −20 degrees.
Normal transition, V3–V4.

Normal voltage.
IWMI, acute (II, III, aVF).

5–25. Normal axis, +5 to −5 degrees.
Early transition, V1.
IWMI, recent (II, III, aVF).
PWMI, recent (V1–V3, note voltage dropoff, V5, V6).

5–26. (ECG of 11/29)
Left axis deviation, −50 to −60 degrees.
Normal transition, V4.
Normal voltage.
A-SWMI, hyperacute (V2–V5).
LAFB.
(ECG of 11/30)
Left axis deviation, −50 to −60 degrees.
Late transition, V6.
Normal voltage, poor R wave progression.
A-SWMI, acute phase (V2–V6).
LAFB.
Note: Technically speaking, this is a non-Q anteroseptal MI.

5–27. Left axis deviation, −55 to −65 degrees.
Normal transition, V4.
Normal voltage, poor R wave progression.
A-SWMI, acute (V2–V3).
LAFB.

5–28. Left axis deviation, −5 to −15 degrees.
Normal transition, V3–V4.
Normal voltage.
IWMI (III, aVF).
Anterior ischemia versus non-Q infarction.

5–29. (ECG of 9/30)
Normal axis, +60 to +70 degrees.
Normal transition, V3.
Normal voltage.
IWMI, hyperacute phase (II, III, aVF with reciprocal changes in I, aVL, V1–V6).
(ECG of 10/1)
Left axis deviation, −35 to −45 degrees.
Early transition, V1.
Normal voltage.
IWMI, acute (II, III, aVF).
PWMI, acute (V1–V3 with voltage dropoff in V5–V6).

5–30. Right axis deviation, +205 to +215 degrees.
Early transition, V1.
Low voltage (14.0 mm).
IWMI (II, III, aVF).
PWMI, age indeterminant (V1–V3).
Possible LWMI, age indeterminant (V5, V6).

5–31. Left axis deviation, −30 to −40 degrees.
Late transition (?).
Normal voltage, poor R wave progression.
A-LWMI, recent (I, aVL, V4–V6).
Possible LAFB.
(ECG of 3/25)
Same findings with supraventricular tachycardia, 214/minute.

5–32. (ECG of 2/23)
Normal axis, +55 to +65 degrees.
Normal transition, V3–V4.
Normal voltage.
Possible IWMI, old (II, III, aVF).
A-SWMI, hyperacute phase (V2–V5).
(ECG of 2/24)
Normal axis, +25 to +35 degrees.
Normal transition, V3–V4.
Low voltage (14.0 mm).
Non-Q AWMI (V2, V3).

On the rhythm strip taken 9/20, (1) what are the complexes marked by arrows and (2) what are the complexes marked by asterisks?

5–33. (ECG of 9/12)
Left axis deviation, −5 to −15 degrees.
Late transition, V4–V5.
Normal voltage.
IWMI, old (III, aVF).
Anterolateral ischemia (V3–V6).
(ECG of 9/19)
Right axis deviation, +115 to +125 degrees.
IWMI, old (III, aVF).
Probable AWMI, acute (V1).
LPFB.
RBBB.
(ECG of 9/20)
Right axis deviation, +100 to +120 degrees.
IWMI, old (III, aVF).
A-SWMI, acute (V1–V3).
LPFB.

RBBB.
Sinus tachycardia, 107–130/min, third-degree AV block. A single escape beat appears in the first strip. The complexes marked by arrows are P waves; the complexes marked by asterisks are pacer artifacts.

5–34. Normal axis, +35 to +45 degrees.
Early transition, V1.
Normal voltage.
PWMI, recent (V1–V3, voltage dropoff in V6).

5–35. (ECG of 11/23)
Normal axis, 0 to −10 degrees.
Normal transition, V2–V3.
Normal voltage.
IWMI, acute (II, III, aVF).
Possible RBBB.
(ECG of 11/24)
Left axis deviation, −5 to −15 degrees.
Early transition, V2.
Normal voltage.
IWMI, acute (II, III, aVF).
Rhythm strip of 2:46 A.M.: Second-degree AV block, type I, 3:2 conduction ratio.
Rhythm strip of 3:50 A.M.: Second-degree AV block, 2:1 to 3:1 conduction ratios.

5–36. (ECG of 7/08)
Normal axis, +70 to +80 degrees.
Late transition (?).
Low voltage (9.5 mm) and poor R wave progression.
LWMI, acute (I, aVL, V5, V6).
A-SWMI, acute (V1–V4).
Sinus rhythm, 100/minute, paired premature ventricular complexes.
(ECG of 7/09)
Right axis deviation, +200 to +210 degrees.
Low voltage (13.0 mm).
A-SWMI, acute (V1–V5).
LPFB.
RBBB.
Sinus tachycardia, 130/min; normal intraventricular conduction changes to RBBB after fourth sinus beat.

5–37. Left axis deviation, −50 to −60 degrees.
Early transition, V1.

PWMI, acute (V1–V3, with voltage dropoff noted V5–V6).
Possible LWMI (I, aVL, V5, V6).
LAFB.

5–38. (ECG of 1/6, 7:05 A.M.)
Normal axis, +60 to +70 degrees.
Late transition, V6.
Normal voltage.
Probable non-Q LWMI, acute (V5, V6).
(ECG of 1/6, 4:19 P.M.)
Right axis deviation, +115 to +120 degrees.
Late transition (?).
Normal voltage.
Non-Q A-LWMI, acute (V3–V6).
LPFB.
(ECG of 1/6, 9:00 P.M.)
Right axis deviation, +100 to +110 degrees.
A-SWMI, acute (V1–V5).
LPFB.
RBBB.

5–39. Left axis deviation, −50 to −60 degrees.
Late transition, V5.
Normal voltage, poor R wave progression.
LWMI, recent (I, aVL, V5, V6).
AWMI, acute (V2–V4).
LAFB.

5–40. (ECG of 10/22)
Right axis deviation, +100 to +110 degrees.
Normal transition, V3.
Normal voltage.
IWMI, hyperacute phase (II, III, aVF, reciprocal changes in I, aVL, V1, V2).
Possible LPFB.
First-degree AV block (PR 0.22).
(ECG of 10/23)
Normal axis, +5 to −5 degrees.
Normal transition, V3.
Normal voltage.
IWMI, acute (II, III, aVF).
Anterior wall ischemia (V2–V6).

5–41. (ECG of 5/06)
Left axis deviation, −60 to −70 degrees.
Late transition, V5.
Normal voltage.
LWMI, hyperacute phase (I, aVL with reciprocal changes in II, III, aVF, V1–V3).

LAFB.
(ECG of 5/08)
Left axis deviation, −50 to −60 degrees.
Late transition (?).
Normal voltage, poor R wave progression.
LWMI, acute (I, aVL).
Probable non-Q A-LWMI (loss of R wave amplitude V3–V6).
LAFB.

5–42. Left axis deviation, −10 to −20 degrees.
Early transition, V2.
Normal voltage.
IWMI, acute (II, III, aVF with reciprocal changes in V1–V5).
First-degree AV block (PR 0.32).

5–43. (ECG of 1/25)
Left axis deviation, −55 to −65 degrees.
Early transition, V2.
A-SWMI, hyperacute phase (V1–V4 with reciprocal changes II, III, aVF).
LAFB.
(ECG of 1/26)
Left axis deviation, −55 to −65 degrees.
A-SWMI, acute (V1–V3).
LAFB.
RBBB.
Ventricular demand pacer, 72/minute; AV dissociation.

5–44. Right axis deviation, +120 to +130 degrees.
Normal voltage.
IWMI, age undetermined (II, III, aVF).
LPFB.
RBBB.

5–45. Left axis deviation, −5 to −15 degrees.
Late transition, V4–V5.
Normal voltage, poor R wave progression.
IWMI, acute (II, III, aVF).
2nd degree, type I sinoatrial block, 3:2 to 4:3 conduction.

5–46. Normal axis, +55 to +65 degrees.
Normal voltage.
Nonspecific intraventricular conduction delay.

5–47. Normal axis, +25 to +35 degrees.
Normal voltage.
LBBB.

5–48. Left axis deviation, −55 to −65 degrees.
Nonspecific intraventricular conduction delay.

5–49. Right axis deviation, +150 to +160 degrees.
Normal voltage.
Probable LPFB.
RBBB.

5–50. Left axis deviation, −40 to −50 degrees.
Early transition, V2.
Normal voltage.
IWMI, acute (II, III, aVF).
Possible PWMI (V1–V2).
Atrial tachycardia, 187/minute with variable AV conduction consistent with Wenckebach conduction of alternate beats.

5–51. Right axis deviation, +135 to +145 degrees.
LPFB.
RBBB.
Sinus tachycardia, 107/minute. Second-degree AV block, Mobitz type II.

5–52. (ECG of 9/10)
Normal axis, +50 to +60 degrees.
AWMI, hyperacute phase (V1–V5).
(ECG of 9/11)
Normal axis, +45 to +55 degrees.
AWMI, acute phase (V1–V3). Note loss of R wave amplitude in leads V2–V4.

5–53. Left axis deviation, −55 to −65 degrees.
LBBB.

5–54. Normal axis, +65 to +75 degrees.
RBBB.
IWMI, acute phase (II, III, aVF).

5–55. Left axis deviation, −10 to −20 degrees.
IWMI, age undetermined (II, III, aVF).
Anterior segment ischemia versus non-Q infarction (T wave inversion, V3–V6).

CHAPTER SIX

CHAMBER ENLARGEMENT AND HYPERTROPHY

COGNITIVE GOALS

1. Identify four factors that influence QRS amplitude and explain how these factors influence the accuracy of the electrocardiogram.
2. Define the terms **sensitivity** and **specificity** and explain how these concepts are related to **false-negative** and **false-positive** results.
3. Give the criteria for the normal P wave.
4. Give the ECG criteria for left atrial abnormality (LAA).
5. Define the term **P mitrale.**
6. Give the ECG criteria for right atrial abnormality (RAA).
7. Define the term **P pulmonale.**
8. Give at least three voltage criteria for left ventricular hypertrophy (LVH).
9. Define the term **strain pattern** and describe the characteristic ECG findings.
10. Describe how ventricular activation time (VAT) is measured.
11. Describe how ventricular activation time is affected by ventricular hypertrophy.
12. Define the term **intrinsicoid deflection.**
13. Discuss the prognostic significance of LVH-ECG.
14. Give the ECG criteria for right ventricular hypertrophy (RVH).
15. Identify three conditions likely to be present with RVH-ECG.

The electrical forces that produce the electrocardiogram originate primarily from the left ventricle, and for this reason some authorities have referred to the normal ECG as a "levocardiogram" (Cooksey et al, 1977). Therefore, left ventricular hypertrophy (LVH), an increase in the left ventricular muscle mass, simply increases its normal electrical preponderance to an even greater extent. On the ECG this increase in muscle mass is reflected by an increase in the amplitude (height) of the QRS complexes. Unfortunately for diagnostic accuracy, the amplitude of the QRS complex is determined by factors other than the sheer electrical potential generated by the ventricles.

Among the factors that determine QRS amplitude are (1) the conductivity of body tissues, (2) the distance of surface electrodes from the heart, (3) the intraventricular pressure and volume, and (4) the body habitus of the subject. Because air and fat are poor electrical conductors, patients with chronic obstructive lung disease or obesity tend to produce ECGs with low voltage, or smaller than average QRS complexes. On the other hand, larger than average QRS complexes are often recorded from young patients with thin chest walls. In the case of the young, asthenic subject, such high-amplitude QRS complexes are frequently lacking in diagnostic significance. An erroneous diagnosis of left ventricular hypertrophy by ECG (LVH-ECG) can be made on many women following mastectomy, owing to the excision of interposed breast tissue (Surawicz, 1986).

Further aggravating the problem of diagnostic accuracy is the fact that chamber enlargement or wall hypertrophy or both do not always occur as an isolated event. On the contrary, dilatation and hypertrophy are responses to increased volume and pressure demands that arise from congenital anomalies, systemic or pulmonary hypertension, and valvular disease. These conditions and their sequelae, such as myocardial infarction or conduction deficits, tend to further muddy the electrocardiographic waters by producing ECG abnormalities of their own. In addition, extensive replacement of functioning myocardium with electrically inert scar tissue or deposits such as amyloid diminishes the heart's electrical forces and results in low voltage ECGs regardless of the actual size of the heart.

Many criteria for determining chamber enlargement or hypertrophy have been advanced. All have important diagnostic limitations and some have fallen out of use. Most authors now discuss the surviving criteria in terms of their **sensitivity** and **specificity.** Briefly stated, sensitivity refers to recognition. If the ECG recognizes a condition each time it occurs, the sensitivity is 100 per cent. If the patient has a condition, but the ECG does not recognize it, a **false-negative** result is obtained. False negatives reflect a failure of sensitivity. Specificity refers to the number of positive diagnoses that are confirmed by other tests. If the diagnosis made from the ECG is corroborated in each case by other means, such as autopsy, echocardiogram, or cardiac catheterization findings, then the specificity is known to be 100 per cent. If the patient does not have a condition even though the ECG indicates that he or she does, a **false-positive** result is obtained. False positives reflect a failure of specificity. Textbooks and articles that correlate ECG criteria with echocardiogram or autopsy findings customarily rate those criteria in terms of their sensitivity and specificity, expressed as percentages. The previously mentioned caveat regarding the imperfections of the ECG as an assessment tool could be repeated here. Although they are fairly specific, most of the criteria for chamber enlargement or hypertrophy are not very sensitive; or, to put it another way, many patients have chamber enlargement or hypertrophy but their ECGs do not reflect that fact. Conversely, a significant number of subjects have chamber enlargement by ECG without evidence of enlargement either by autopsy or echocardiogram. To achieve maximum application, ECG findings should always be correlated with the patient's total clinical picture. Owing to its serious limitations, the ECG is being replaced by the echocardiogram as the preferred tool for diagnosing and monitoring chamber enlargement.

Atrial abnormalities

The normal sinus P wave assumes the shape of a truncated pyramid with rounded contours. It does not exceed 2.5 millimeters in height (2.5 small squares) and its duration does not exceed 0.11 second. Normally the P wave is not pointed or notched. The normal P wave axis in the frontal plane ranges from +40 to +60 degrees and is therefore usually tallest in lead II and upright in leads I, II, and aVF and precordial leads V4 to V6 (Schamroth, 1980). Normal waves are shown in Figure 3–2 and panel **A** of Figure 5–5.

Because the left atrium is activated slightly later than the right, its electrical potentials account for the inscription of the last half of the P wave. Dilatation or delayed conduction or both through the left atrium may result in P wave changes that are labeled **left atrial abnormality** or **left atrial enlargement.** Left atrial abnormality (LAA) is now the preferred term. The criteria for left atrial abnormality consist of (1) increased P wave duration, (2) notching of the P wave, and (3) an increase in the P terminal force. **Increased duration** is reflected by P wave width of 0.12 second or more (panels **A** through **D** in Fig. 6–1). Although very slight **notching** of the P wave is an occasional finding in normal ECGs, a "peak to peak" interval of 0.04 second or more is distinctly abnormal (note **1** and **2** in panels **A** and **C;** panel **D** illustrates a peak to peak interval of 0.06 second). The **P terminal force** in lead V1 is the product of the depth of the terminal negative deflection of the P wave in millimeters and its duration in seconds. If the terminal part of the P wave in lead V1 is greater than 1

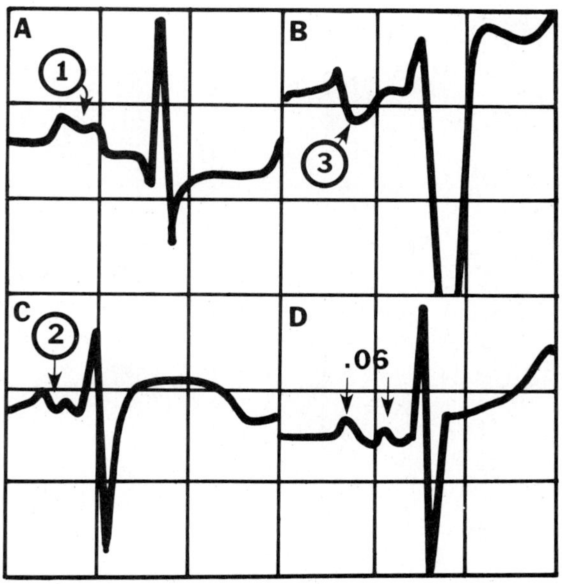

Figure 6–1. The electrocardiogram of left atrial abnormality.

millimeter in depth (one small square) and at least 0.04 second wide (one small square), the P wave is abnormal (Chou, 1986). Panel **B** in Figure 6–1 illustrates an abnormal P terminal force (**3**).

The term **P mitrale** is frequently used to describe P waves that are both notched and of abnormal width. As this designation implies, such P waves were once thought to be characteristic of tracings from patients with mitral valve disease, particularly mitral stenosis. The ECG findings of left atrial abnormality have been found to correlate with (1) left atrial enlargement, (2) right atrial enlargement, (3) left ventricular hypertrophy, (4) coronary artery disease, and (5) impaired left ventricular function (Rios, 1977; Surawicz, 1986).

Because the right atrium is depolarized first, its electrical potentials determine the formation of the first half of the P wave. Increased potentials from the right atrium increase the height of the P wave but do not prolong its duration. **Right atrial abnormality** or **right atrial enlargement** is diagnosed when the P waves in lead II or aVF are 2.5 millimeters or more in height and of normal duration (0.11 second or less) and/or when the initial positive portion of the P wave in lead V1 is 1.5 millimeters or more tall. Since tall, pointed P waves with an axis of +70 degrees or greater, and therefore usually tallest in lead II or aVF, are often observed in the tracings of patients with severe lung disease, they have acquired the name **P pulmonale.**

The ECG in Figure 6–2, recorded on admission to an emergency room, was from a 53-year-old woman who had had a total right pneumonectomy in her teens. She entered in severe respiratory distress with a $PaCO_2$ of 130. Note that the P waves in leads II and aVF exceed the upper limit of normal (4.5 and 3.0 millimeters, respectively) and that the P wave in V1 is 2.5 millimeters tall. Occasionally the right atrial abnormality (RAA) pattern is seen in patients with left-sided heart disease, so the pattern cannot be regarded as highly specific.

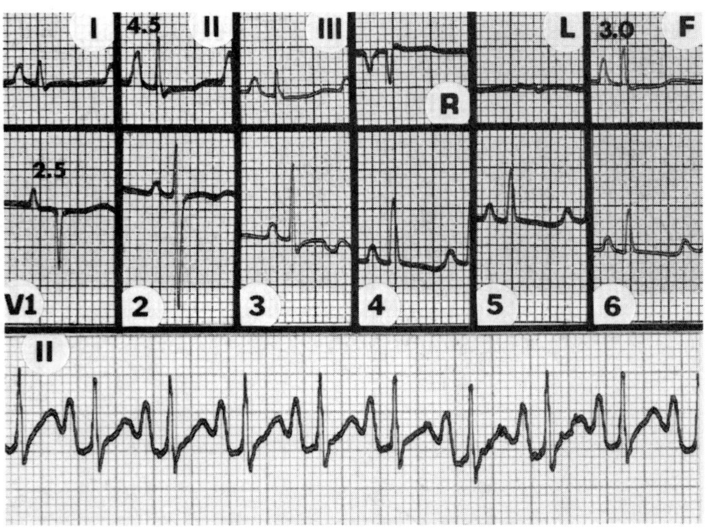

Figure 6–2. The electrocardiogram of right atrial abnormality.

Left ventricular hypertrophy

The diagnosis of left ventricular hypertrophy by ECG (LVH-ECG) is made primarily on the basis of (1) **increased QRS amplitude** and is supported by the additional findings of (2) **secondary ST segment and T wave changes** and (3) **prolonged ventricular activation time.** Unfortunately, none of the ECG criteria taken individually is a very sensitive indicator of LVH. As noted previously, enlargement of the left ventricular muscle mass is reflected on the ECG mainly by an increase in QRS amplitude—particularly in the precordial leads because they are closer to the heart. Ordinarily LVH produces no marked alteration of the mean QRS axis, nor does it produce any distinctive deformity of the QRS complex, as seen with infarction or bundle branch block.

Many individual ECG criteria as well as several more or less complex scoring systems for diagnosing LVH have been proposed. The various individual criteria and the scoring systems are thoroughly discussed and evaluated in many standard texts. Some of the more widely recognized criteria are listed below:

Frontal plane leads
R wave in I + S wave in III = 25 mm
R wave in aVL = 11 mm
R wave in aVF = 20 mm

Horizontal plane leads
S wave in V1 + R wave in V5 or V6 = 26 mm
R wave in V5 or V6 = 26 mm
Largest precordial S wave + largest precordial R wave = 45 mm
Secondary ST segment and T wave abnormalities
Delayed onset of intrinsicoid deflection (prolonged QR interval) in V6

Factors such as age, race, sex, body habitus, and electrode position negatively affect the specificity of voltage criteria with the result that none of the individual voltage criteria has greater than 46 per cent overall accuracy (Surawicz, 1986). It should be noted that the computerized ECG machines in use in the majority of larger American hospitals routinely scale the precordial leads to **half size** when high-amplitude QRS complexes are encountered. This reduction in scale is indicated on the tracing and must, of course, be taken into account if the amplitude of the precordial complexes is to be determined accurately.

Several of the voltage criteria diagnostic of LVH are shown in Figure 6–3. Note that the precordial leads are one-half scale **(½).** The S wave in V1 is 27½ millimeters deep and the R wave in V5 is 25 millimeters tall. Taking into account that the precordial leads are half scale, the total amplitude of both complexes is 105 mm: (27.5 × 2) + (25 × 2) = 105. Although the voltage criteria for LVH are met in the horizontal plane leads, none of the criteria is met in the frontal plane leads in this tracing. This is in keeping with the observation that high voltage in the precordial leads is a far more common

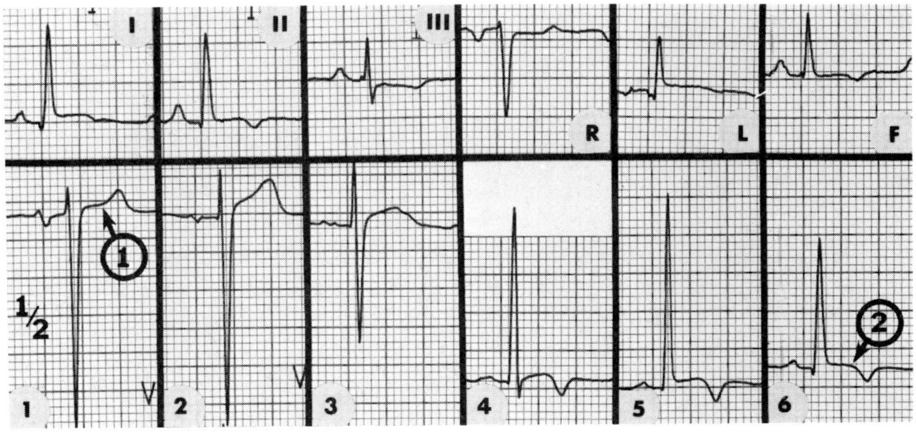

Figure 6–3. The electrocardiogram of left ventricular hypertrophy with "strain."

finding than high voltage in the limb leads (Chou, 1986), although high voltage in the frontal plane leads (limb leads) is more specific for diagnosing LVH-ECG.

Frequently, but not always, subjects with LVH-ECG manifest changes in the ST segment and T wave that occur secondarily to ventricular hypertrophy. These changes are thought to represent, at least in part, conduction delay through the thickened ventricular wall or to reflect ischemia due to an increase in the diameter of myocardial muscle fibers. The ST segments may exhibit elevation or depression. Frequently, ST segments exhibit **upward concavity** in the right precordial leads, V1 and V2 (**1** in Fig. 6–3), and **upward convexity** in the left precordial leads, V5 and V6 (**2** in Fig. 6–3). The T waves are often opposite in polarity to the QRS complexes; that is, negative QRS complexes are followed by positive T waves, and positive QRS complexes are followed by negative T waves (compare leads V1 to V3 with leads V4 to V6 in Fig. 6–3). Taken together, these ST segment and T wave changes are often called the **strain pattern,** a term that has become firmly embedded in ECG terminology despite the fact that "strain" characterizes a physical, not an electrical, event. Tracings such as the one in Figure 6–3 are often read "left ventricular hypertrophy with strain." When present, secondary ST-T abnormalities add further support to the diagnosis of LVH.

Ventricular activation time (VAT) is related to the speed of impulse conduction through the bundle branches or through the ventricular muscle itself, or through both. Therefore, delayed conduction due to bundle branch block or to increased thickness of the ventricular wall will result in a prolonged ventricular activation time, making it an expected finding in both the aforementioned conditions.

The VAT is determined by measuring the **QR interval,** from the beginning of the QRS complex to the peak of the R wave. The end of the VAT is marked by the inscription of the **intrinsicoid deflection,** the descending limb of the R

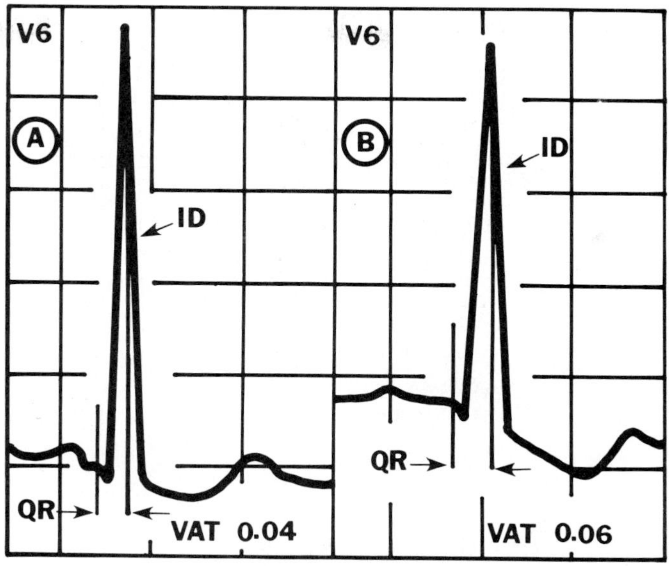

Figure 6–4. Ventricular activation times in left ventricular hypertrophy.

wave (**ID** in Fig. 6–4). The normal QR interval (or VAT) is 0.035 second in lead V1 and 0.045 second in lead V6.

Because it faces the left ventricular muscle mass, lead V6 reflects increased VAT due to left ventricular hypertrophy. Figure 6–4 shows two QRS complexes taken from lead V6. In both diagrams, the QR intervals, measured from the beginning of the QRS complex to the peak of the R wave, are indicated by arrows. Diagram **A** shows a QRS complex with an essentially normal QR interval (0.04 second) but increased voltage (24 millimeters) and secondary repolarization changes. Diagram **B** illustrates increased VAT (0.06 second), increased voltage (20 millimeters), and secondary repolarization changes reflected by the deformed, downsloping ST segment.

Despite the shortcomings of LVH-ECG as a specific marker of ventricular hypertrophy compared with more accurate means of detection such as echocardiography, it has proved to be a fairly reliable indicator of cardiovascular pathology in general. The conclusion of Kannel that LVH-ECG should "be regarded as a grave prognostic sign carrying a high risk of clinically overt coronary heart disease and of premature death" has been amply borne out by the results of subsequent investigations (Kannel et al, 1970). In addition to having an expectedly higher incidence of hypertension, subjects with LVH-ECG also have more frequent occurrence of left ventricular dysfunction and at least a five-fold increase in their risk for sudden death and are at substantially higher risk of heart failure, myocardial infarction, and stroke (Hamby et al, 1980; Kannel and Schatzkin, 1984; Kannel and Abbott, 1986). Results of recent studies indicate that patients with LVH-ECG also have a high incidence of complex ventricular arrhythmias even when other possible factors are accounted for, a finding that may explain their increased propensity for sudden death (Levy et al, 1987; McLenachan et al, 1987). Patients with LVH-ECG by voltage criteria whose tracings also demonstrate left atrial abnormality (LAA) or secondary ST-T wave changes ("strain"), or both, appear to be at greater risk for cardiovascular morbidity and mortality than patients with LVH-ECG by voltage criteria alone.

Left axis deviation, frequently noted in conjunction with the ECG findings of LVH, is not a reliable sign of ventricular hypertrophy per se. In the setting of LVH-ECG, left axis deviation is thought to represent left anterior fascicular block due to fibrosis or infarction. In addition, poor R wave progression in the right to midprecordial leads (V1 to V4) is often noted in cases of LVH-ECG, with leads V1 to V3 sometimes showing pure QS complexes. These findings can lead to a mistaken diagnosis of anterior wall infarction. Occasionally, abnormal Q waves are recorded in the inferior leads, particularly in leads III and aVF, in cases of LVH, resulting in yet another pseudoinfarction pattern (Goldberger, 1979).

Right ventricular hypertrophy

If the reliability of the criteria for left ventricular hypertrophy is suspect, the dependability of the individual criteria for right ventricular hypertrophy can only be considered worse. In fact, the sensitivity of the individual criteria for RVH is as low as or less than 20 per cent (Chou, 1986). This is largely due to the fact that the normally predominant left ventricular potentials must be overshadowed by right ventricular forces before RVH becomes apparent on the ECG. Such a dramatic shift in the balance of electrical forces may take place suddenly, as in the case of massive pulmonary embolism, but the findings of RVH-ECG more commonly represent longstanding and severe pulmonary or cardiac disease.

Some of the generally accepted criteria for RVH are given below:

Frontal plane leads
Right axis deviation of at least +110 degrees

Horizontal plane leads
R:S ratio in V1 greater than 1.0
R wave in V1 = 7 mm
S wave in V1 less than 2 mm
qR or qRS pattern in V1
S wave in V5 or V6 = 7 mm
rSR′ in V1 with R′ greater than 10 mm
R in V1 + S in V5 or V6 greater than 10.5 mm

Because lead V1 most directly faces the mass of the right ventricle, an increase in right ventricular electrical forces will be reflected most in that lead. Some authors distinguish between as many as three electrocardiographic types of RVH based on the QRS morphology in V1. These are **type A,** consisting of a large R wave; **type B,** represented by an equiphasic RS complex; and **type C,** which consists of an rSr′ or rSR′ pattern essentially identical to the pattern observed in right bundle branch block (Cooksey, 1977).

Type A RVH, shown in Figure 6–5, is considered by most authorities to represent right ventricular pressure overloading such as occurs in subjects with severe isolated pulmonic stenosis. Type C RVH, consisting of an rSR′ pattern in V1, is felt to represent volume overloading such as occurs in cases of atrial septal defect.

In severe cases, such as those found among children and young adults with congenital cardiac anomalies, a strain pattern like that described in connection with LVH may appear in lead V1. In some patients with congenital heart disease, tall R waves in V1 are accompanied by peaked P waves with an axis in the range of +30 to +40 degrees; these P waves have been christened **P congenitale** (compare Fig. 6–5).

Figure 6–5, recorded from a 14-year-old subject with congenital heart disease, illustrates several of the features of RVH in addition to P congenitale. The mean QRS axis is in the range of +120 degrees, the R wave in V1 is 12 millimeters in height, and the sum of the R wave in V1 and the S wave in V6 is 17 millimeters. The ST segment and T wave in V1 show a typical strain pattern. Although the individual criteria for RVH lack specificity, finding combinations of them, such as in this tracing, greatly increases the probability of making a correct diagnosis.

Three conditions in particular are likely to produce RVH-ECG: severe **mitral stenosis** with pulmonary hypertension, chronic **cor pulmonale,** and **congenital heart disease** such as pulmonary stenosis or atrial septal defect. It must be remembered, however, that patients with severe valvular disease, right- or left-sided, may have completely normal ECGs.

Right axis deviation, an expected finding in subjects with RVH, is a normal feature in ECGs of infants and young children. In the adult population some persons, particularly those with a tall, slender habitus, tend to have a rightwardly directed QRS axis. Lateral wall infarction can shift the axis rightward

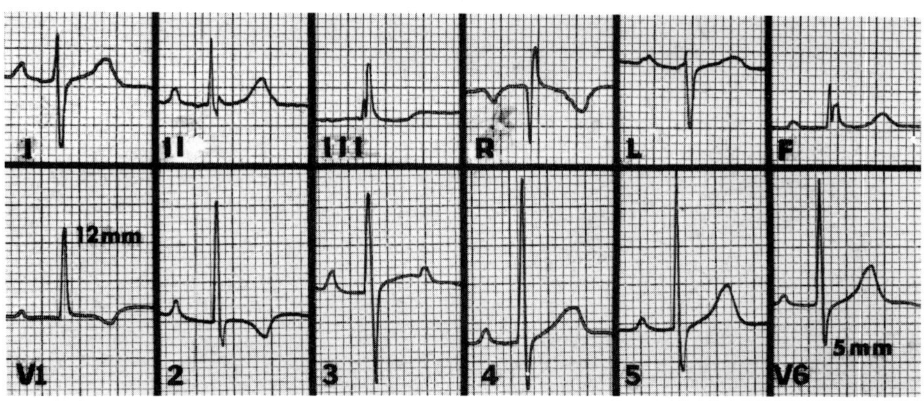

Figure 6–5. The electrocardiogram of right ventricular hypertrophy.

owing to the loss of some left ventricular forces. Right axis deviation is, of course, the sine qua non of left posterior fascicular block.

References

Chou, T-C. **Electrocardiography in Clinical Practice,** 2nd ed. Grune & Stratton, New York, 1986, pp 27–31, 49, 68.

Cooksey, JD, Dunn, M, and Massie, E. **Clinical Vectorcardiography and Electrocardiography,** 2nd ed. Year Book Medical Publishers, Chicago, 1977, pp 172–177.

Goldberger, AL. **Myocardial Infarction: Electrocardiographic Differential Diagnosis,** 2nd ed. CV Mosby, St Louis, 1979, pp 45–46.

Hamby, R, et al. **Am Heart J** 100:794–801, 1980.

Kannel, WB, et al. **Ann Intern Med** 72:813–822, 1970.

Kannel, WB, and Abbott, RD. **Am Heart J** 111:391–397, 1986.

Kannel, WB, and Schatzkin, A. **Progr Cardiovasc Dis** 26:324–327, 1984.

Levy, D, et al. **Am J Cardiol** 60:560–565, 1987.

Marriott, HJL. **Practical Electrocardiography,** 7th ed. Williams & Wilkins, Baltimore, 1983, p 83.

McLenachan, JM, et al. **N Engl J Med** 317:787–792, 1987.

Rios, JC (ed): **Clinical Electrocardiographic Correlations.** FA Davis, Philadelphia, 1977, pp 29–30.

Schamroth, L. **The Disorders of Cardiac Rhythm,** 2nd ed. Vol. I. Blackwell Scientific Publications, Oxford, 1980, p 23.

Surawicz, B. **J Am Coll Cardiol** 8:711–724, 1986.

SELF-ASSESSMENT

Multiple Choice

1. False-negative results reflect a failure of:

   a. sensitivity.

   b. specificity.

2. Factors which determine QRS amplitude include:

   a. the conductivity of body tissues.

   b. body habitus.

   c. the voltage of the electrical potentials generated by the ventricles.

   d. all of the above.

3. The normal P wave does not exceed ______ millimeters in height and ______ second in duration.

   a. 3.5, 0.11

   b. 1.5, 0.12

   c. 2.5, 0.11

   d. 2.0, 0.11

4. Notching of the P wave is diagnostically significant when it reaches or exceeds:

   a. 0.02 second.

   b. 0.03 second.

   c. 0.04 second.

   d. 0.05 second.

5. The term P mitrale is often used to designate P waves that are:

   a. more than 2.5 mm in height in lead II, III, or aVF.

   b. abnormally notched.

   c. abnormally notched and of abnormal duration.

   d. greater than 2.5 mm in height in lead I.

6. In left or right ventricular hypertrophy with strain, the orientation of the T wave is ______ that of the QRS complex in leads facing the enlarged ventricle, and the ST segments in those leads exhibit ______.

   a. opposite, convexity.

   b. opposite, concavity.

   c. the same as, convexity.

   d. the same as, concavity.

7. Ventricular activation time is reflected by the ______ interval, which normally does not exceed ______ second in lead V6.

   a. PR, 0.045

   b. QT, 0.12

   c. QR, 0.035

   d. QR, 0.045

8. Criteria for right ventricular hypertrophy in the frontal plane leads include:

   a. R wave in aVL = 11 mm.
   b. R wave in aVF = 20 mm.
   c. QS complexes in V1 to V3.
   d. right axis deviation in excess of +110 degrees.

9. The finding of left ventricular hypertrophy by ECG (LVH-ECG) identifies a population at increased risk of:

   a. sudden death.
   b. pulmonary embolism.
   c. coronary artery disease.
   d. both a and c.

10. In left ventricular hypertrophy, high voltage in the ______ leads is the more common finding, although high voltage in the ______ leads is more specific for diagnostic purposes.

   a. limb, precordial
   b. precordial, limb

Practice Strips

For the following ECGs, determine the axis and any abnormalities that appear.

6-1.

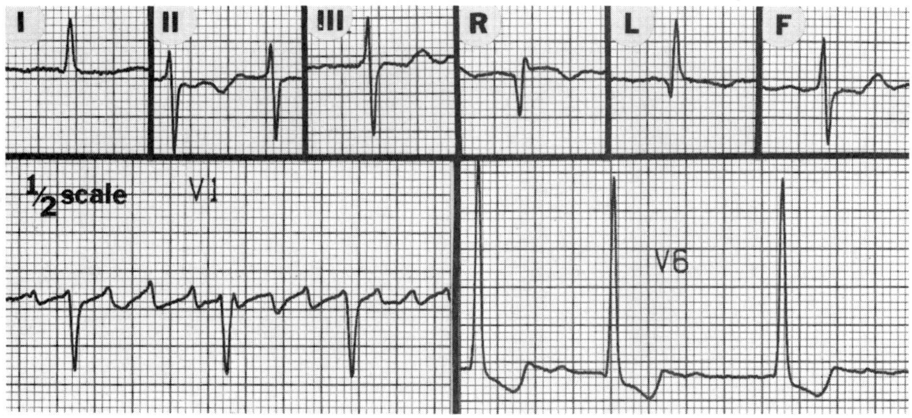

6-2.

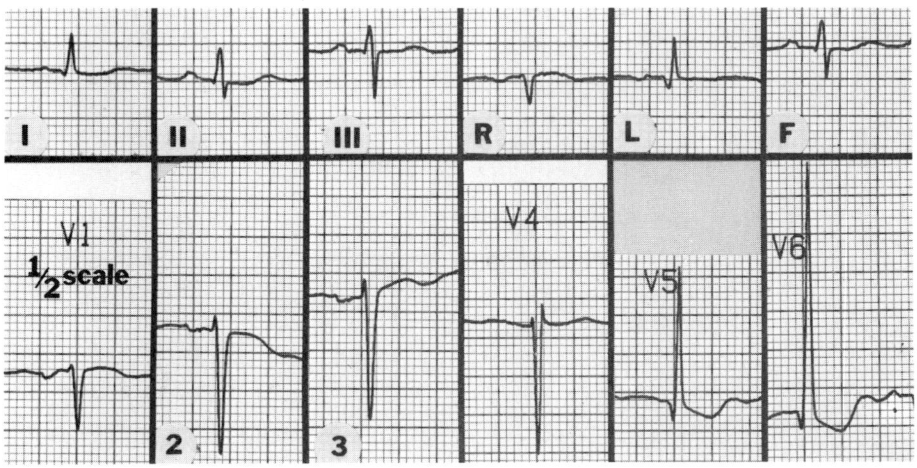

6-3.

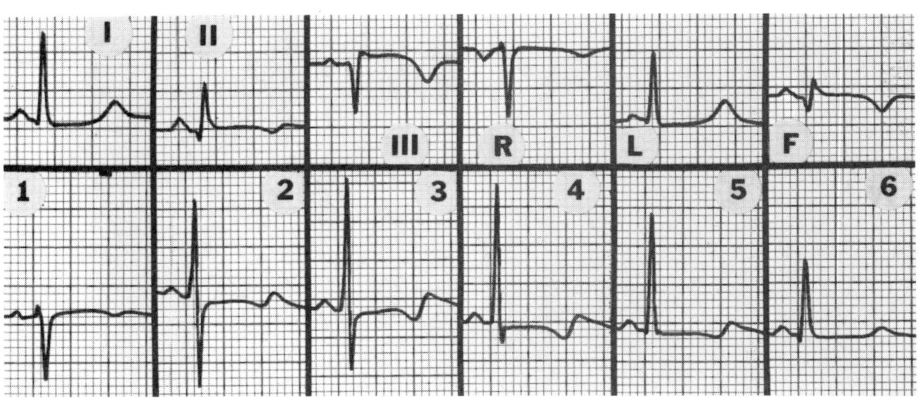

6-4.

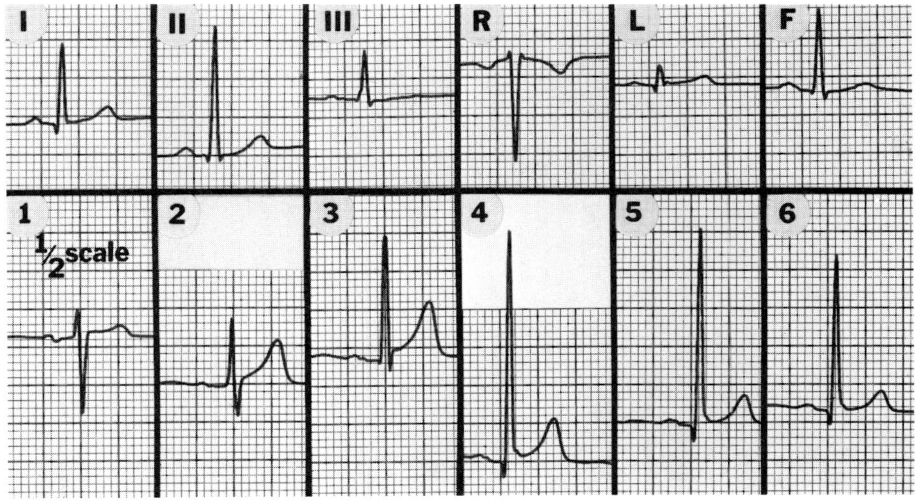
I
II
III
R
L
F
1
½ scale
2
3
4
5
6

6-5.

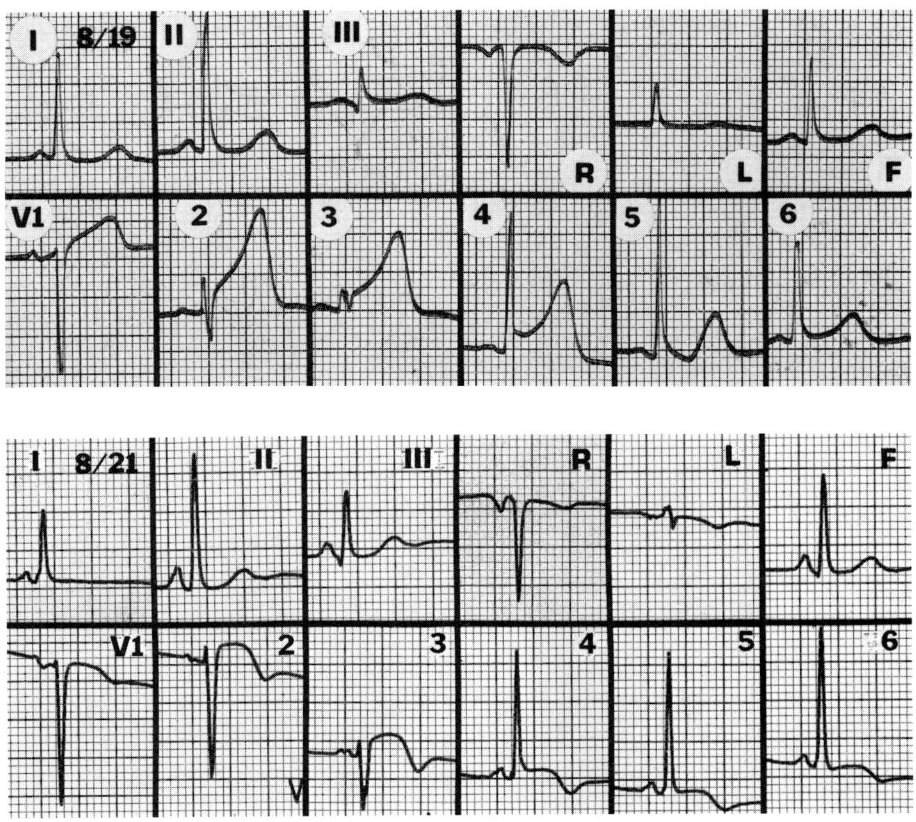
I 8/19
II
III
R
L
F
V1
2
3
4
5
6
I 8/21
II
III
R
L
F
V1
2
3
4
5
6

6-6.

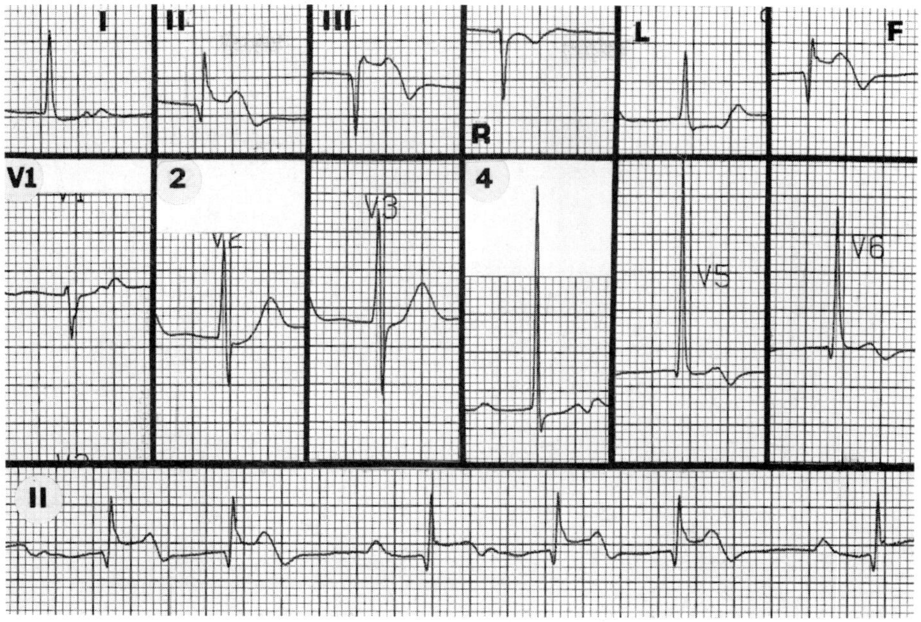
I
II
III
R
L
F
V1
2
V3
4
V5
V6
II

6-7.

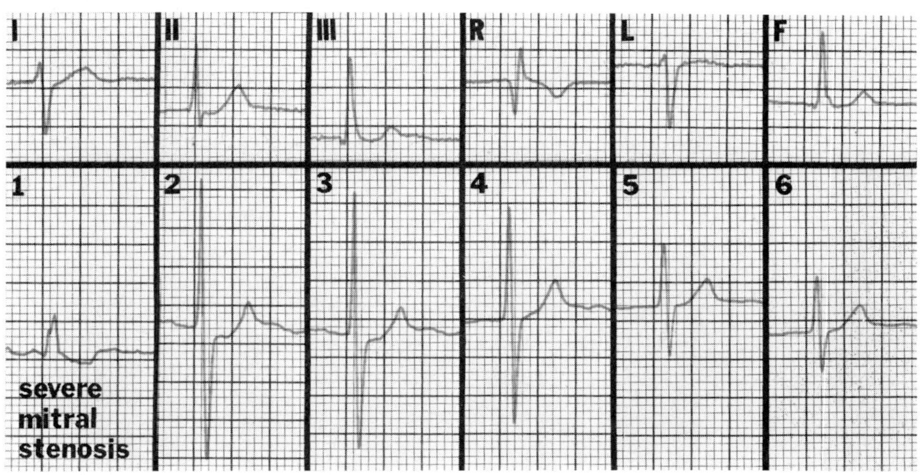
I
II
III
R
L
F
1
2
3
4
5
6
severe mitral stenosis

6-8.

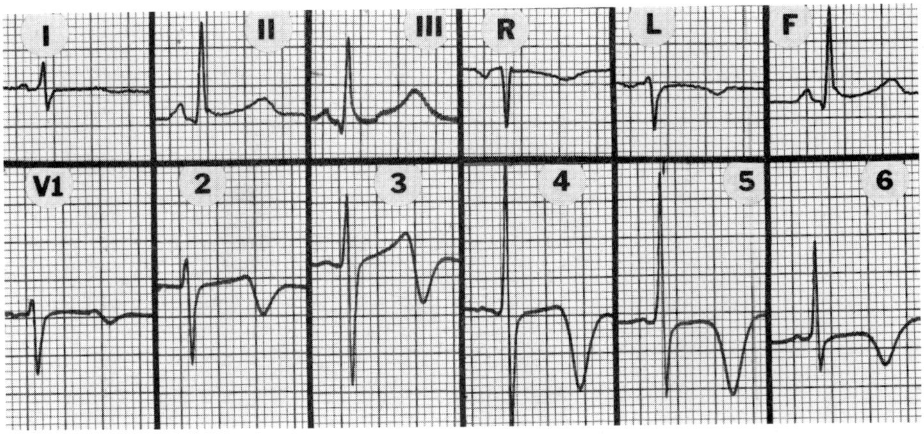
I
II
III
R
L
F
V1
2
3
4
5
6

6-9.

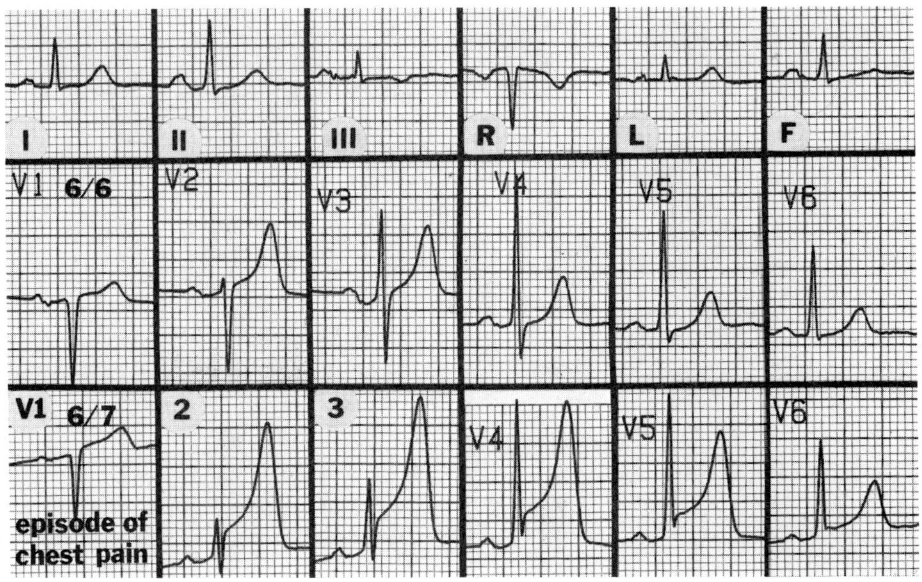
I
II
III
R
L
F
V1 6/6
V2
V3
V4
V5
V6
V1 6/7
2
3
V4
V5
V6
episode of chest pain

6-10.

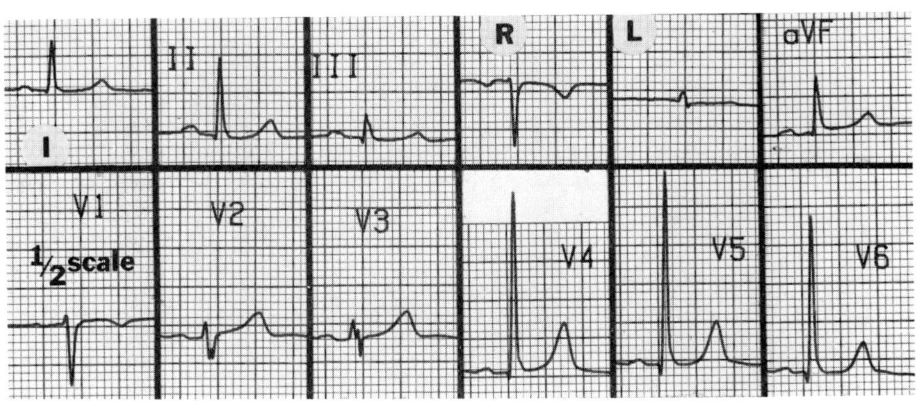
I
II
III
R
L
aVF
V1
½ scale
V2
V3
V4
V5
V6

6-11.

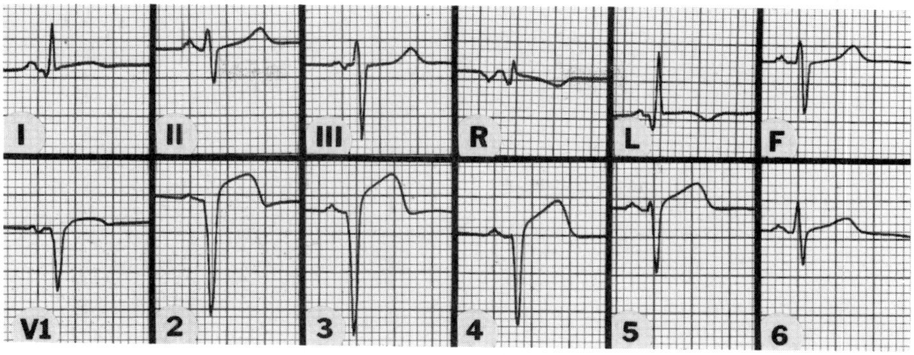

6-12.

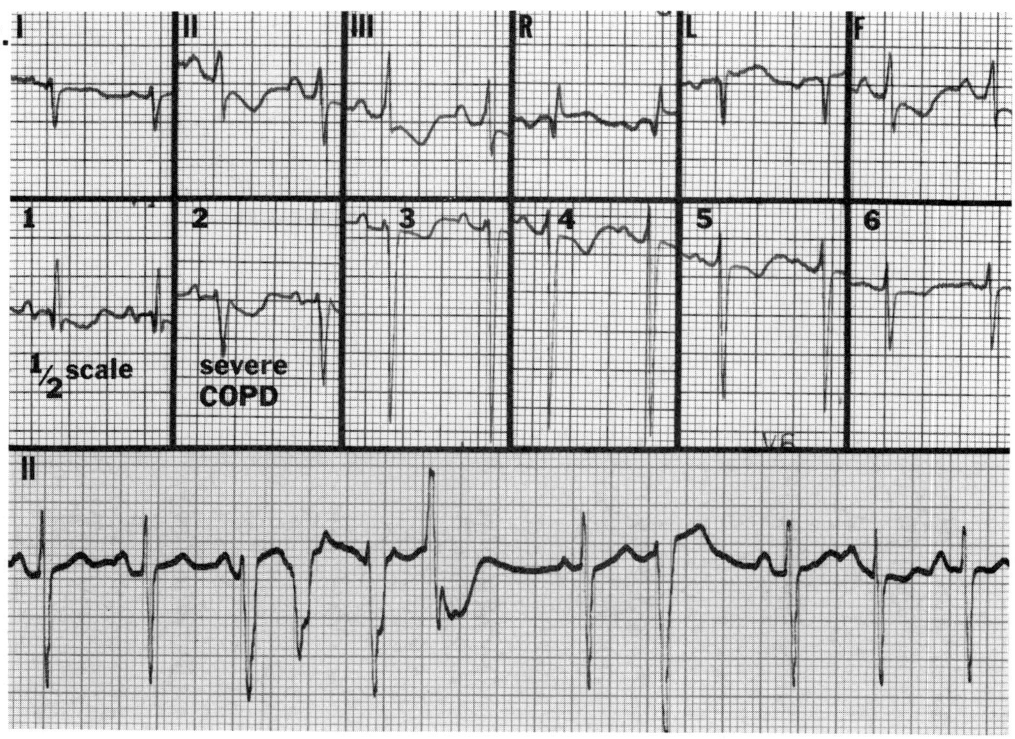

6-13.

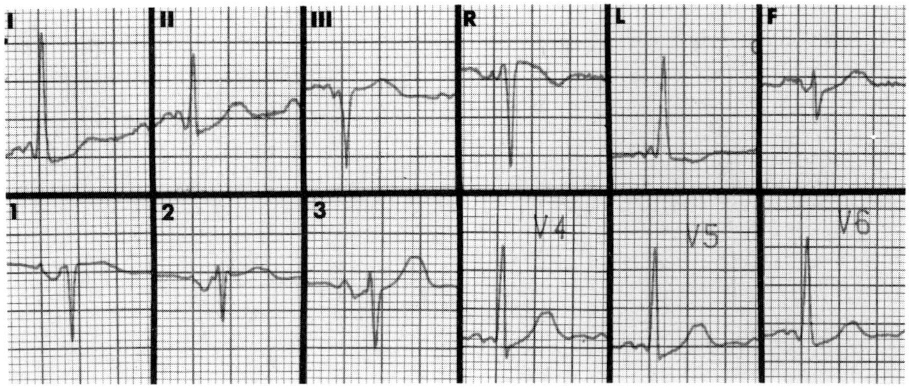

6-14.

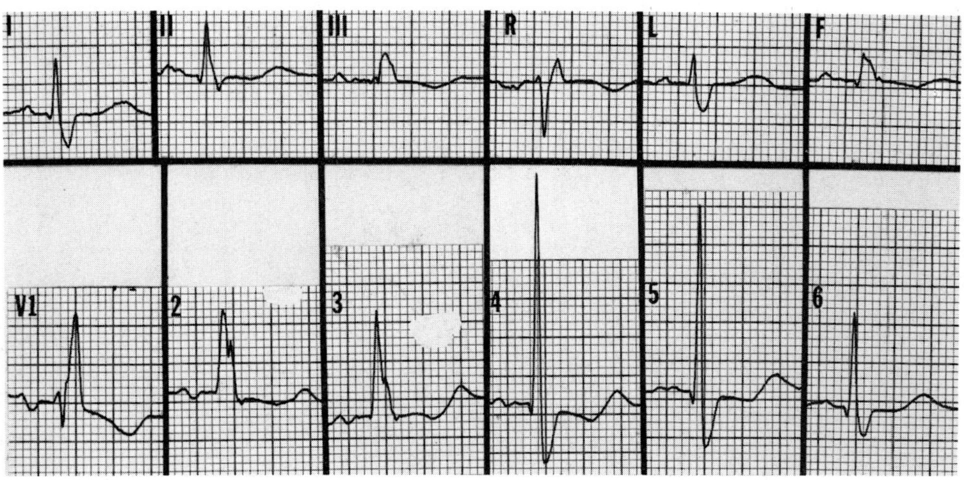

6-15.

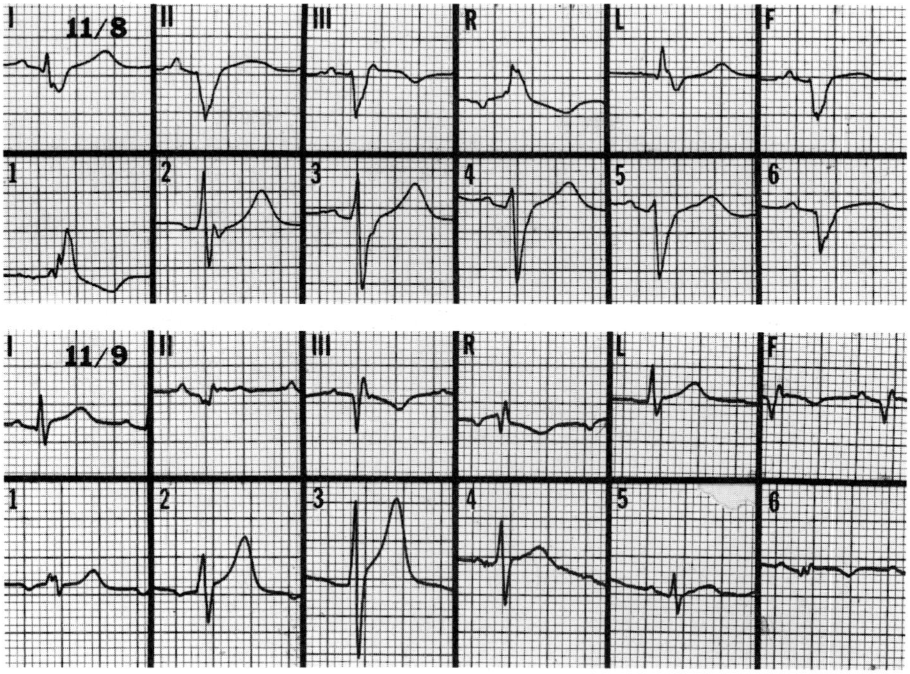
I 11/8
II
III
R
L
F
1
2
3
4
5
6
I 11/9
II
III
R
L
F
1
2
3
4
5
6

6-16.

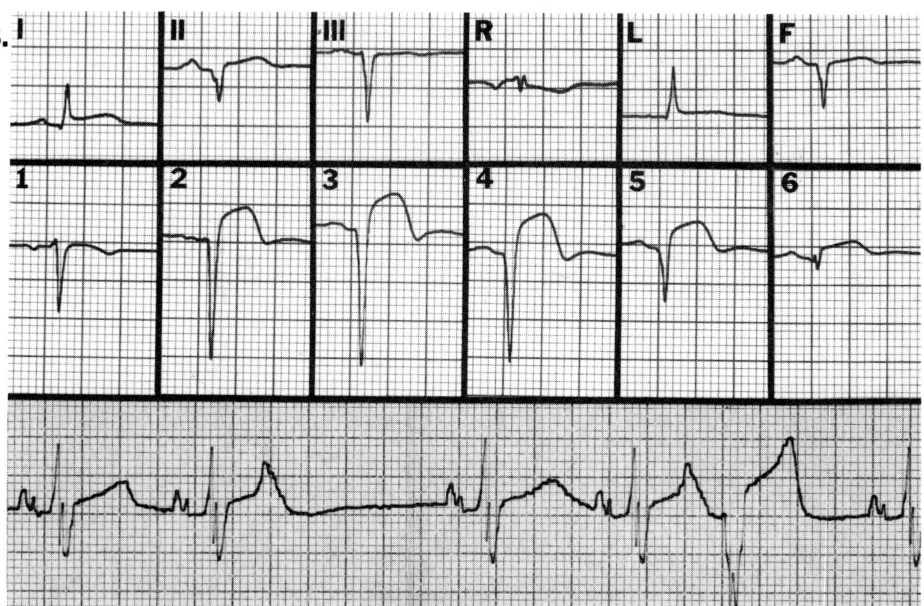
I
II
III
R
L
F
1
2
3
4
5
6

6-17.

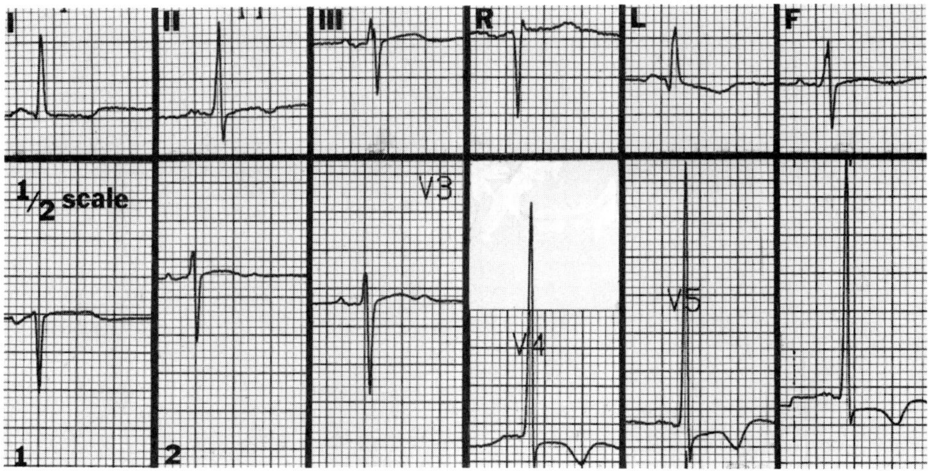
I
II
III
R
L
F
1/2 scale
V3
V4
V5
1
2

6-18.

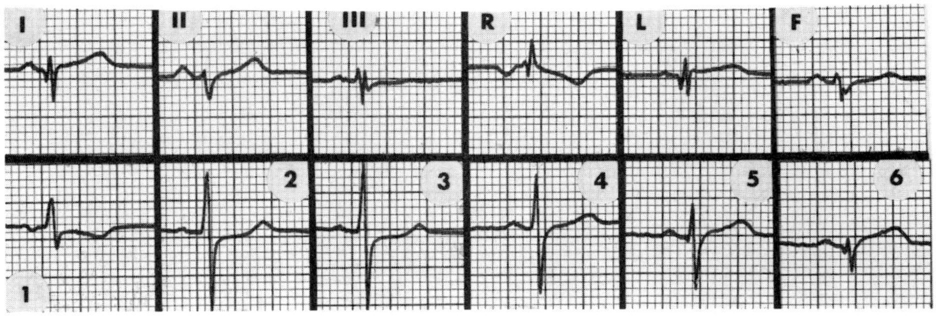
I
II
III
R
L
F
1
2
3
4
5
6

6-19.

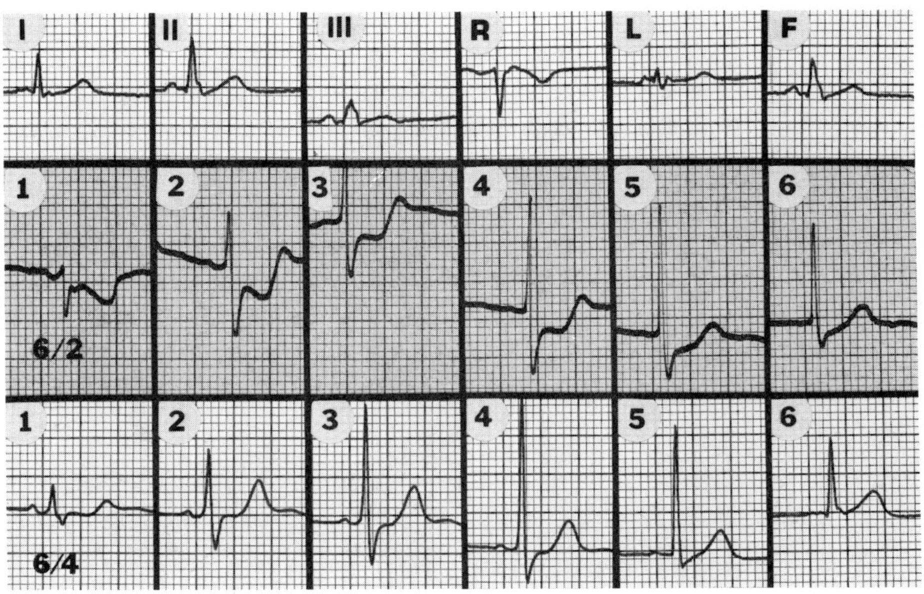
I
II
III
R
L
F
1
2
3
4
5
6
6/2
1
2
3
4
5
6
6/4

6-20.

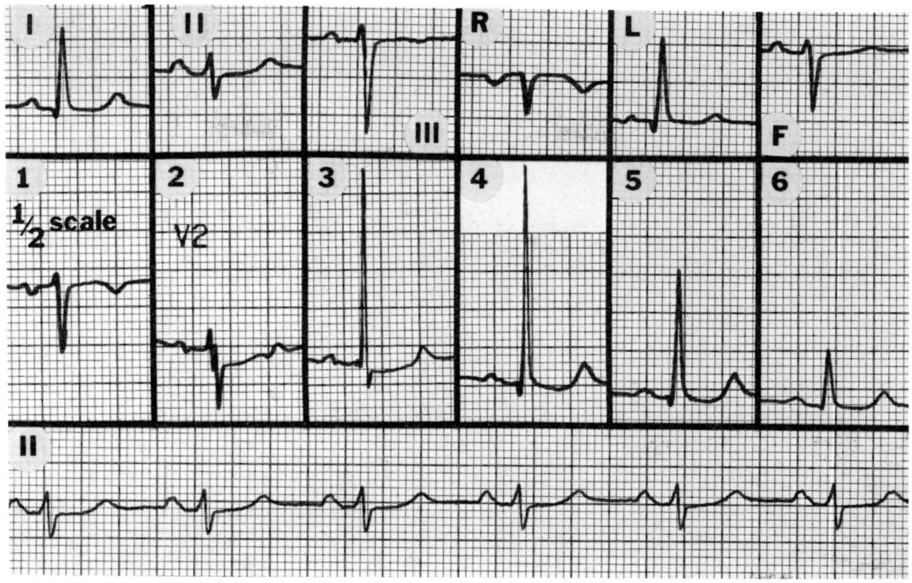
I
II
III
R
L
F
1
1/2 scale
2
V2
3
4
5
6
II

6-21.

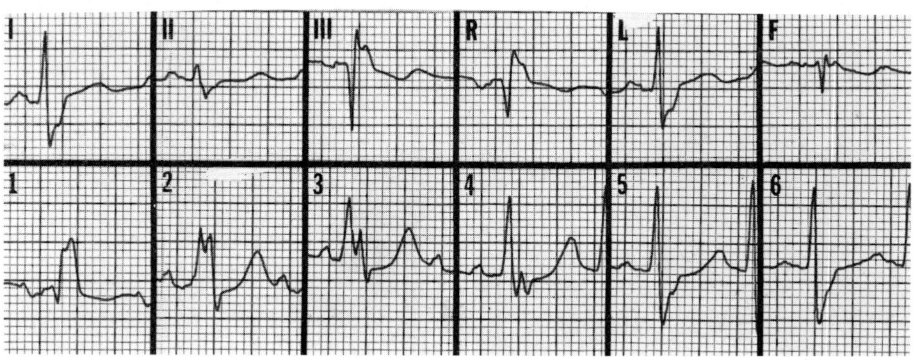
I
II
III
R
L
F
1
2
3
4
5
6

6-22.

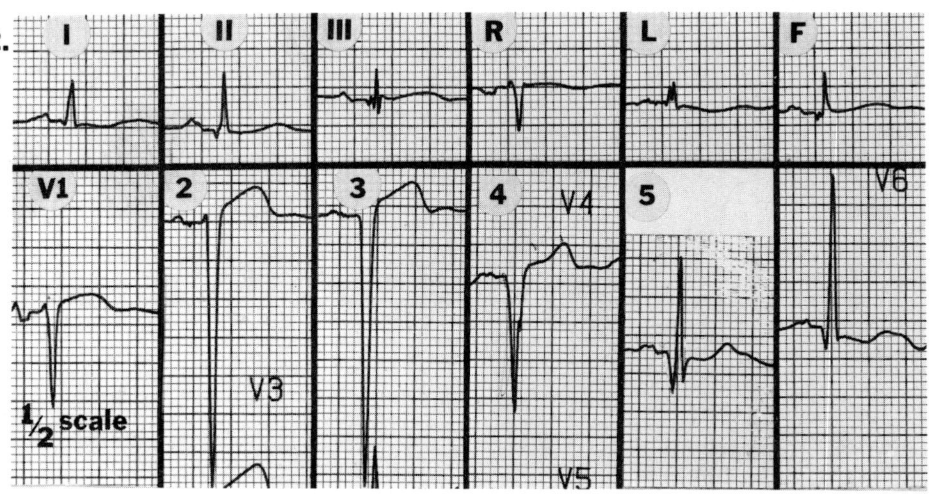
I
II
III
R
L
F
V1
1/2 scale
2
V3
3
4
V4
V5
5
V6

6-23.

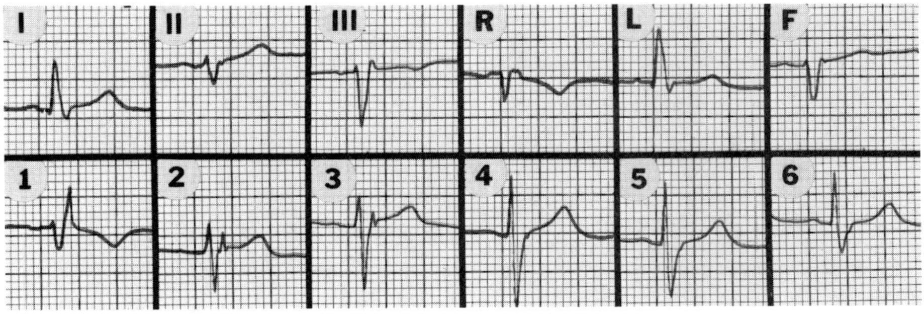
I
II
III
R
L
F
1
2
3
4
5
6

6-24.

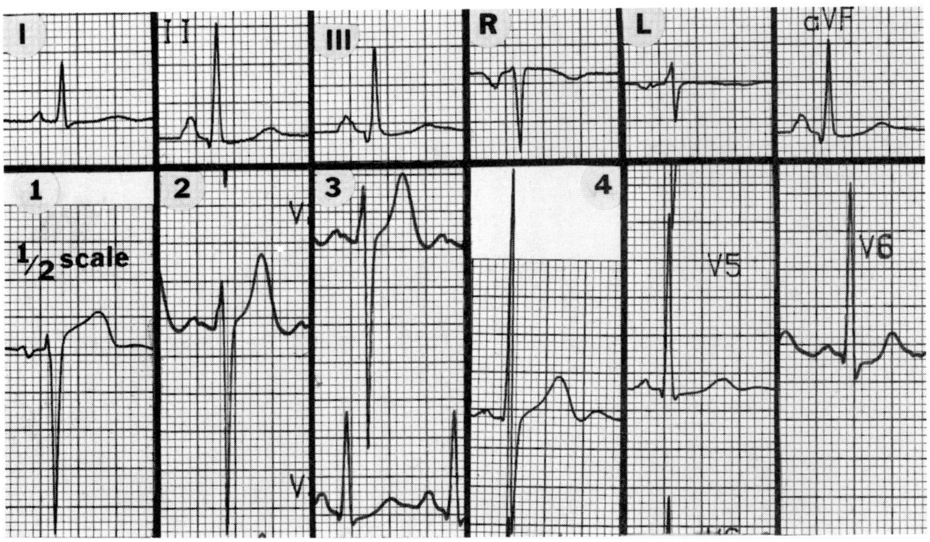
I
II
III
R
L
aVF
1
½ scale
2
3
4
V5
V6

6-25.

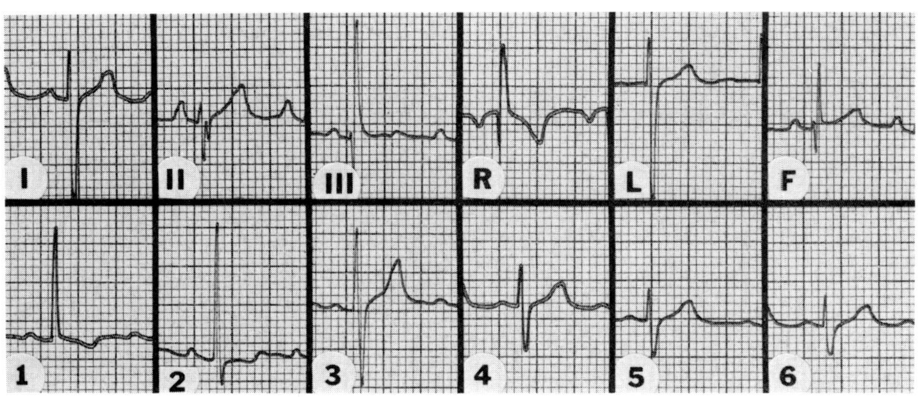
I
II
III
R
L
F
1
2
3
4
5
6

6-26.

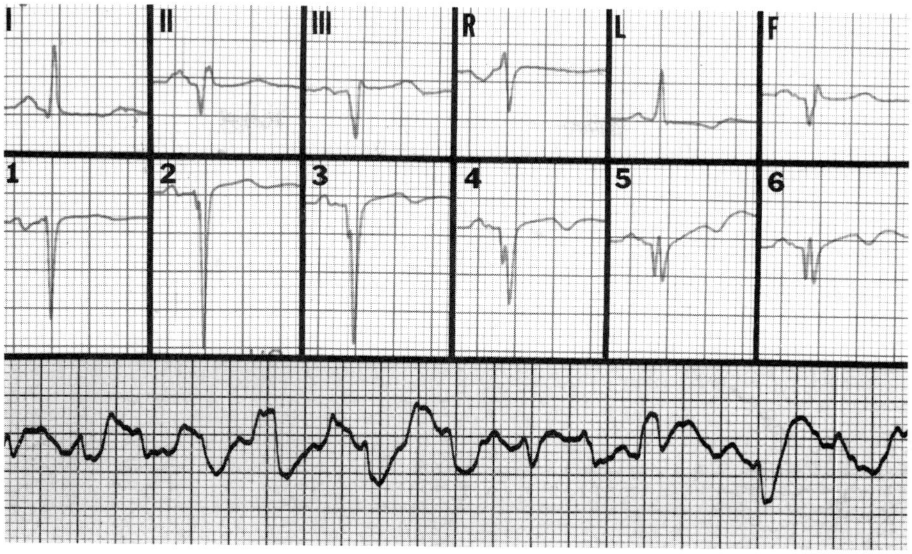
I
II
III
R
L
F
1
2
3
4
5
6

6-27.

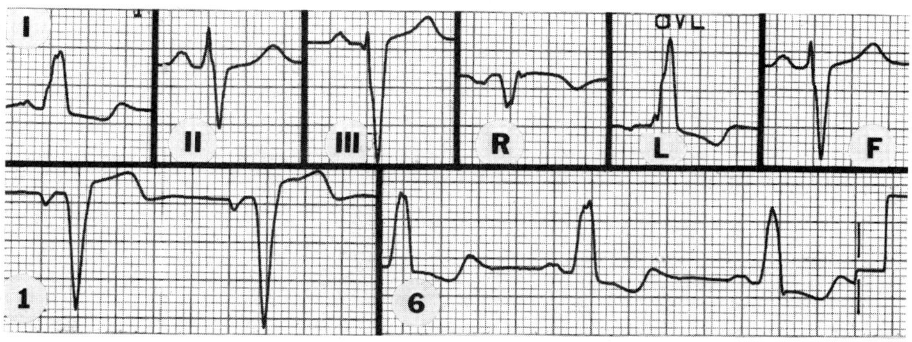
I
II
III
R
aVL
L
F
1
6

6-28.

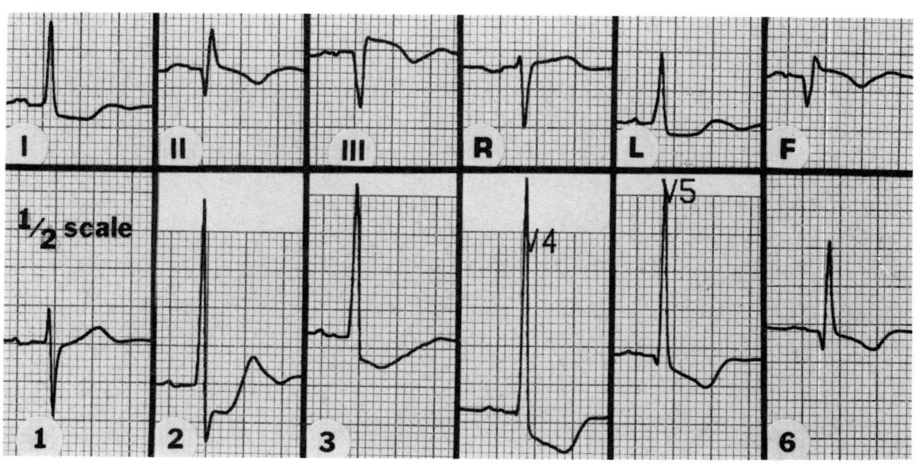
I
II
III
R
L
F
½ scale
V4
V5
1
2
3
6

6-29.

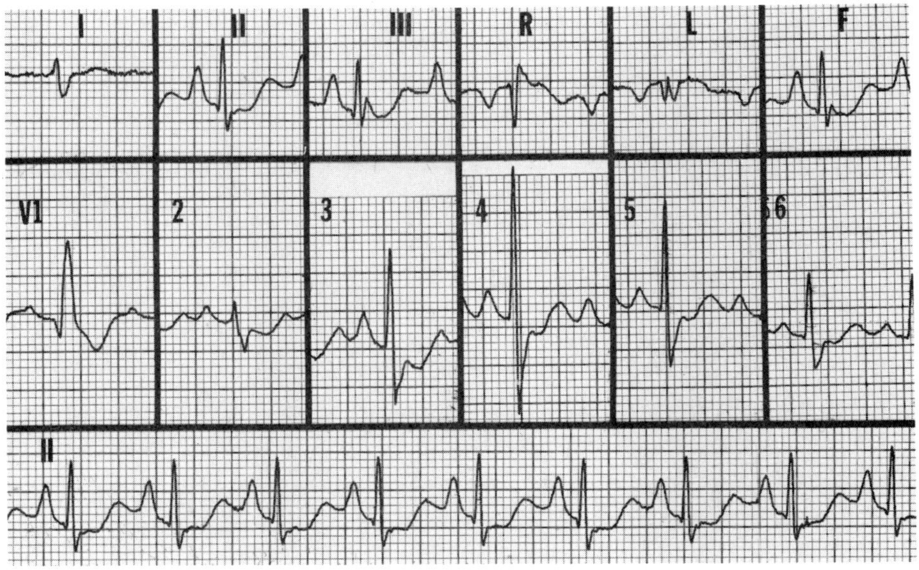
I
II
III
R
L
F
V1
2
3
4
5
6
II

6-30.

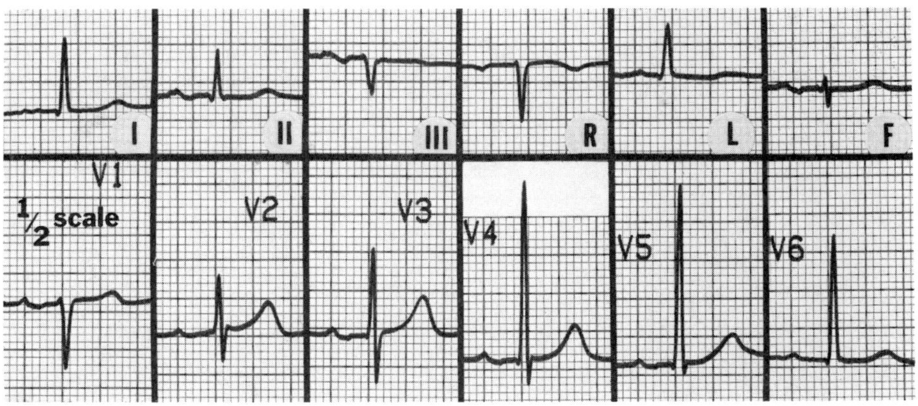
I
II
III
R
L
F
V1
1/2 scale
V2
V3
V4
V5
V6

6-31.

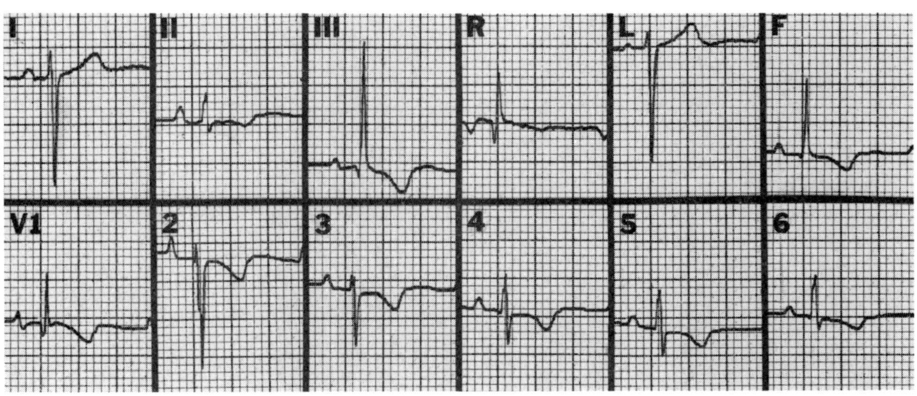
I
II
III
R
L
F
V1
2
3
4
5
6

6-32.
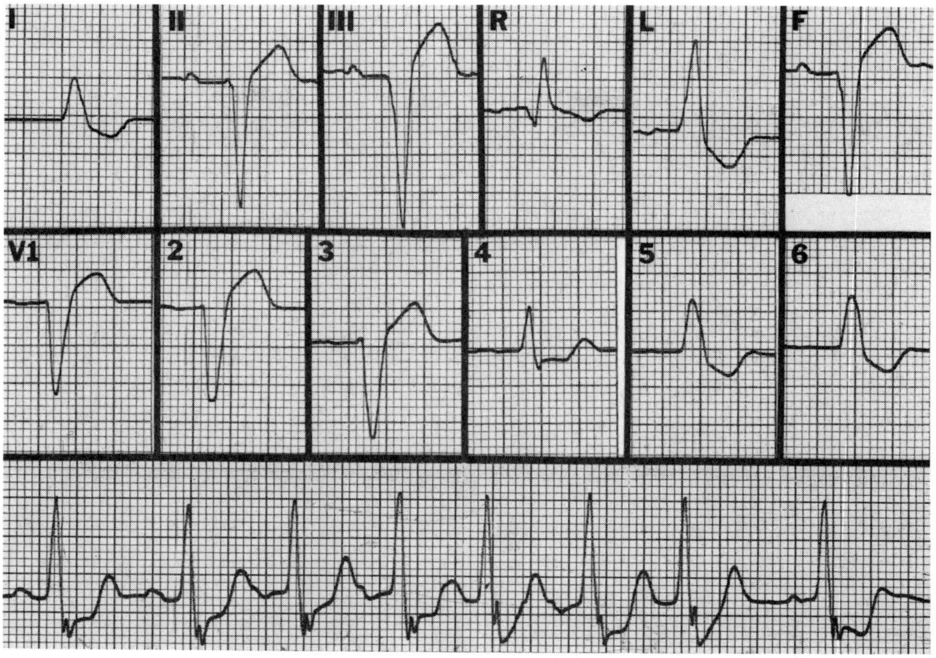

6-33.
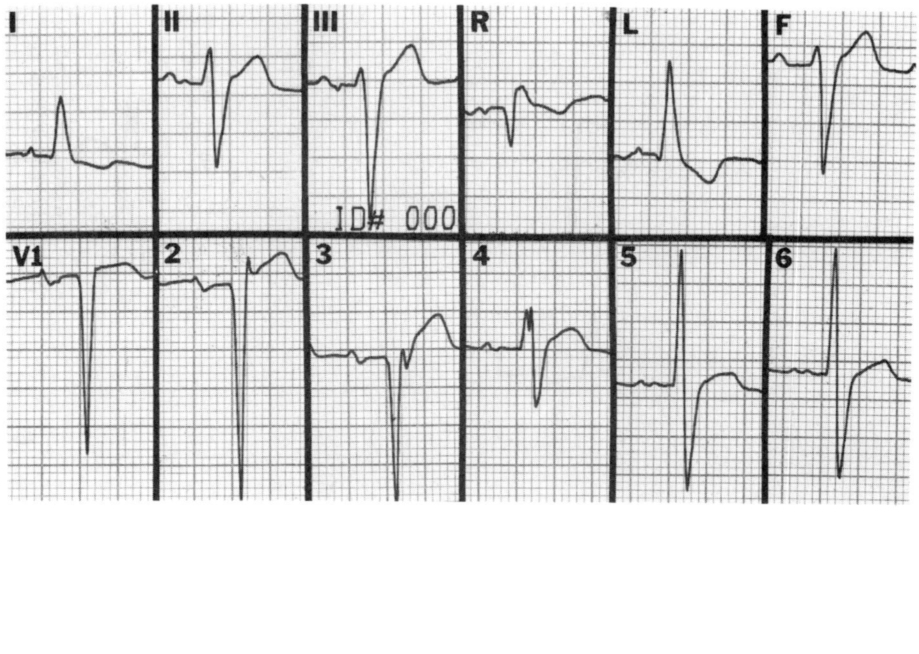

6-34.

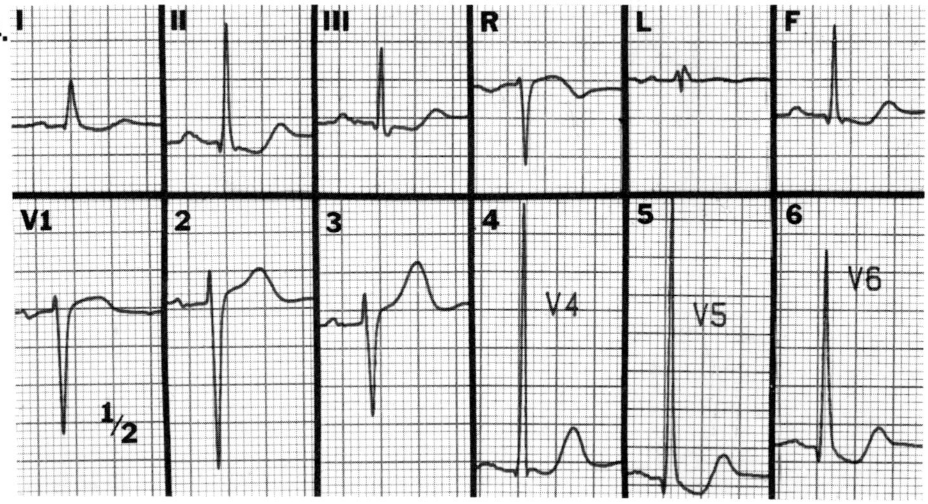

6-35.

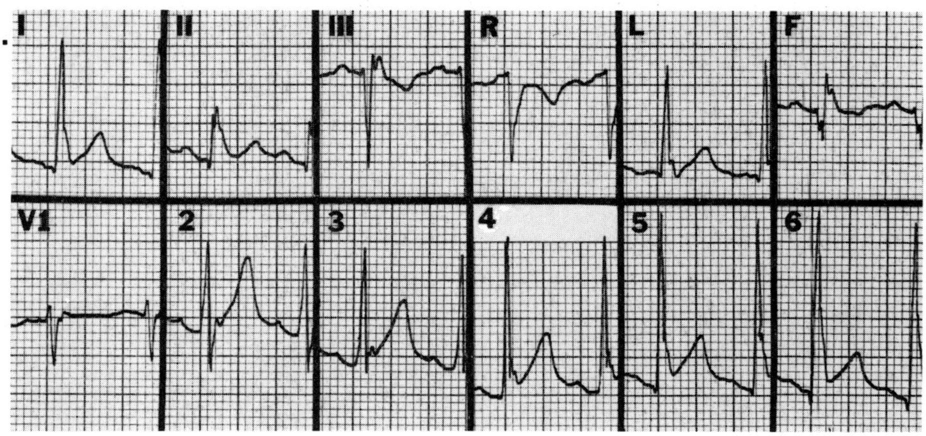

6-36.

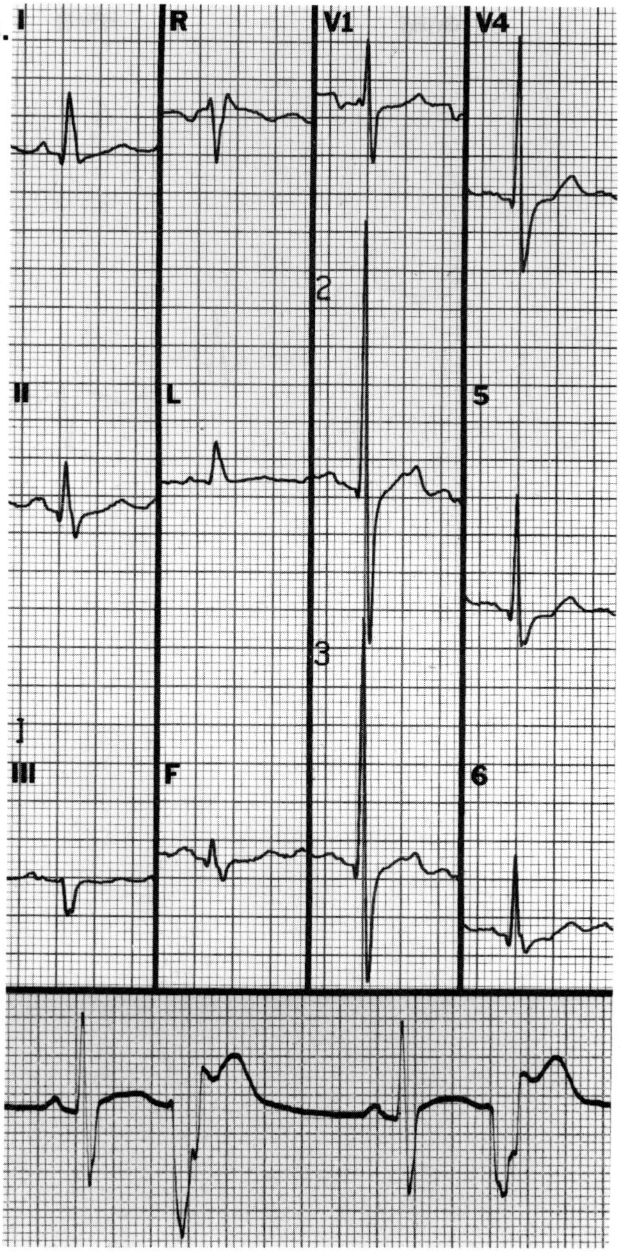

6-37.

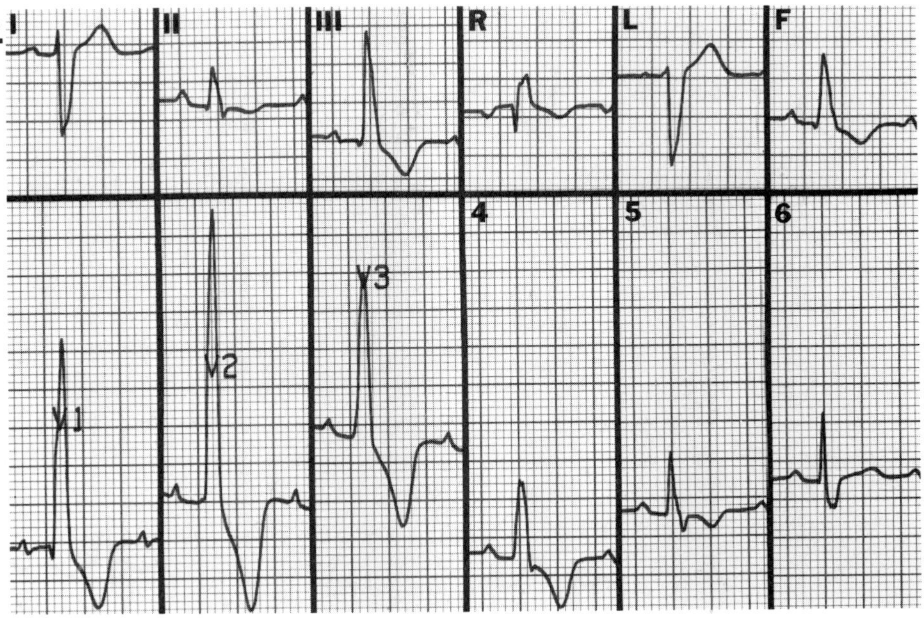

6-38.

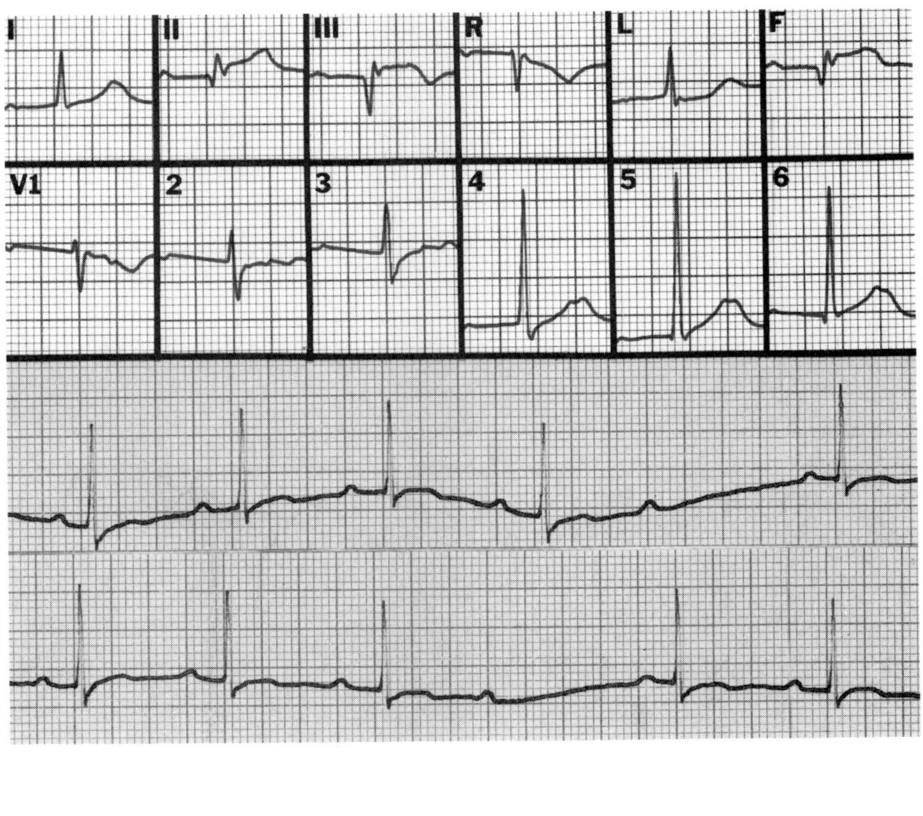

6-39.

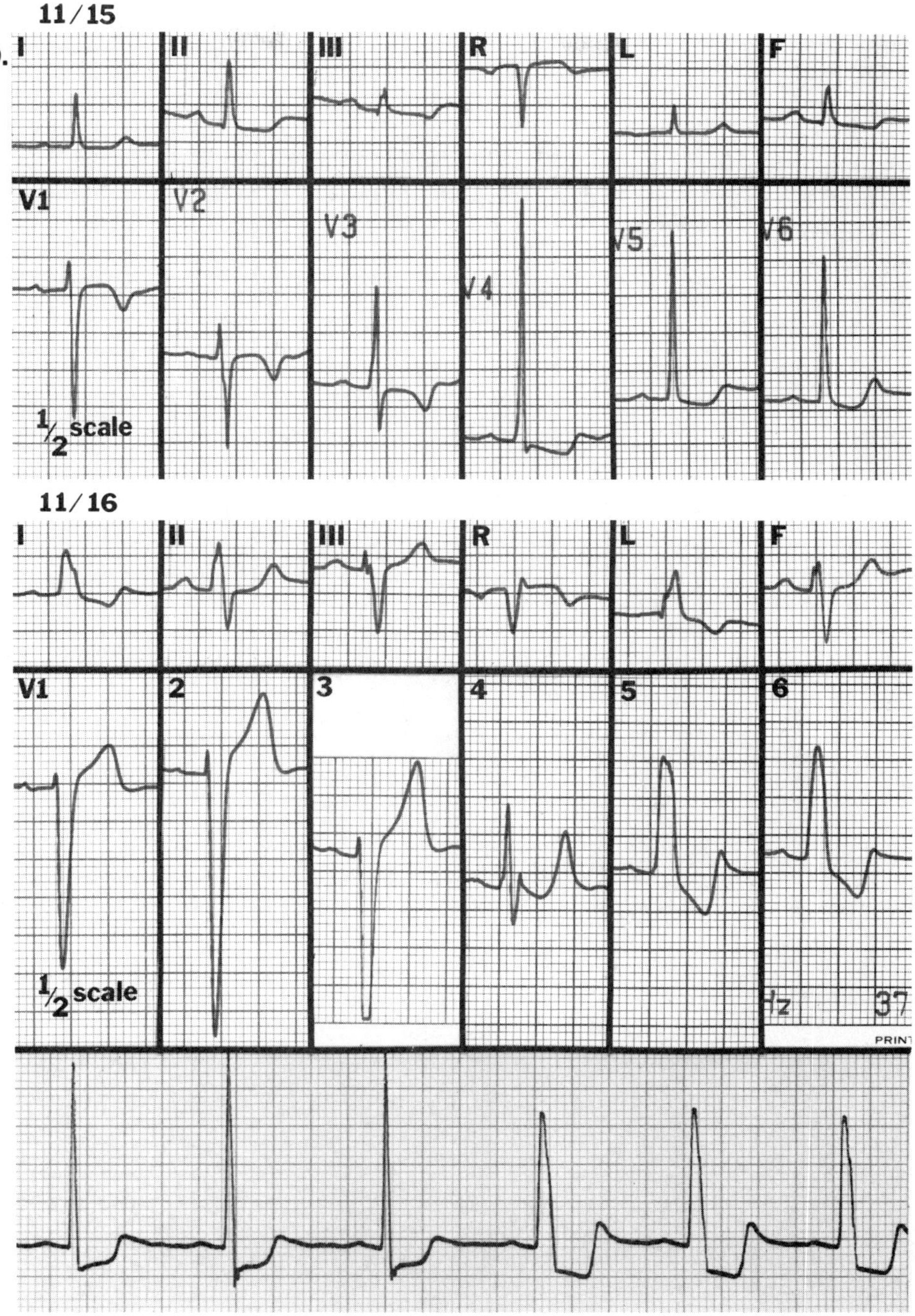
11/15
I
II
III
R
L
F
V1
V2
V3
V4
V5
V6
1/2 scale
11/16
I
II
III
R
L
F
V1
2
3
4
5
6
1/2 scale

6-40.

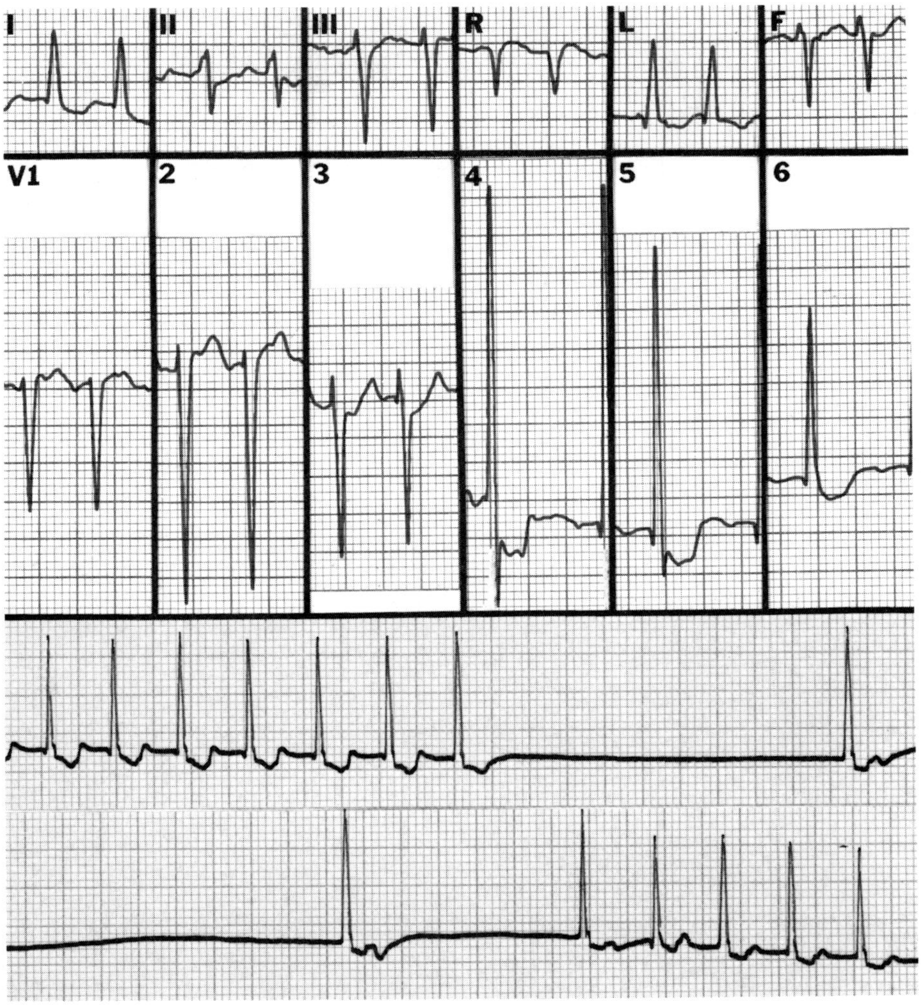

ANSWER KEY

Multiple Choice

1. a
2. d
3. c
4. c
5. c
6. a
7. d
8. d
9. d
10. b

Practice Strips

6–1. Left axis deviation, −10 to − 20 degrees.
Possible old LWMI (aVL).
LVH.
Atrial flutter.

6–2. Left axis deviation, −10 to −20 degrees.
Late transition, V4–V5.
LVH.

6–3. Normal axis, +5 to −5 degrees.
Early transition, V2.
IWMI, acute (II, III, aVF).
Possible PWMI (V2, V3).

6–4. Normal axis, +50 to +60 degrees.
Early transition, V2.
LVH.

6–5. (ECG of 8/19)
Normal axis, +45 to +55 degrees.
A-SWMI, hyperacute phase (V1–V5).
(ECG of 8/21)
Normal axis, +55 to +65 degrees.
Poor R wave progression.
Non-Q acute AWMI (V1–V5).

Right atrial abnormality (II).
LVH.

6–6. Normal axis, +5 to −5 degrees.
Early transition, V2.
IWMI, acute (II, III, aVF).
LVH.
Second-degree AV block, type I, 3:2 to 4:3 conduction ratios.

6–7. Right axis deviation, +115 to +125 degrees.
Early transition, V1.
RVH.

6–8. Normal axis, +65 to +75 degrees.
Non-Q AWMI (V1–V6) versus anterior wall ischemia.

6–9. (ECG of 6/6)
Normal axis, +50 to +60 degrees.
Probable anterior wall ischemia (pointed, symmetrical T wave).
(ECG of 6/7)
AWMI, hyperacute phase versus ischemia (V2–V6).

6–10. Normal axis, +50 to +60 degrees.
LVH.

6–11. Left axis deviation, −45 to −55 degrees.
Poor R wave progression.
Late transition, V6.
LAFB.
A-SWMI, acute (V1–V5).

6–12. Right axis deviation, +125 to +135 degrees.
Early transition, V1.
Right atrial abnormality.
RVH.
Sinus tachycardia, 107/minute with frequent premature ventricular complexes.

6–13. Left axis deviation, −10 to −20 degrees.
Left atrial abnormality.
LVH (frontal lead criteria).

6–14. Right axis deviation, +105 to +115 degrees.
RBBB.
Left atrial abnormality.

6–15. (ECG of 11/18)
Extreme right axis deviation, +205 to +215 degrees.
LPFB.
RBBB.
IWMI, old (II, III, aVF).
Left atrial abnormality.
(ECG of 11/19)
Left axis deviation, −15 to −25 degrees.
IWMI, recent (II, III, aVF).
PWMI, recent (V1–V3).
Left atrial abnormality.

6–16. Left axis deviation, −60 to −70 degrees.
Poor R wave progression.
Late transition (?).
LAFB.
AWMI (V2–V6).
IWMI (II, III, aVF).
Left atrial abnormality.
Sinus rhythm, 75/minute, premature atrial complexes, conducted aberrantly and nonconducted.

6–17. Normal axis, +25 to +35 degrees.
LVH.

6–18. Extreme right axis deviation, +210 to +220 degrees.
Low voltage (14.5 mm).
Early transition, V1.
PWMI, recent (V1–V3).
Probable LWMI (I, aVL, V6).

6–19. (ECG of 6/2)
Normal axis, +60 to +70 degrees.
Anterior ischemia (V1–V4).
(ECG of 6/4)
Early transition, V1.
PWMI (V1–V3).

6–20. Left axis deviation, −40 to −50 degrees.
LAFB.
Left atrial abnormality.
LVH.
Sinus rhythm, 72/minute.

6–21. Right axis deviation, +160 to +170 degrees.
LPFB.

RBBB.
Probable IWMI (III, aVF).
Left atrial abnormality.

6–22. Normal axis, +50 to +60 degrees.
Poor R wave progression.
AWMI, old (V3–V5).
Left atrial abnormality.
LVH.

6–23. Left axis deviation, −25 to −35 degrees.
Probable LAFB.
RBBB.
Possible IWMI, old (II, aVF).

6–24. Normal axis, +65 to +75 degrees.
Right atrial abnormality (II).
Left atrial abnormality (V1–V3).
LVH.

6–25. Right axis deviation, +150 to +160 degrees.
Early transition, V1.
Right atrial abnormality (II).
RVH.

6–26. Normal axis, 0 to +10 degrees.
Poor R wave progression.
IWMI, old (II, III, aVF).
AWMI, old (V2–V6).
Left atrial abnormality.
Ventricular fibrillation.

6–27. Left axis deviation, −60 to −70 degrees.
LAFB.
LBBB.

6–28. Left axis deviation, −10 to −20 degrees.
Early transition, V2.
IWMI, recent (II, III, aVF).
Anterior ischemia (V2–V4).
Left atrial abnormality.
LVH.

6–29. Right axis deviation, +95 to +115 degrees
RBBB.
Right atrial abnormality.

Probable RVH.
Sinus tachycardia, 112/minute.

6–30. Normal axis, +5 to +15 degrees.
Early transition, V2
Left atrial abnormality.
LVH.
First-degree AV block (PR 0.23).

6–31. Right axis deviation, +130 to +140 degrees.
Right atrial abnormality.
RVH.

6–32. Left axis deviation, −55 to −65 degrees.
Poor R wave progression.
LAFB.
LBBB.
Left atrial abnormality (III).
First-degree AV block (PR 0.22).
Sinus rhythm, 86/minute, paroxysmal atrial tachycardia.

6–33. Left axis deviation, −55 to −65 degrees.
Poor R wave progression.
LAFB.
NSIVCD.
Probable AWMI, recent (V2, V3).
Left atrial abnormality.
LVH.

6–34. Normal axis, +55 to +65 degrees.
Left atrial abnormality.
LVH.

6–35. Normal axis, +5 to −5 degrees.
Early transition, V2.
Possible IWMI, recent (III, aVF).
NSIVCD.
LVH (frontal plane criteria).

6–36. Normal axis, +5 to +15 degrees.
Early transition, V1.
NSIVCD.
Left atrial abnormality.
LVH.
Ventricular bigeminy.

6–37. Right axis deviation, +130 to +140 degrees.
Early transition, V1.
RBBB.
RVH.

6–38. Left axis deviation, 0 to −10 degrees.
IWMI, acute (II, III, aVF).
First-degree AV block (PR 0.26).
Sinus rhythm, 81/minute, second-degree AV block, type I, 5:4 conduction ratio.

6–39. (ECG of 11/15)
Normal axis, +35 to +45 degrees.
Probable anterior ischemia (V1–V3).
LVH.
(ECG of 11/16)
Left axis deviation, −15 to −25 degrees.
LBBB.
Sinus rhythm, 75/minute, normal intraventricular conduction alternating with LBBB.

6–40. Left axis deviation, −30 to −40 degrees.
Probable LAFB.
LVH.
Atrial fibrillation in 12-lead.
Supraventricular tachycardia, 167/minute with pauses of more than 2.0 seconds (tachy-brady syndrome).

CHAPTER SEVEN

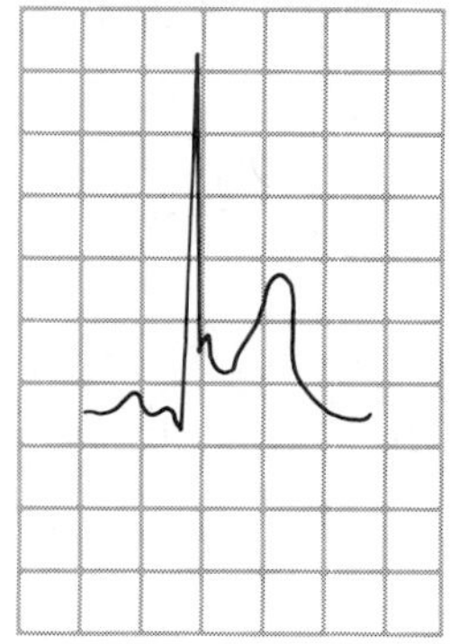

ACUTE PERICARDITIS

COGNITIVE GOALS

1. Identify the single pathognomonic finding of acute pericarditis.
2. List the ECG criteria for acute pericarditis.
3. Identify three important differences that distinguish the ECG of acute pericarditis from the ECG of acute myocardial infarction.
4. Define the term **PR segment** and discuss how PR segment depression can be detected.
5. Give the ECG criteria for early repolarization.
6. Identify the ECG features of early repolarization that may result in misidentifying this syndrome with the hyperacute phase of myocardial infarction.
7. Identify the age, race, and sex of the patient population in which the early repolarization syndrome is most frequently seen.

Many popular electrocardiography texts fail to discuss the diagnostic criteria of acute pericarditis, and most of those that do place it in the miscellany. Relegating the condition to the "boondocks" of the nursing and medical literature tends to create the impression that it is rare or of little clinical importance. This section, included specifically to disabuse both novice and veteran alike, addresses pericarditis as an important differential diagnosis that must be made in cases of both de novo and recurrent chest pain. The ECG is an important tool in making that diagnosis.

Acute pericarditis, a common though usually transitory affliction, is a frequent complication of open heart surgery and myocardial infarction. It poses an important clinical problem for two reasons: it is often the cause of intense physical discomfort, and it predisposes the patient to atrial tachyarrhythmias. The pain of pericarditis can closely mimic angina and, like angina, can radiate, particularly to the intrascapular area and the base of the neck. Unlike angina, pericardial pain is often aggravated by deep inspiration and rotation of the trunk and relieved to some extent by sitting up or leaning forward. The pain is often sharp, with a stabbing quality that generates intense anxiety (Fowler, 1980).

The single pathognomonic finding of pericarditis is the classic three-component friction rub. The three rapidly consecutive sounds are produced by atrial systole, ventricular systole, and movement associated with ventricular diastolic filling. Best heard at the lower left sternal border, the friction rub has a superficial quality sometimes likened to the squeaking of wet shoe leather or the crunching of footsteps in snow. Rubs may be transient, soft, of less than three components, or obscured by adventitious breath sounds or murmurs. In many cases, no rub can be auscultated. Fortunately, diagnostic ECG changes often appear before pain, rubs, troublesome atrial arrhythmias, or even in the complete absence of symptoms.

Electrocardiographic criteria

The ECG findings in acute pericarditis include (1) **ST segment elevation,** (2) **PR segment depression,** (3) late **T wave inversion,** and (4) **atrial arrhythmias.** The occurrence of supraventricular tachycardias in patients following open heart surgery should always elicit a search for signs and symptoms of pericarditis. These arrhythmias often respond more rapidly to treatment with low doses of steroids than to standard antiarrhythmic drugs.

The ECG in Figure 7–1 was obtained from a patient post–coronary artery bypass. The patient's chief complaints were aching precordial pain and malaise. The tracing shows widespread ST segment elevation, particularly in leads I, II, aVF, and in the lateral precordial leads, V5 and V6. The ST elevation differs from that of ischemic myocardial injury in that it is **not isolated to discrete segments,** and it exhibits a typical **upward concavity** (**1** in Fig. 7–1) as opposed to the upward convexity or coving usually seen during ischemia. In several leads, particularly II and V6, **notching** is discernible at the junction of the QRS and ST segment **(2)**. It is also noted that reciprocal ST depression, such as would be expected in a case of ischemia, is completely lacking. Equally important is the observation that there is **no T wave inversion during the acute phase.** Usually the T waves remain upright until ST segment elevation subsides

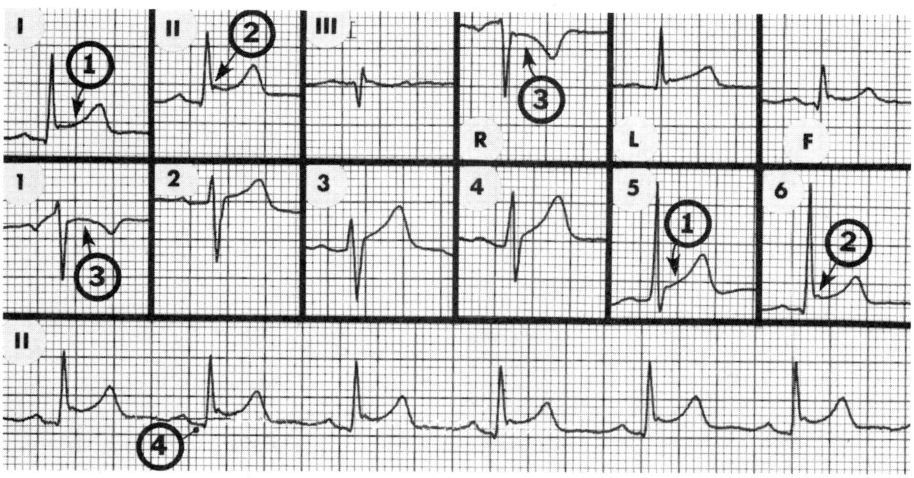

Figure 7–1. The electrocardiogram of acute pericarditis. Note PR segment depression in lead II.

and the ST segment has returned to baseline. Only as pericarditis enters its postacute phase does T wave inversion become an obvious feature. **In uncomplicated pericarditis, pathologic Q waves never occur** (Chung, 1980; Hurst et al, 1982). Negative T waves are noted only in those leads in which negative T waves are an expected finding, aVR and V1 **(3).**

Depression of the PR segment, the interval between the end of the P wave and the beginning of the QRS complex, is a common, but subtle, sign that is most often seen in lead II and the precordial V leads. The isoelectric line, or T-P interval, can be used as a point of reference. When compared with the isoelectric line in this way, PR segment depression **(4)** tends to become more noticeable. In some cases, PR segment depression may be the only ECG finding (Bruce and Spodick, 1980).

Inversion of the T wave generally takes place after the ST segment elevation has returned to baseline, a finding in marked contrast to T wave behavior in cases of ischemia and infarction in which T wave inversion occurs early, while the ST segment is still elevated (Spodick, 1974; Conner, 1983).

Early repolarization

Early repolarization is a normal variant of very striking appearance that closely resembles both acute pericarditis and the hyperacute phase of myocardial infarction. The pattern is most often observed in young, thin-chested adults, particularly black men. There is almost never any clinical or laboratory evidence of heart disease.

The features of early repolarization, illustrated in Figure 7–2, include (1) **ST segment elevation,** particularly in the lateral precordial leads; (2) **concave upward ST segments,** which are virtually identical to those seen in cases of pericarditis **(1)**; and (3) **notching of the J point (2)**, which is also reminiscent of pericarditis. The characteristic (4) **tall T waves** of the syndrome closely mimic the vaulting T waves of hyperacute infarction (Goldberger, 1979). In marked

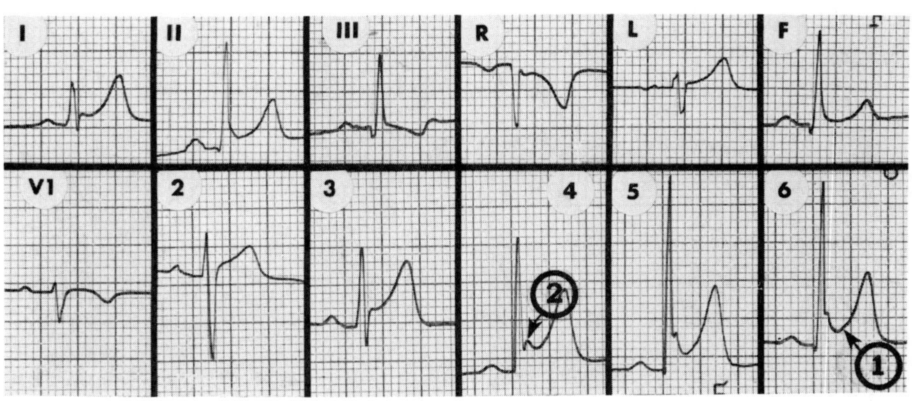

Figure 7–2. The electrocardiogram of the early repolarization syndrome.

contrast to the evolution of the pericarditis and infarction patterns, the ECG findings of early repolarization are stable over long periods of time.

The differential diagnosis of early repolarization can almost always be made by integrating the ECG findings with the history and physical examination. Although the syndrome has been documented in all age and ethnic groups, it shows a definite predilection for black males 20 to 40 years of age. In otherwise asymptomatic subjects, it should be considered an innocent, incidental finding.

References

Bruce, MA, and Spodick, DH. **J Electrocardiol** 13:61–66, 1980.

Chung, EK. **Electrocardiography: Practical Applications with Vectorial Principles,** 2nd ed. Harper & Row, New York, 1980, p 617.

Conner, RP. **Crit Care Nurse** 3:40–42, 1983.

Fowler, NO. **Cardiac Diagnosis and Treatment,** 3rd ed. Harper & Row, New York, 1980, pp 978–986.

Goldberger, AL. **Myocardial Infarction, Electrocardiographic Differential Diagnosis,** 2nd ed. CV Mosby, St. Louis, 1979, pp 141–148.

Hurst, JW, et al. **The Heart,** 5th ed. McGraw-Hill, New York, 1982, pp 1371–1393.

Spodick, DH. **Am J Cardiol** 33:470–474, 1974.

SELF-ASSESSMENT

Multiple Choice

1. The pain of pericarditis is:

   a. often modified by changes in the patient's position.
   b. relieved by nitroglycerin preparations.
   c. frequently referred to the jaws and ears.
   d. crushing in quality.

2. The only ECG abnormality in some cases of acute pericarditis is:

   a. abnormal Q waves.
   b. vaulting T waves.
   c. PR segment depression.
   d. T wave inversion.

3. The single pathognomonic finding in acute pericarditis is:

   a. ST segment elevation.
   b. J point depression.
   c. atrial arrhythmias.
   d. a three-component friction rub.

4. Notching of the J point is observed in:

   a. acute pericarditis.
   b. fascicular block.
   c. early repolarization.
   d. both **a** and **c.**

5. The ECG pattern of acute pericarditis can be distinguished from the pattern of acute infarction by:

   a. the lack of T wave inversion.
   b. the failure of ECG changes to localize to a particular segment.
   c. the lack of reciprocal changes.
   d. all of the above choices.

6. The ECG pattern of early repolarization is:

   a. generally stable over time.
   b. associated with a predilection for rapid atrial arrhythmias.
   c. often noted in young, black men.
   d. both **a** and **c.**

Practice Strips

Identify the net QRS axis and any abnormalities in the following ECGs:

7-1.

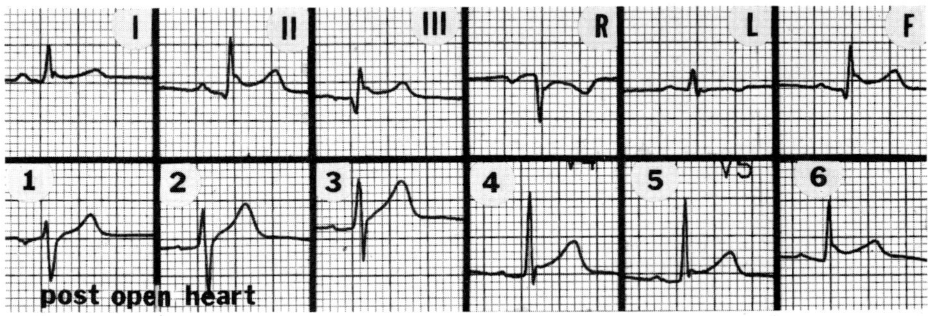

7-2.

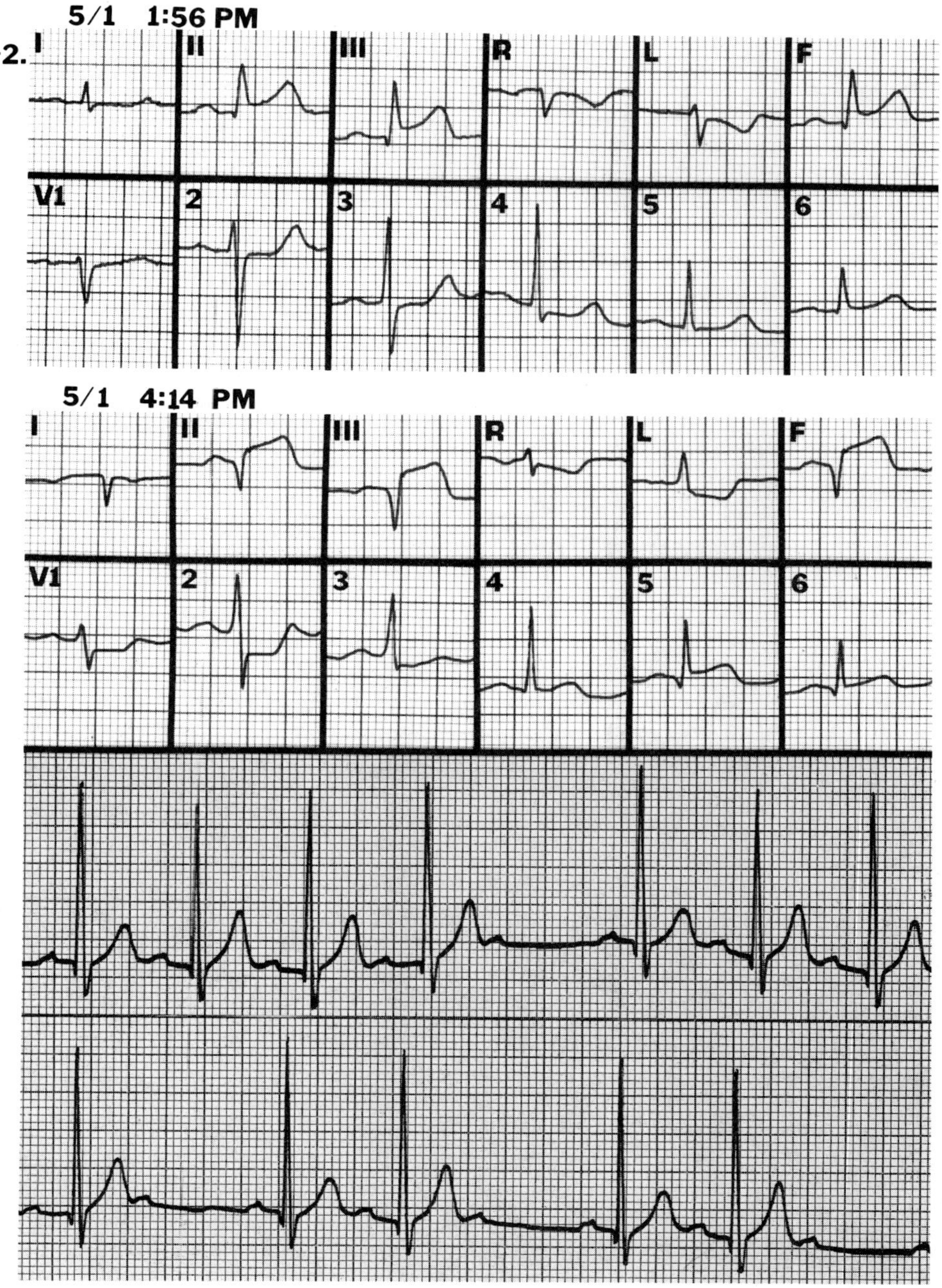

7-3.

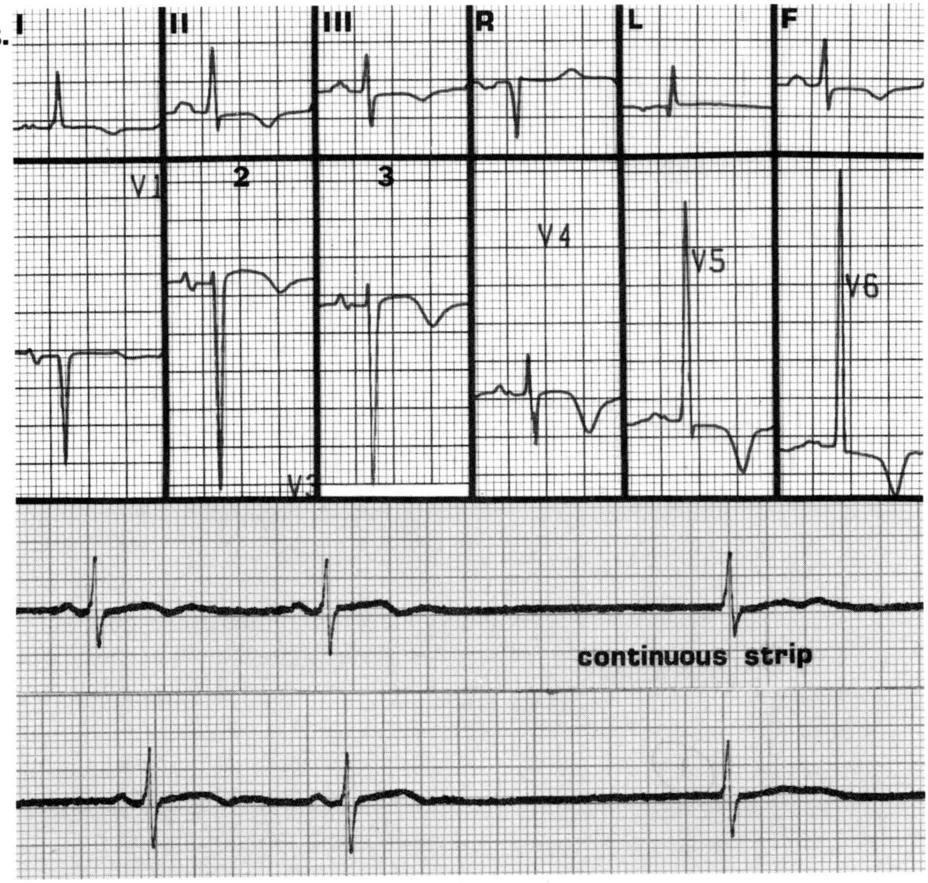
I
II
III
R
L
F
V1
2
3
V4
V5
V6
V3
continuous strip

7-4.

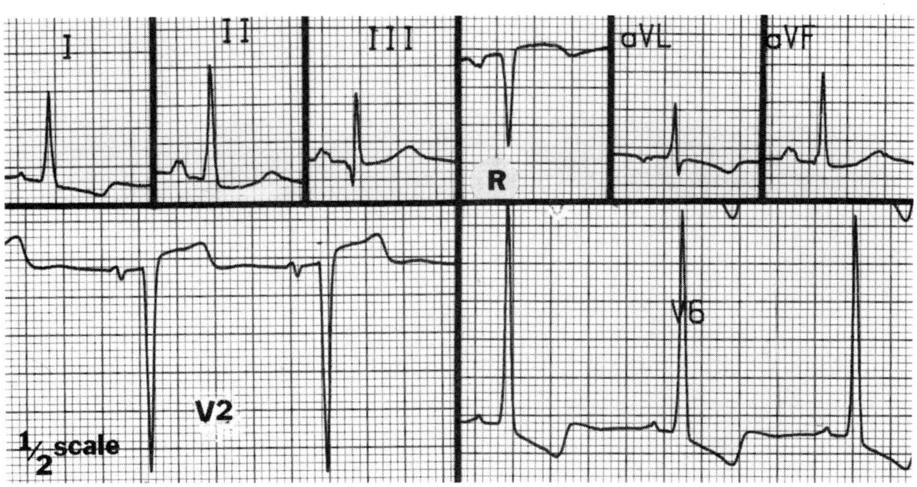
I
II
III
aVL
aVF
R
V6
V2
½ scale

7-5.

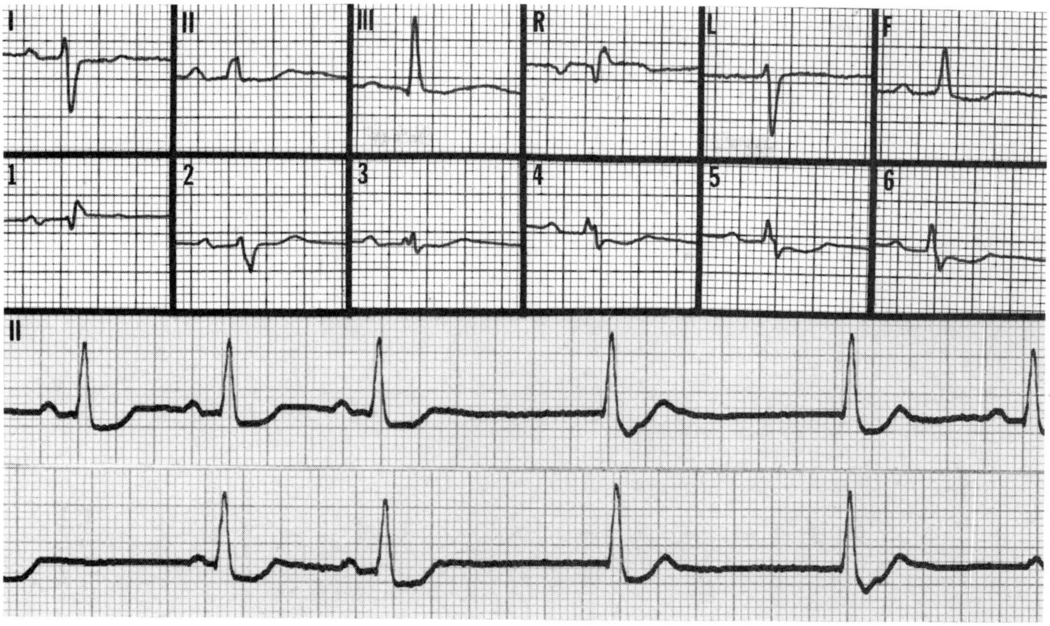

7-6.

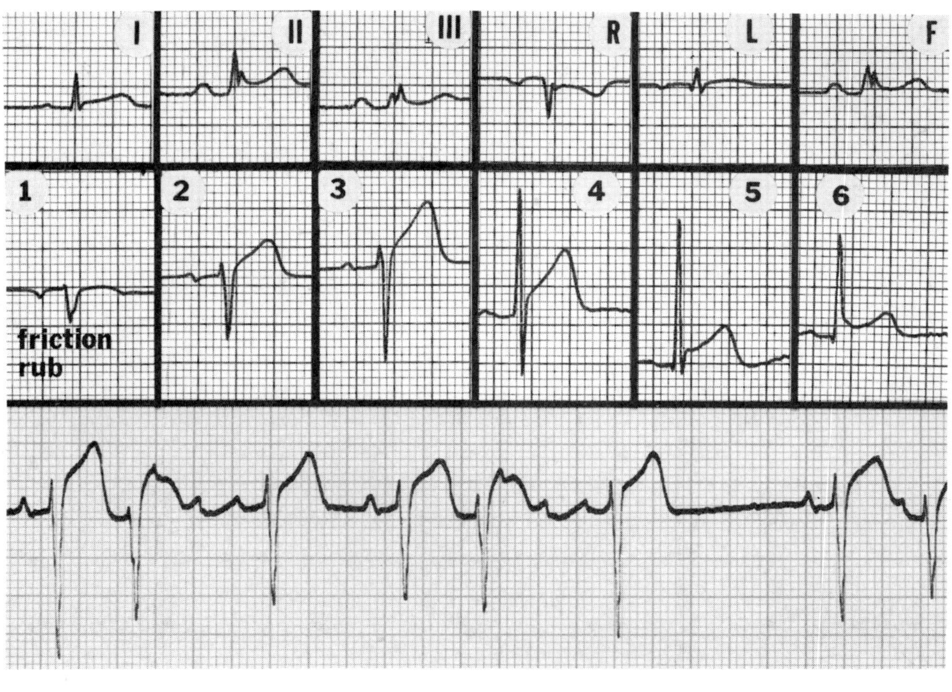

7-7.

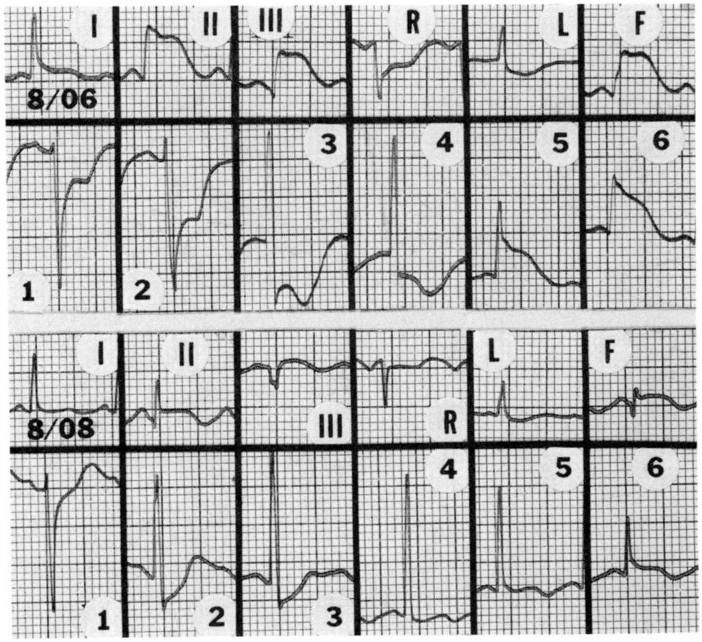
I
II
III
R
L
F
8/06
1
2
3
4
5
6
I
II
III
R
L
F
8/08
1
2
3
4
5
6

7-8.

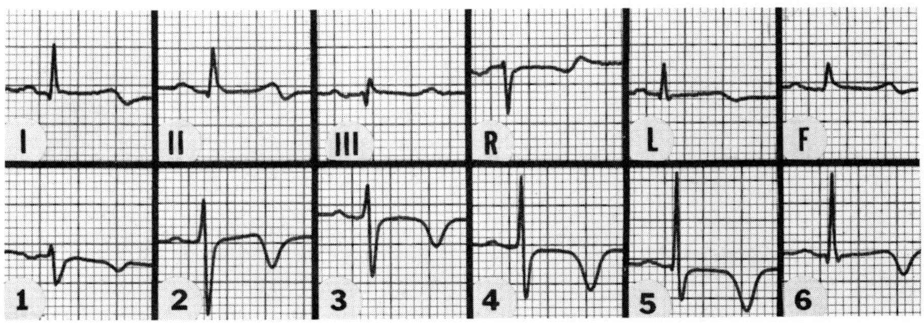
I
II
III
R
L
F
1
2
3
4
5
6

7-9.

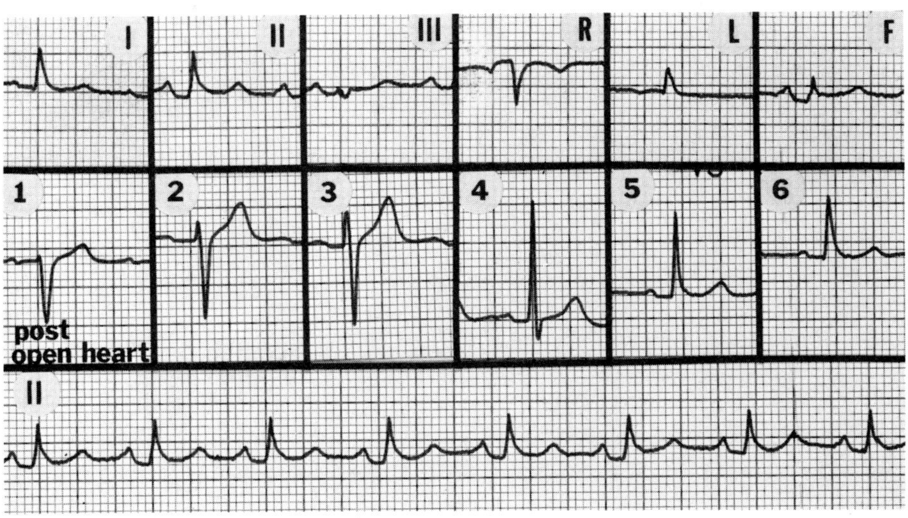
I
II
III
R
L
F
1
2
3
4
5
6
post
open heart
II

7-10.

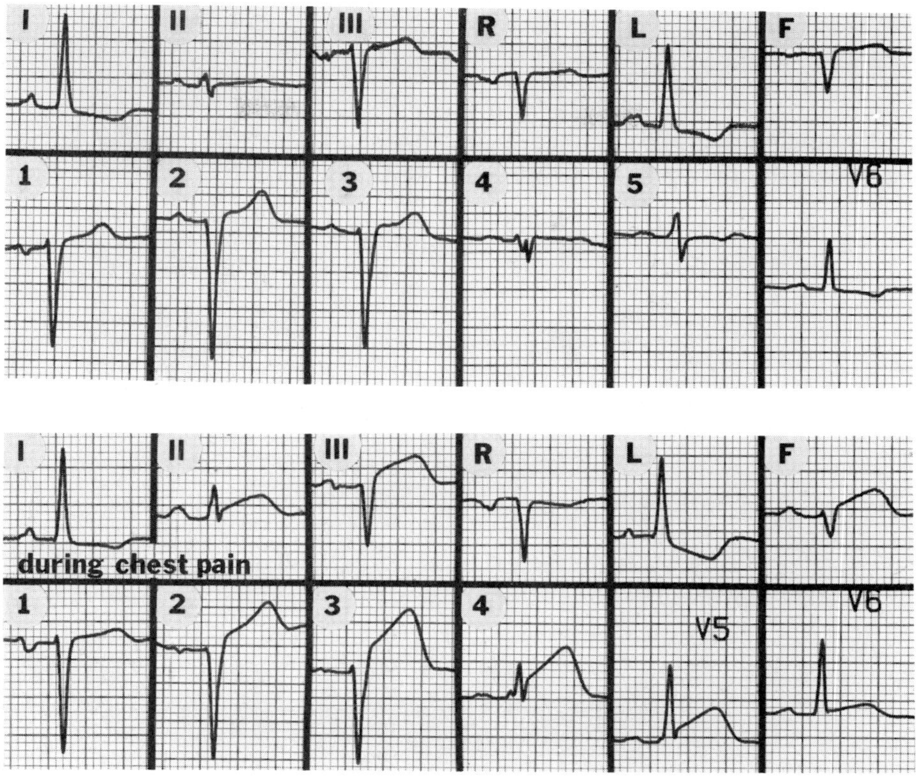
I
II
III
R
L
F
1
2
3
4
5
V6
during chest pain
V5

7-11.

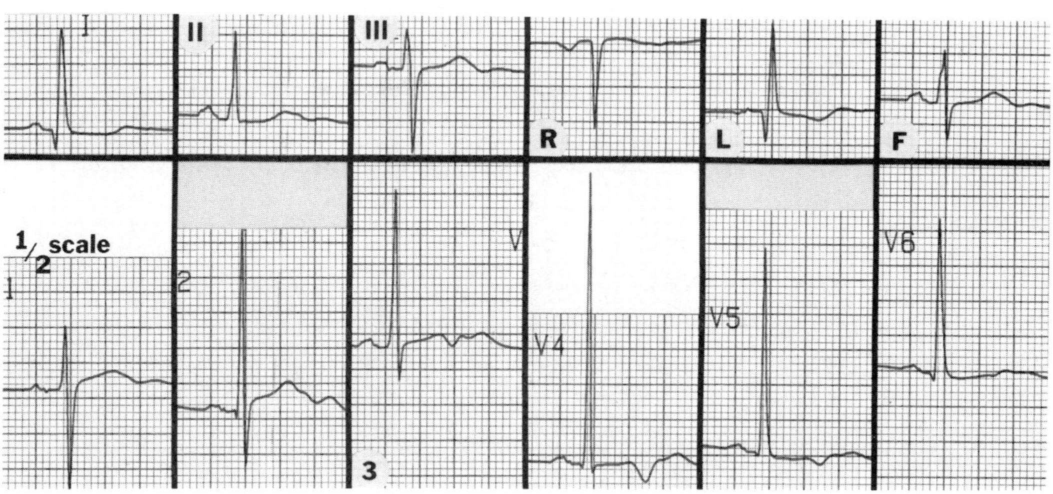
I
II
III
R
L
F
1/2 scale
1
2
3
V4
V5
V6

7-12.

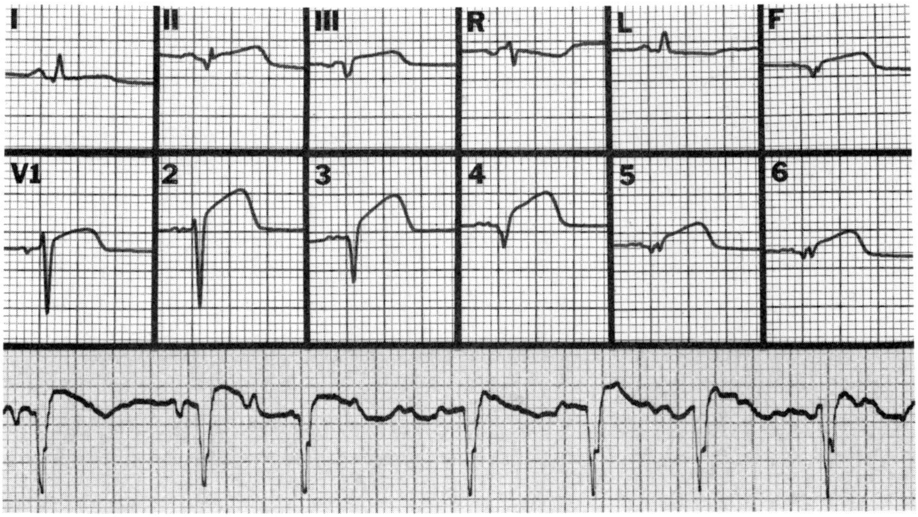
I
II
III
R
L
F
V1
2
3
4
5
6

7-13.

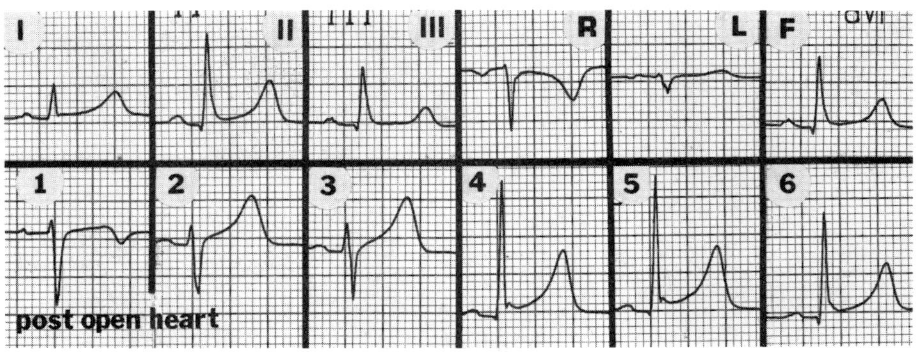
I
II
III
R
L
F
1
2
3
4
5
6
post open heart

7-14.

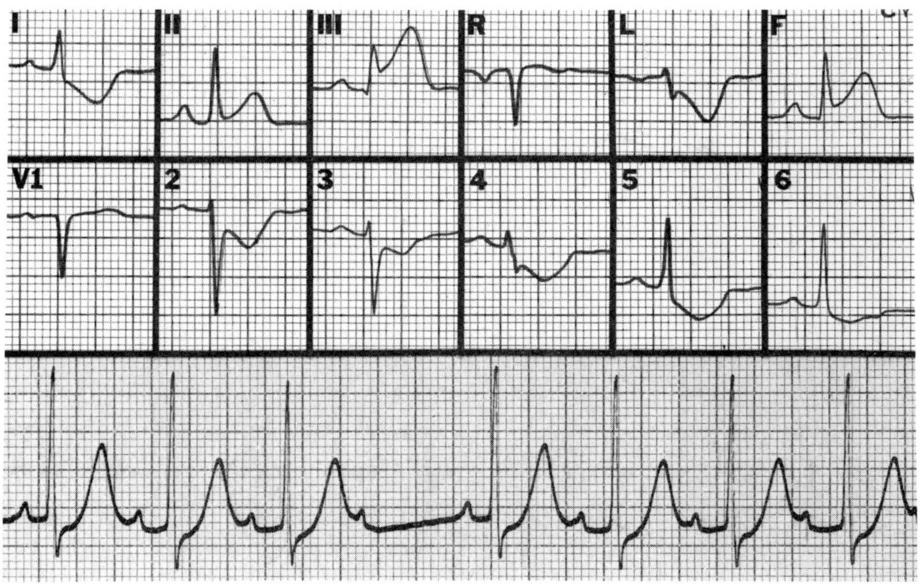
I
II
III
R
L
F
V1
2
3
4
5
6

7-15.

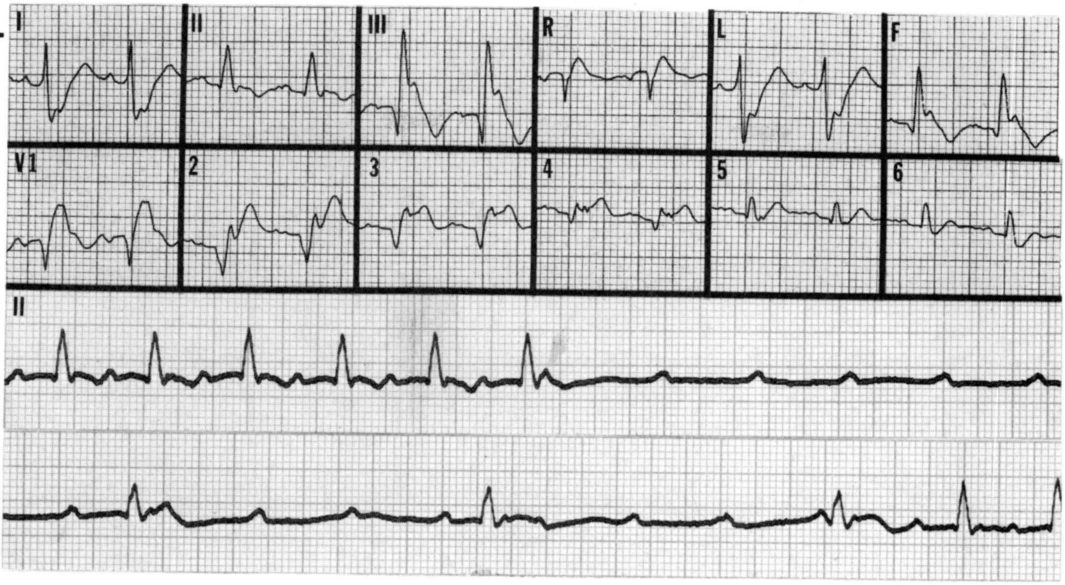

7-16.

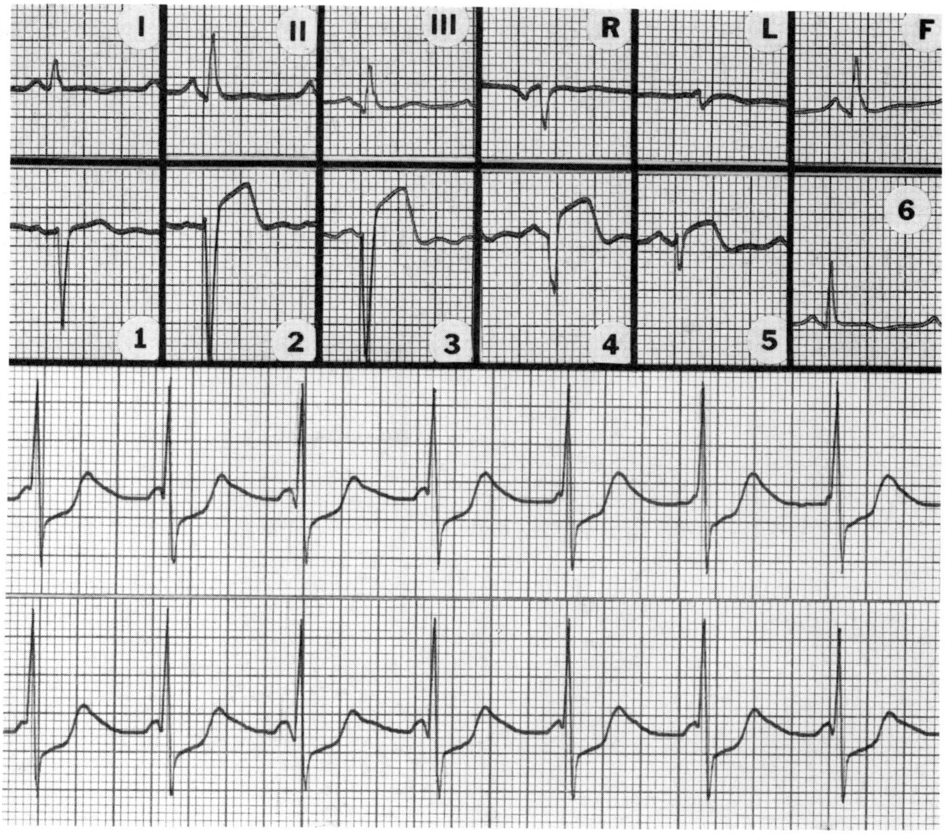

7-17.

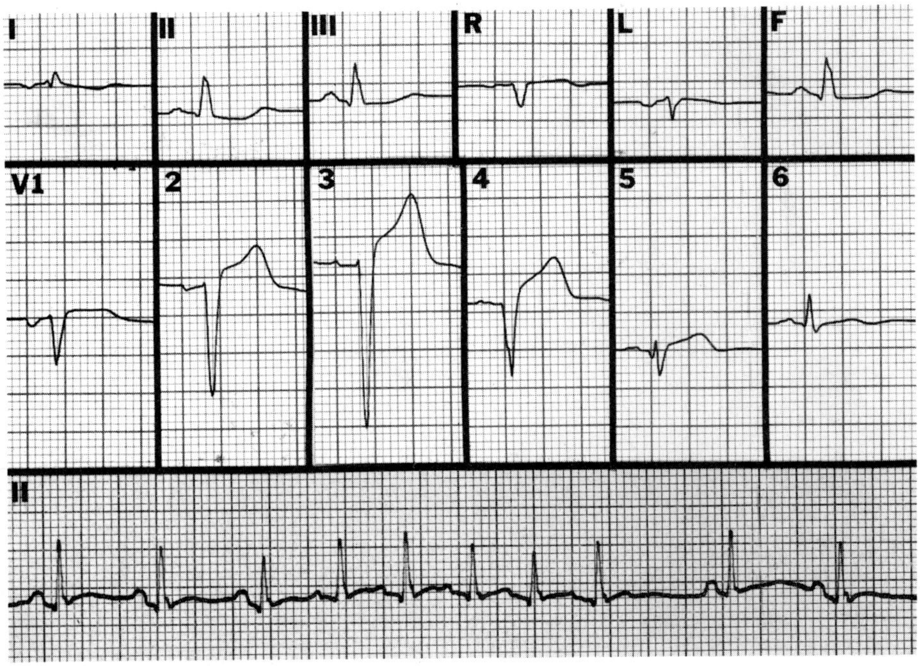

7-18.

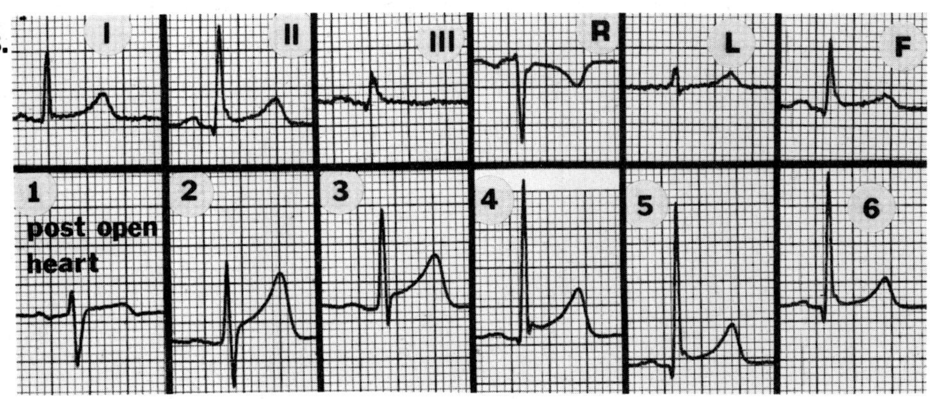

7-19.
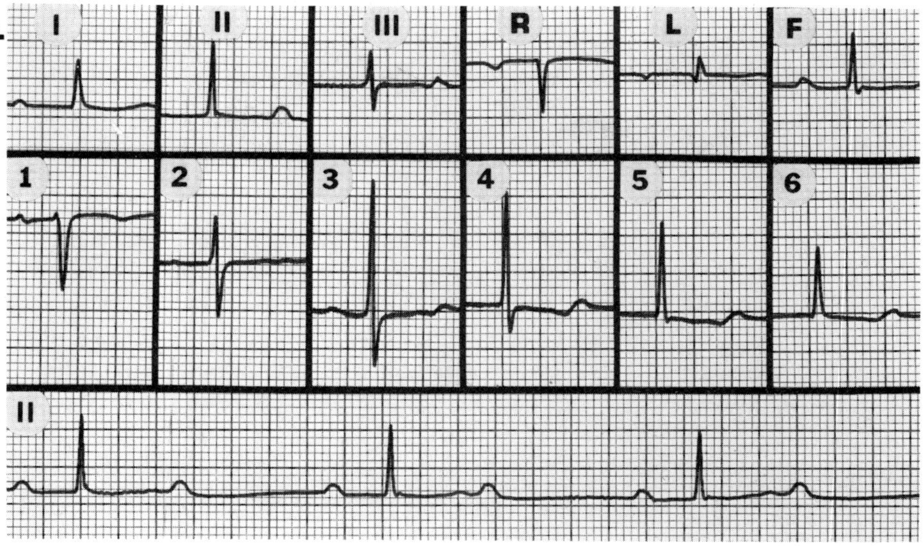

In this case precordial leads V1 to V3 are illustrated. In each of the precordial leads, the first complex is a **premature ventricular complex (PVC).** How are these ectopic beats diagnostically significant?

7-20.
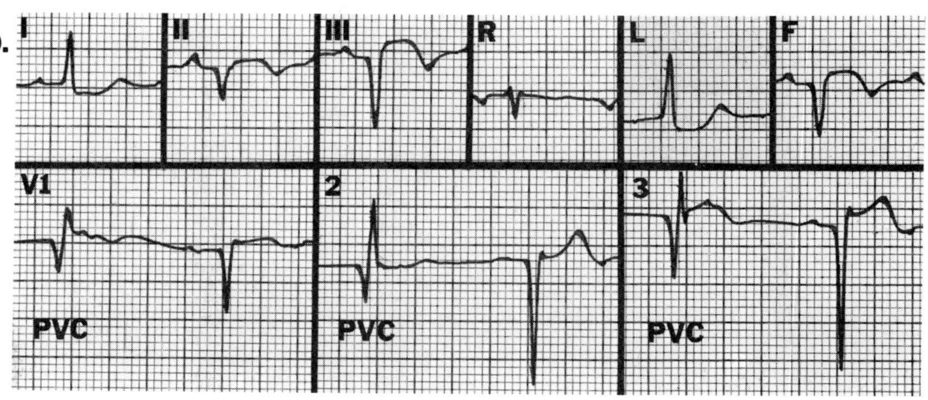

7-21.

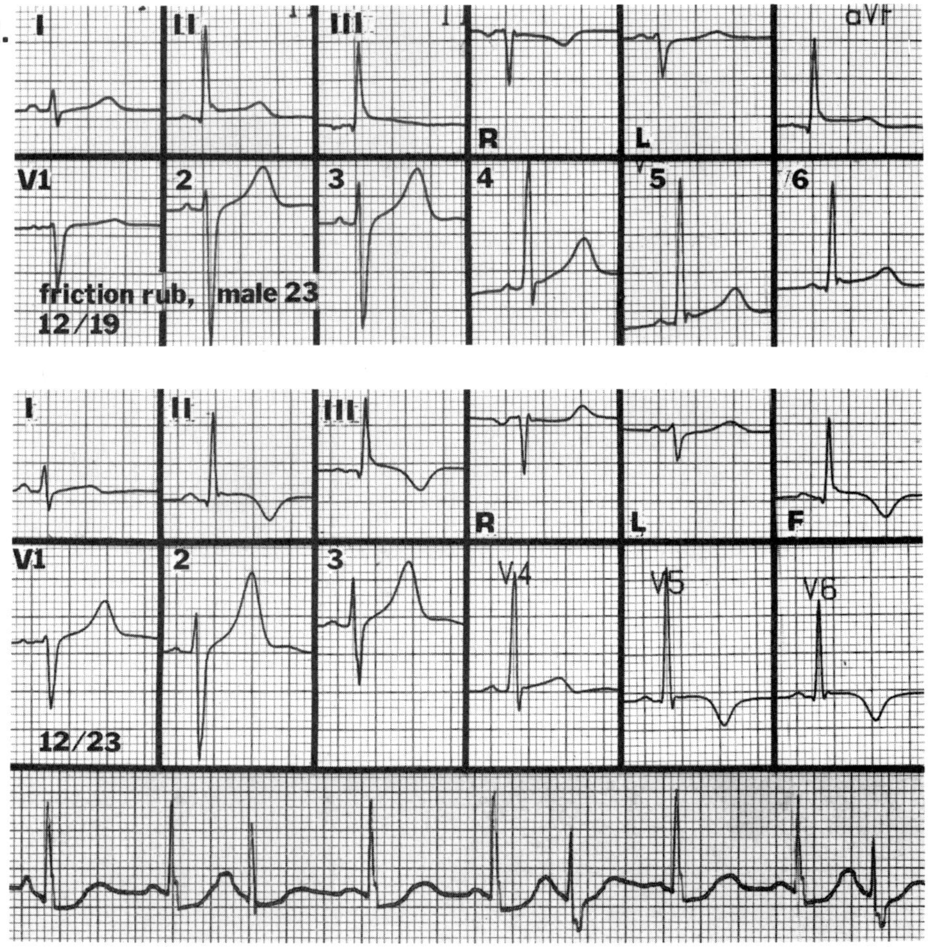
I
II
III
R
L
aVF
V1
2
3
4
5
6
friction rub, male 23
12/19
I
II
III
R
L
F
V1
2
3
V4
V5
V6
12/23

7-22.

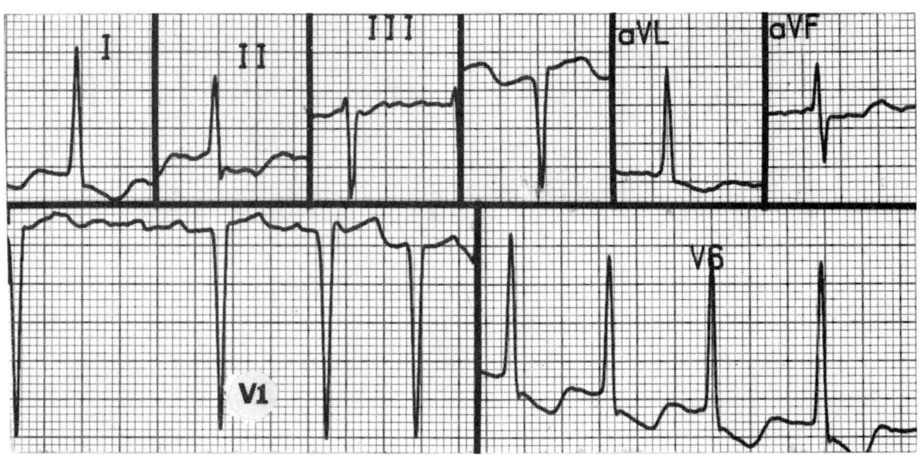
I
II
III
aVL
aVF
V1
V6

7-23.

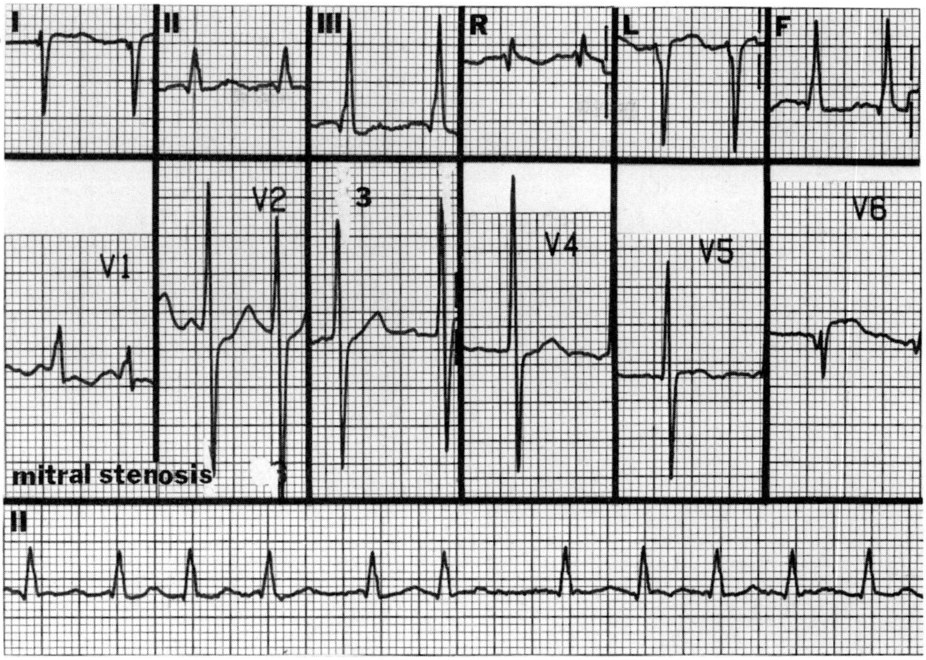
I
II
III
R
L
F
V1
V2
3
V4
V5
V6
mitral stenosis
II

7-24.

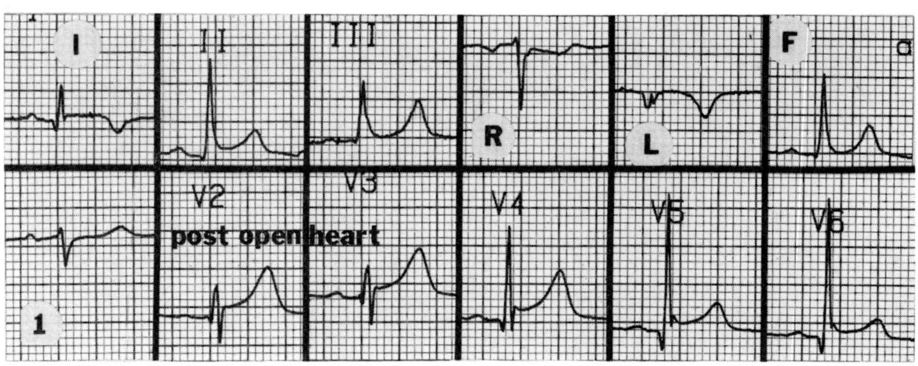
I
II
III
R
L
F
a
1
V2
V3
post open heart
V4
V5
V6

7-25.

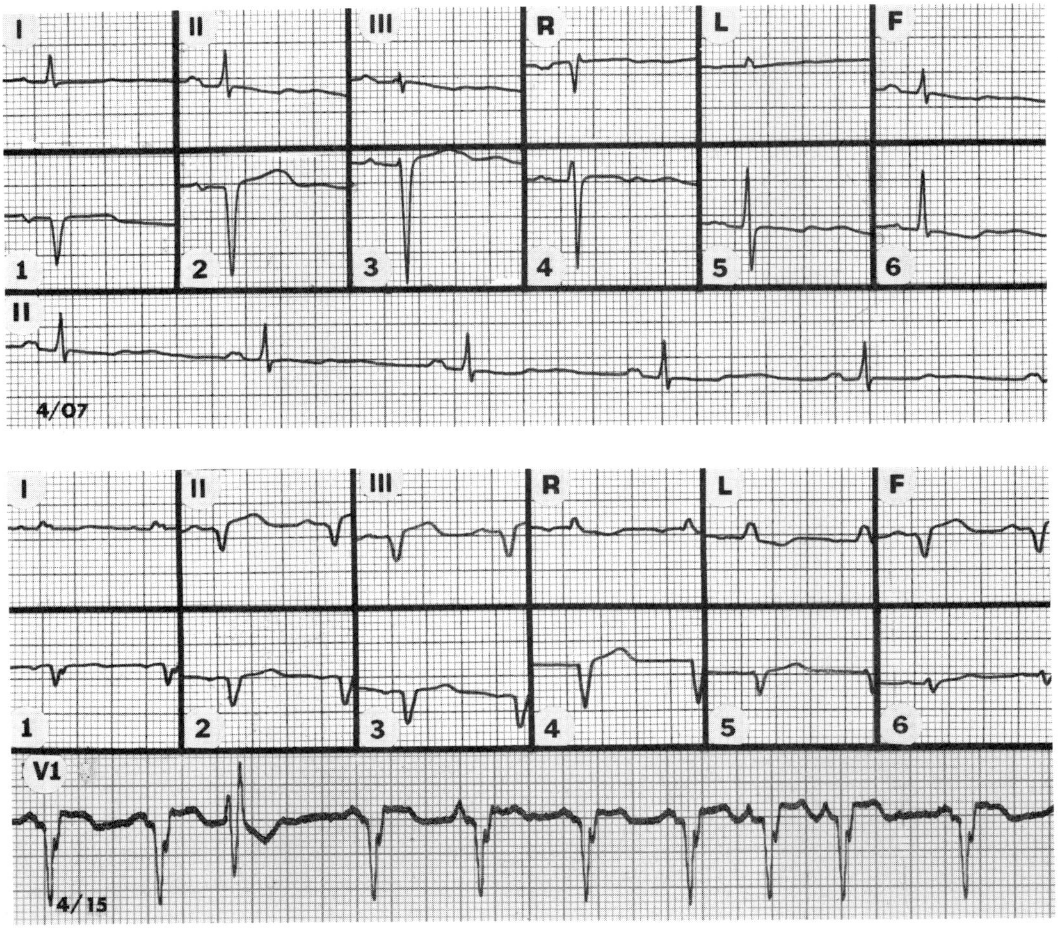

7-26.

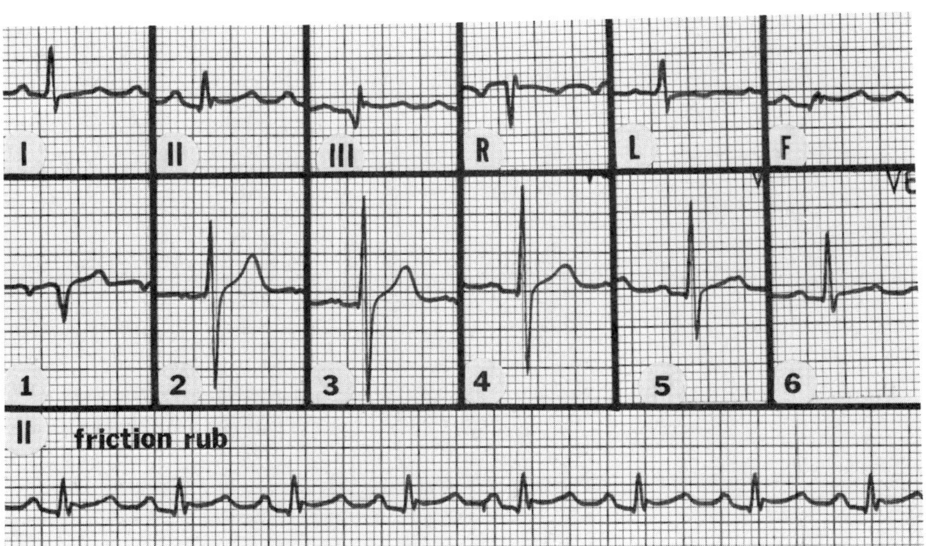

7-27.

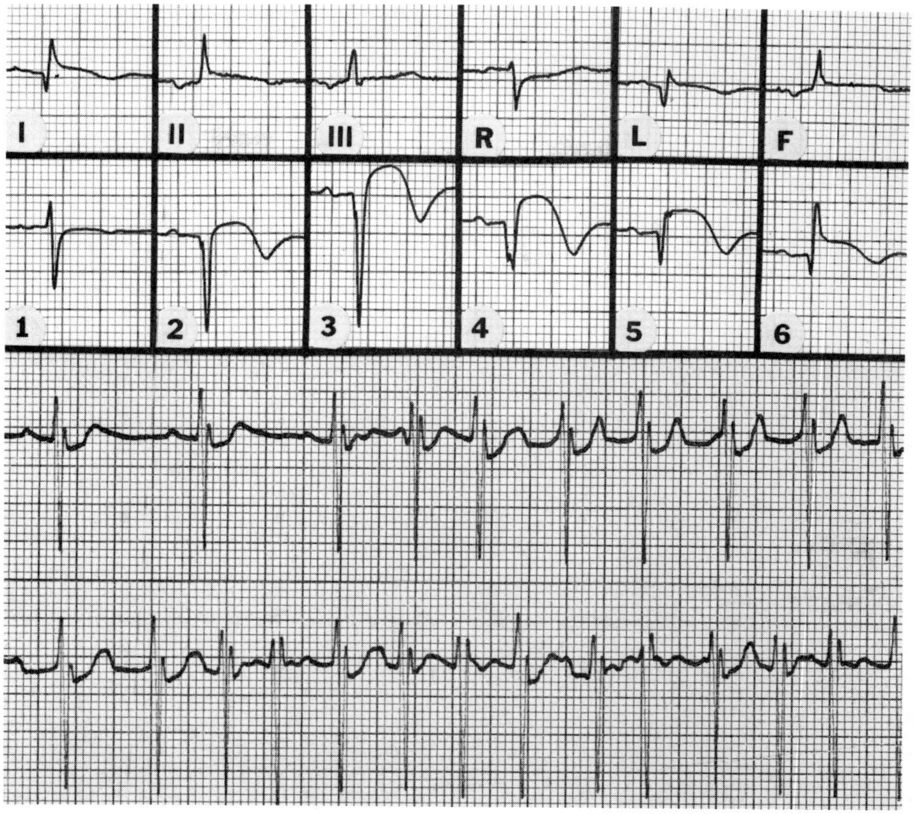

7-28.

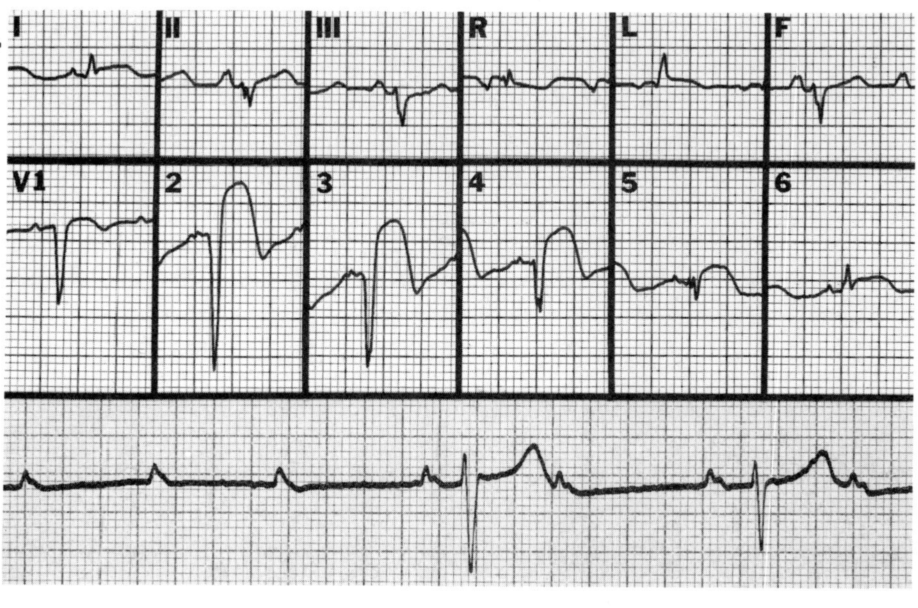

7-29.

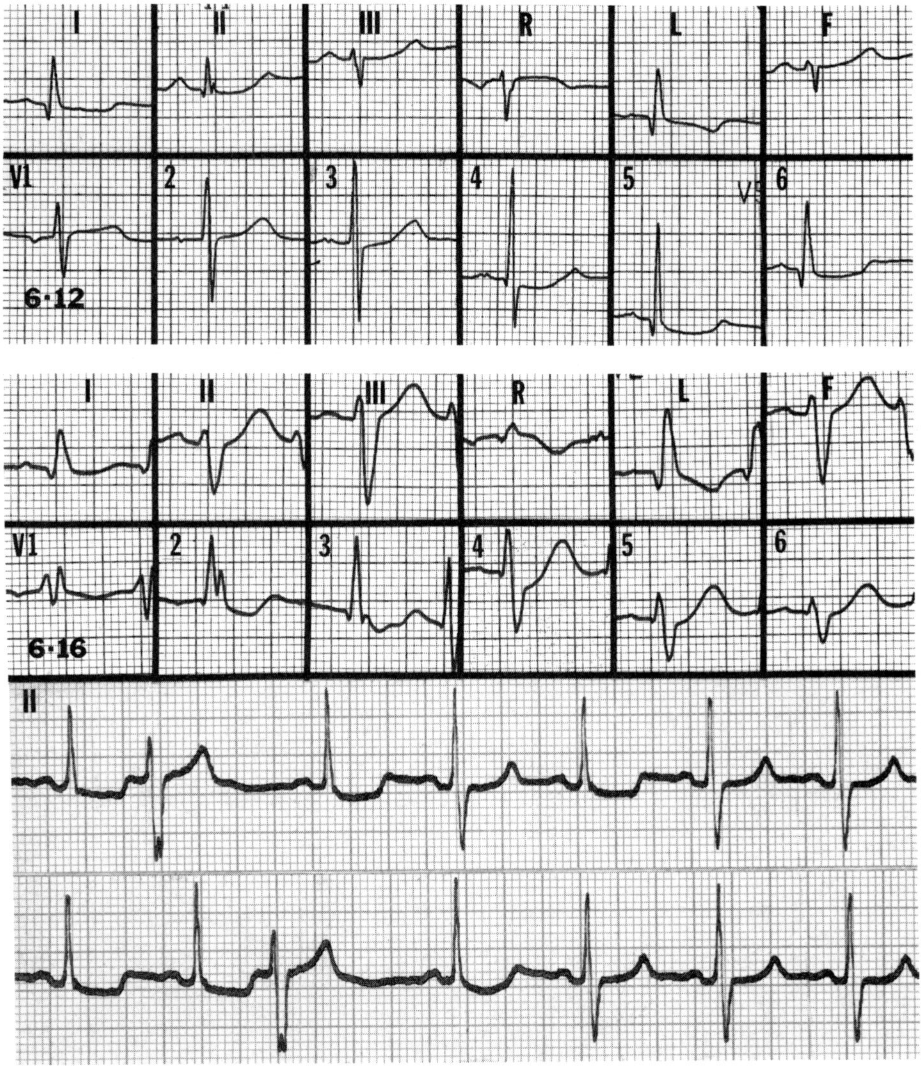

7-30.

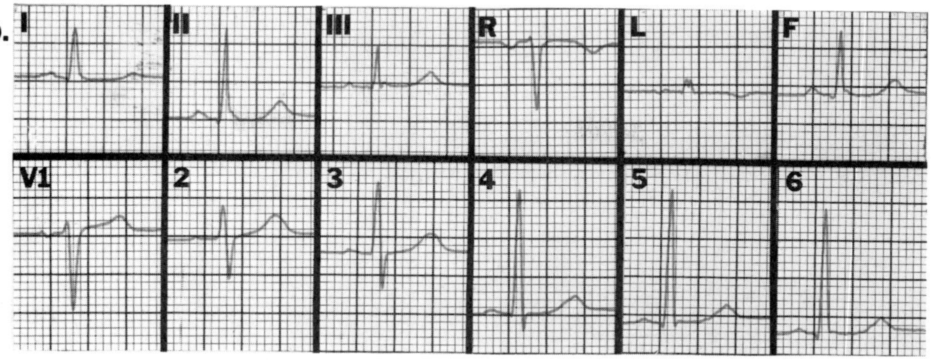
I
II
III
R
L
F
V1
2
3
4
5
6

7-31.

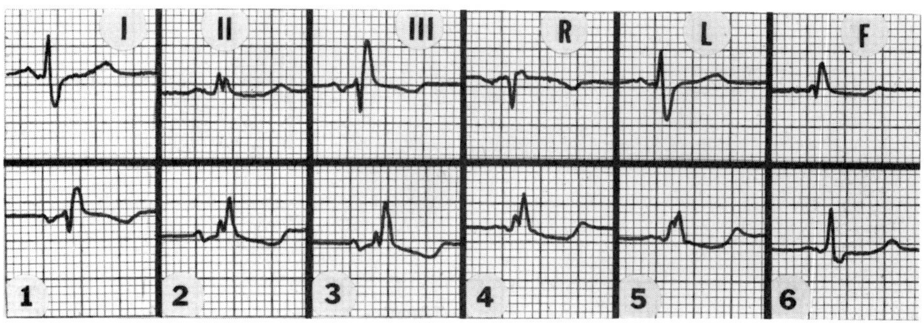
I
II
III
R
L
F
1
2
3
4
5
6

7-32.

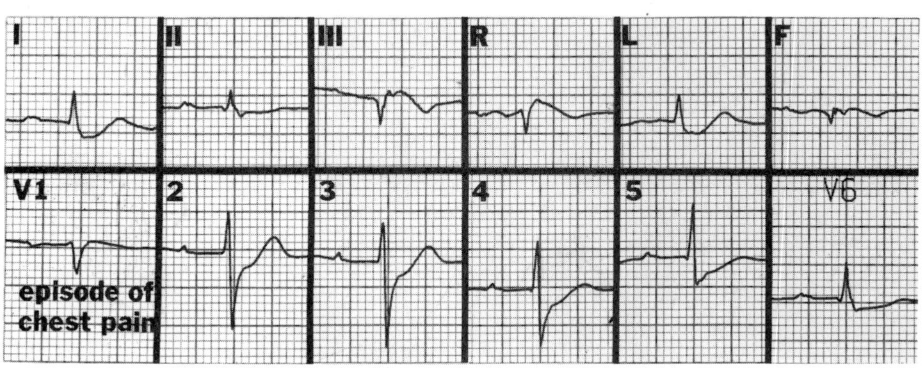
I
II
III
R
L
F
V1
2
3
4
5
V6
episode of
chest pain

7-33.

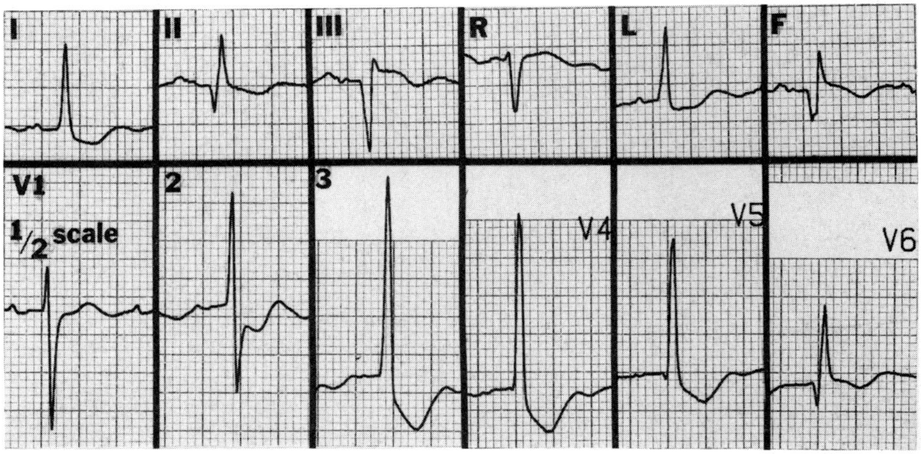
I
II
III
R
L
F
V1
1/2 scale
2
3
V4
V5
V6

7-34.

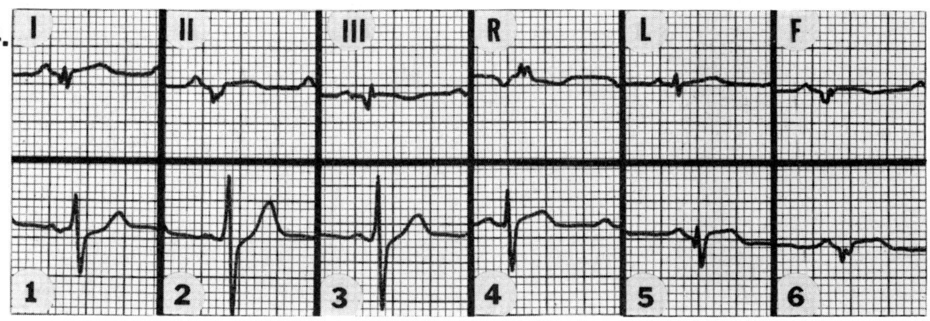
I
II
III
R
L
F
1
2
3
4
5
6

7-35.

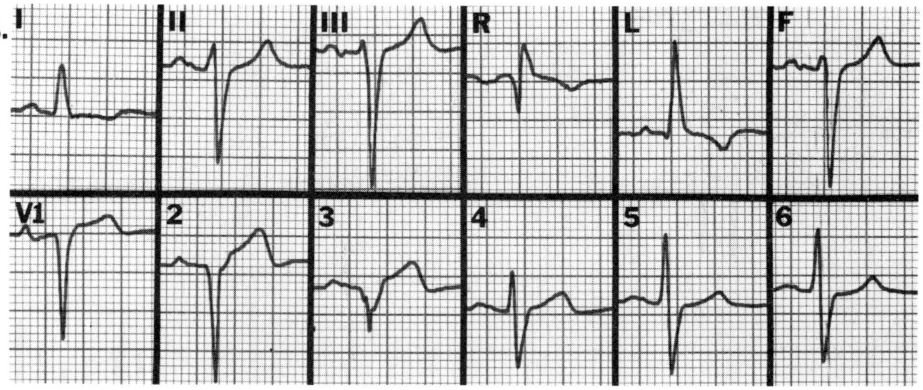
I
II
III
R
L
F
V1
2
3
4
5
6

7-36.

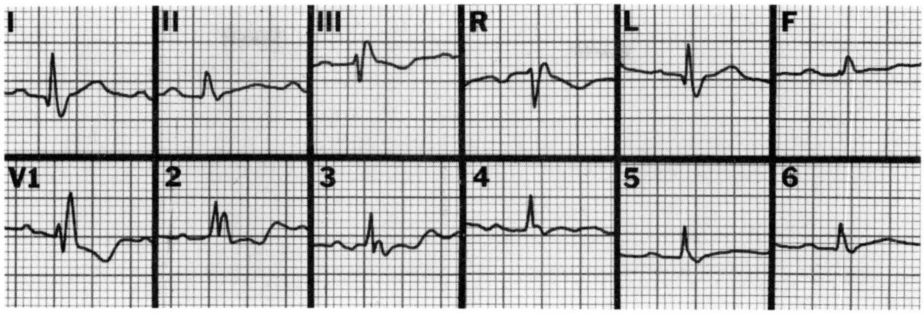

7-37.

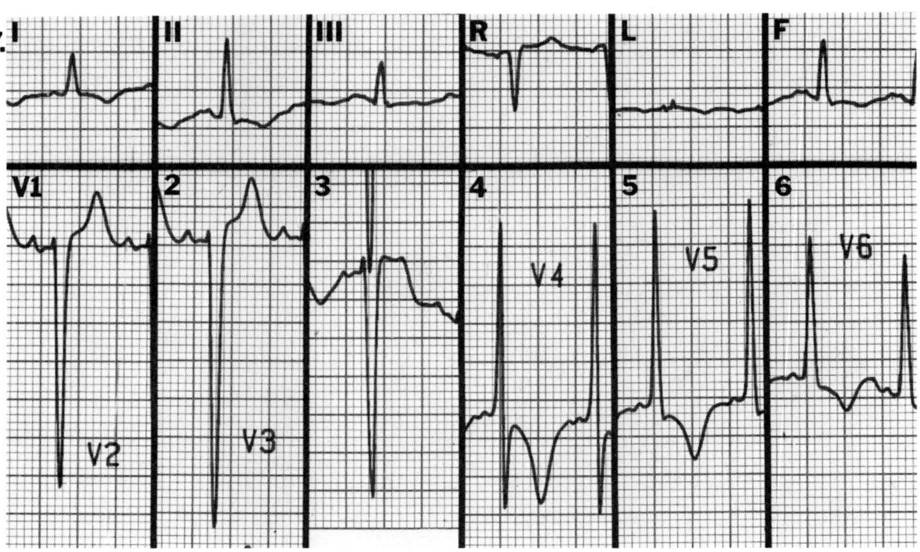

7-38.

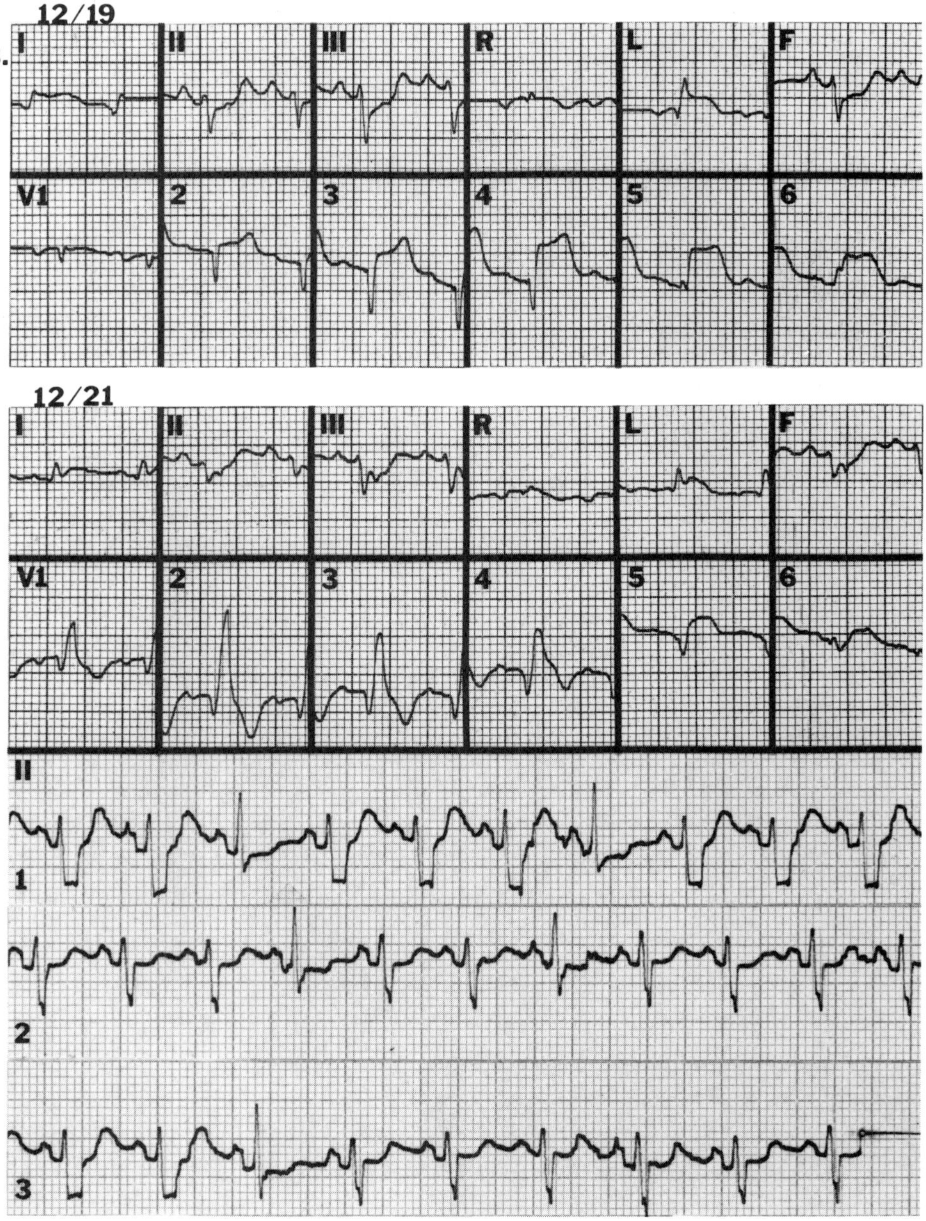

7-39.

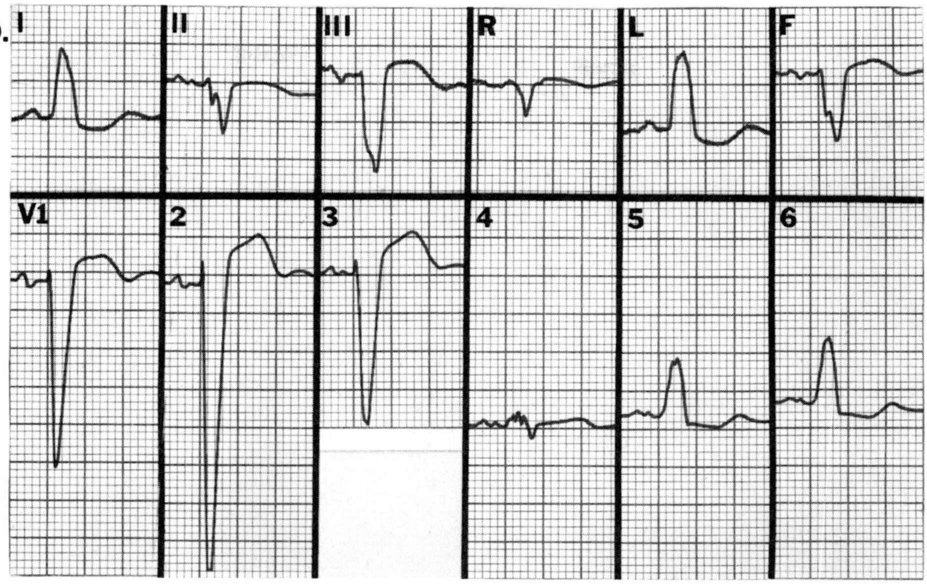

7-40.

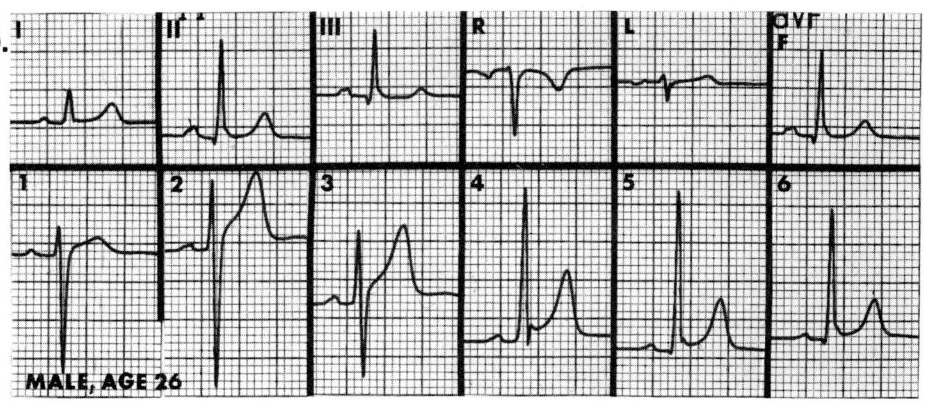

7-41.

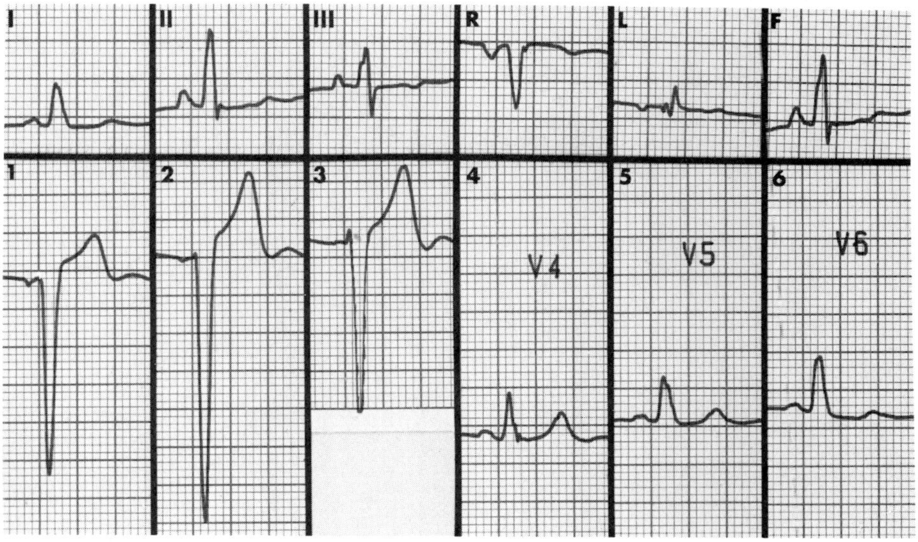

7-42.

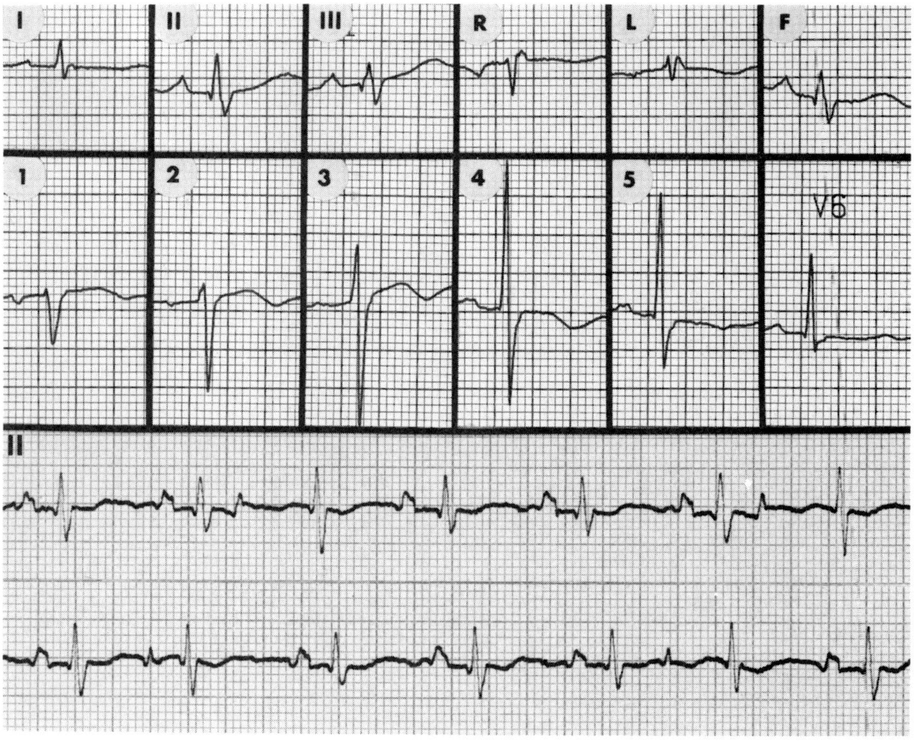

7-43.

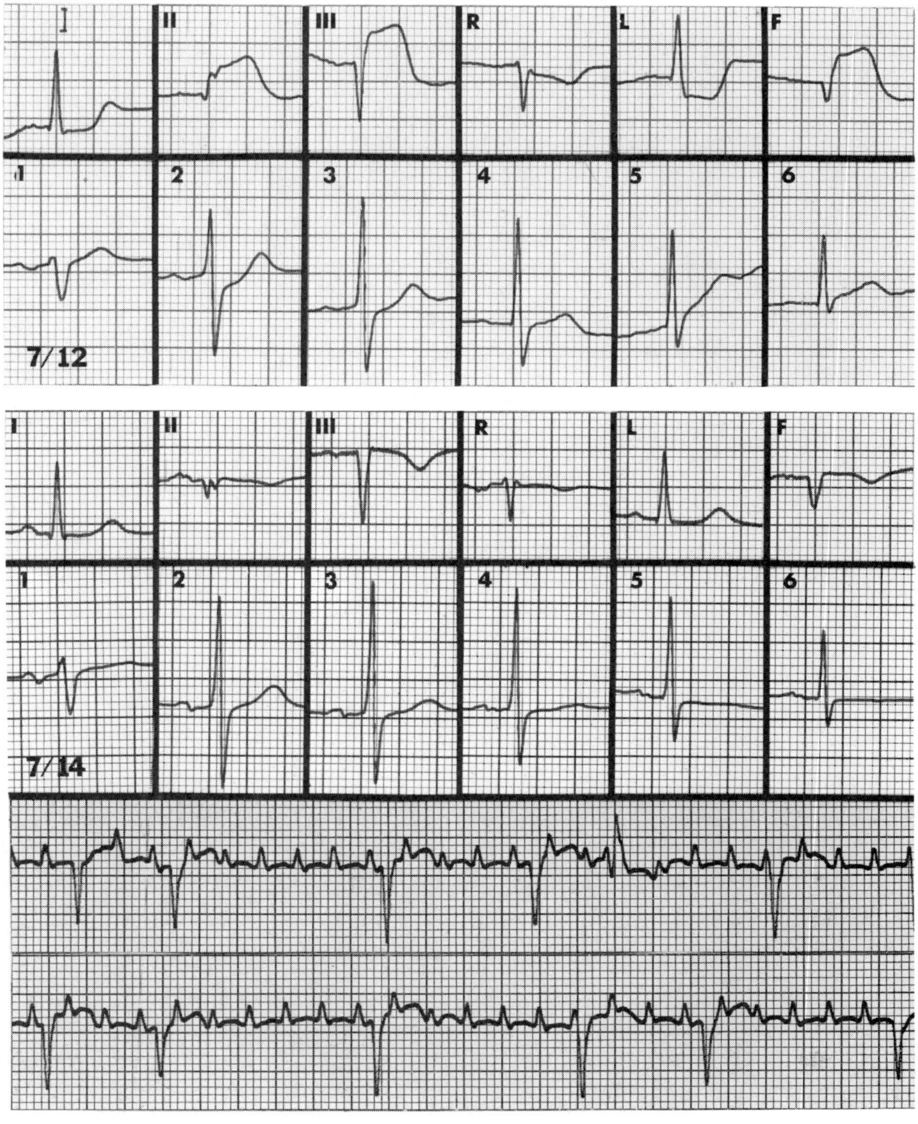

7-44.

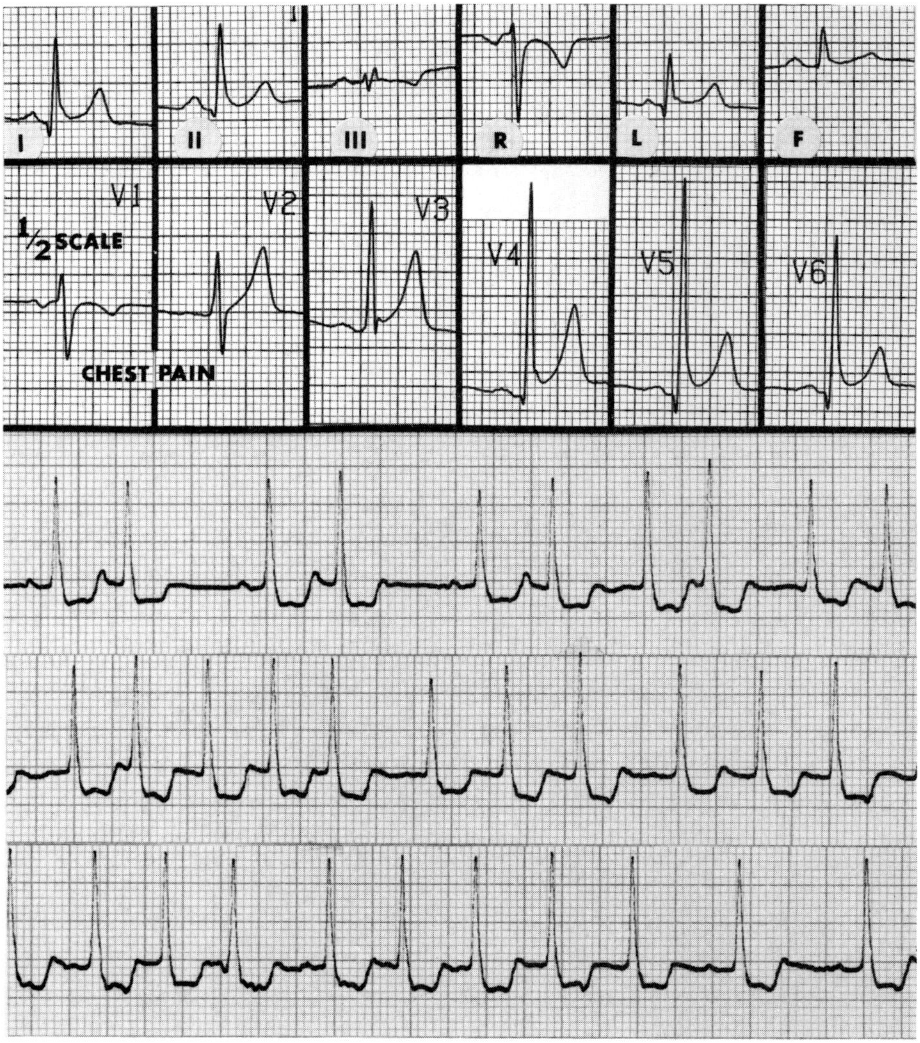
I
II
III
R
L
F
V1
V2
V3
V4
V5
V6
½ SCALE
CHEST PAIN

7-45.

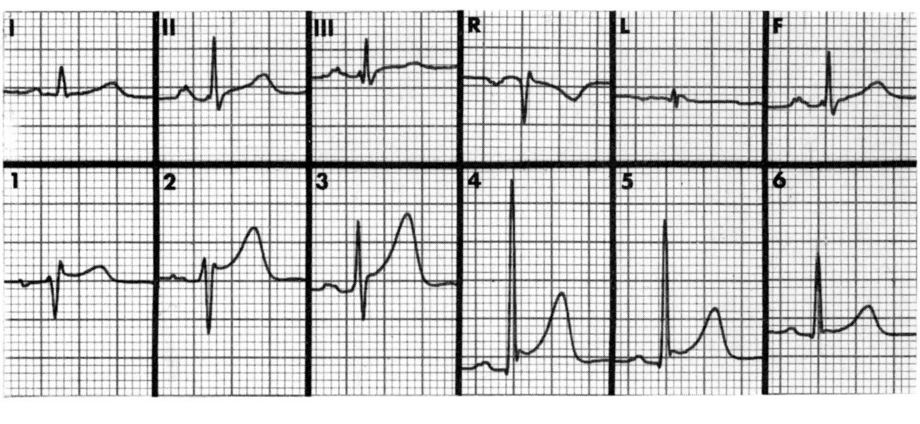
I
II
III
R
L
F
1
2
3
4
5
6

7-46.

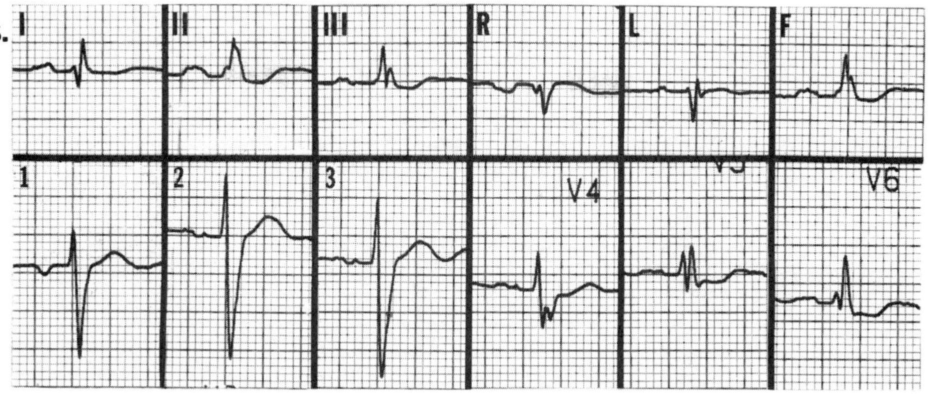

7-47.

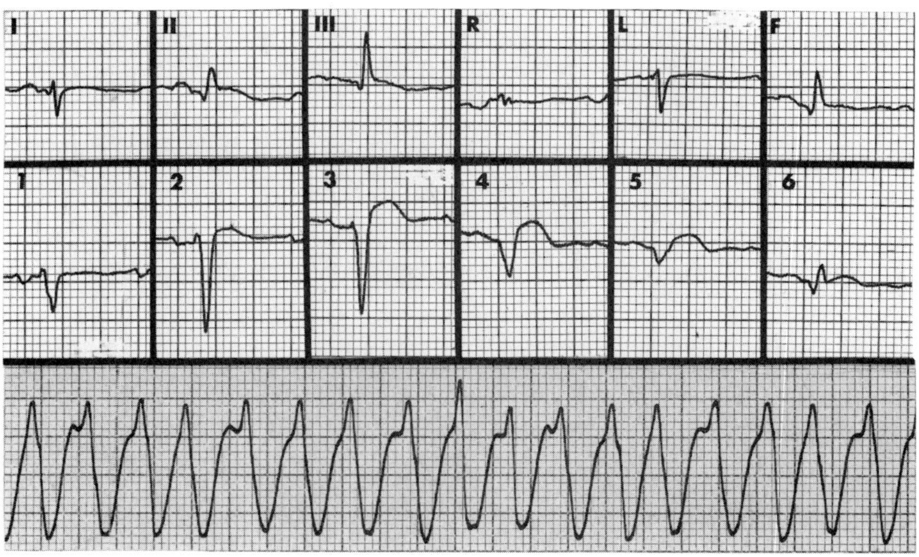

7-48.

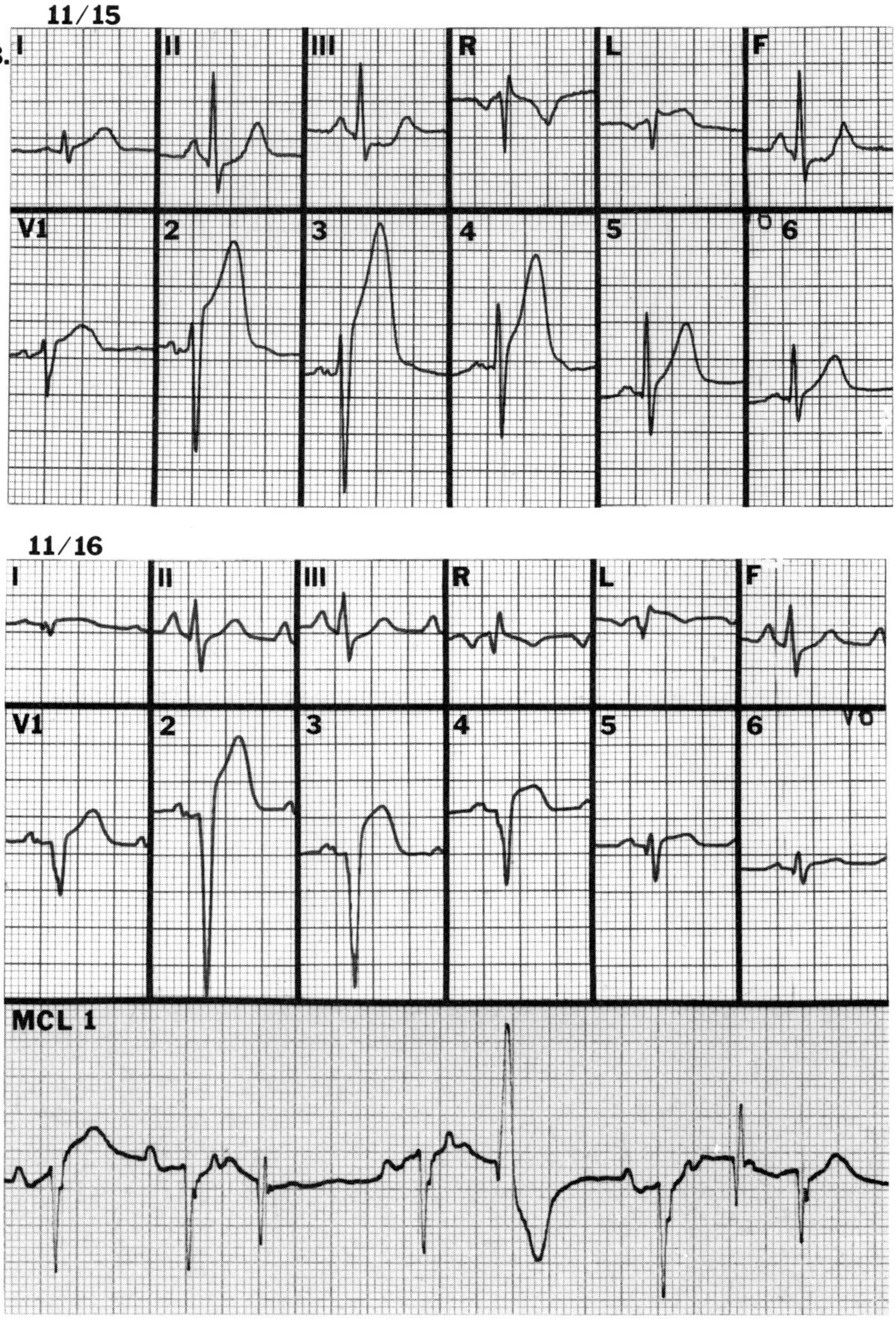

7-49.

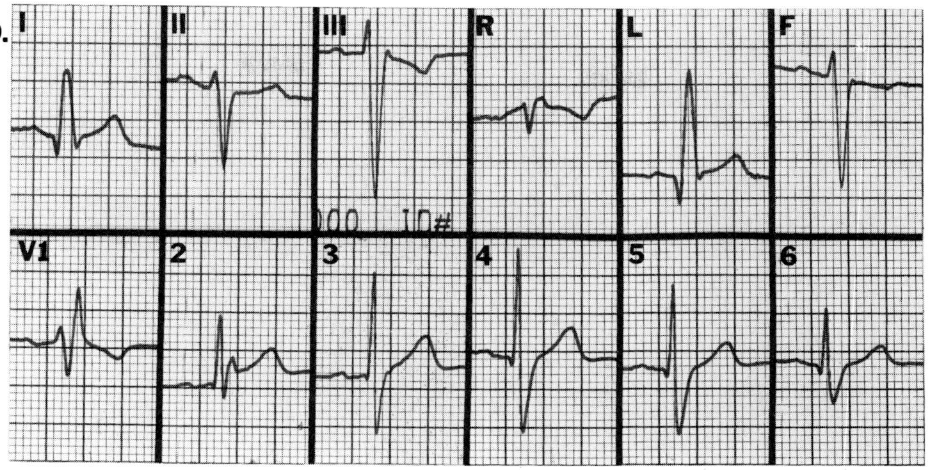

7-50.

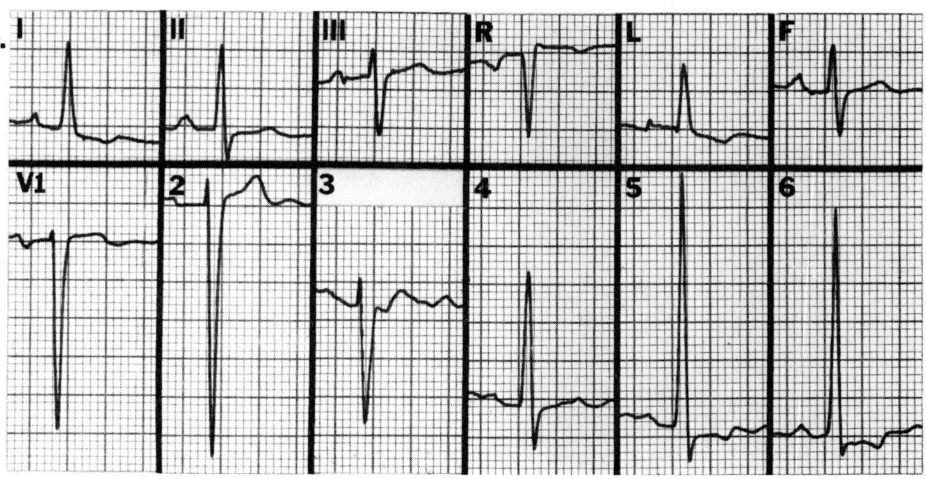

ANSWER KEY

Multiple Choice

1. a
2. c
3. d
4. d
5. d
6. d

Practice Strips

7–1. Normal axis, +60 to +70 degrees.
IWMI, old (III, aVF).
Acute pericarditis.

7–2. (ECG of 5/01, 1:56 P.M.)
Normal axis, +75 to +85 degrees.
IWMI, hyperacute phase (II, III, aVF).
(ECG of 5/01, 4:14 P.M.)
Left axis deviation, −50 to −60 degrees.
IWMI, acute phase (II, III, aVF).
PWMI (V1–V3).
Sinus rhythm, 100/minute, second-degree AV block, type I (Wenckebach) with 5:4 to 3:2 conduction ratios.

7–3. Normal axis, +20 to +30 degrees.
Left atrial enlargement.
Left ventricular hypertrophy.
Sinus bradycardia, 50/minute, sinoatrial block with junctional escape beats.

7–4. Normal axis, +40 to +50 degrees.
LVH.

7–5. Right axis deviation, +115 to +125 degrees.
LPFB.
RBBB.
First-degree AV block (PR 0.22 second).
Sinus rhythm, 78/minute, sinoatrial block, type II, with junctional escape beats.

7–6. Normal axis, +55 to +65 degrees.
Acute pericarditis.
Sinus rhythm, premature atrial complex initiating a brief run of atrial flutter.

7–7. (ECG of 8/06)
Normal axis, +15 to +25 degrees.
IWMI, hyperacute (II, III, aVF).
Lateral wall ischemia (V5, V6).
(ECG of 8/08)
Normal axis, +10 to +20 degrees.
Low voltage (14.0 mm).
Early transition (V2).
IWMI, acute (II, III, aVF).
Possible PWMI, acute (V2, V3).
Lateral wall ischemia (V5, V6).

7–8. Normal axis, +30 to +40 degrees.
Anterior wall ischemia versus non-Q MI (V1–V6).

7–9. Normal axis, +30 to +40 degrees.
Acute pericarditis (note PR segment depression, lead II).

7–10. Left axis deviation, −10 to −20 degrees.
Poor R wave progression.
AWMI, old (QS in V4).
(ECG during chest pain)
Anterior (V2–V6) and inferior (II, III, aVF) ischemia.

7–11. Normal axis, 0 to −10 degrees.
Early transition (V2).
Possible LWMI (I, aVL).
Left atrial abnormality.
LVH.

7–12. Left axis deviation, −10 to −20 degrees.
Low voltage (7.0 mm).
Poor R wave progression.
AWMI, acute (V3–V6).
Sinus rhythm, 70/minute, premature atrial complex initiating atrial fibrillation.

7–13. Normal axis, +55 to +65 degrees.
Acute pericarditis.

7–14. Normal axis, +55 to +65 degrees.
Poor R wave progression.
Late transition (V4–V5).

IWMI, hyperacute (II, III, aVF).
Sinus rhythm, 100/minute, second-degree AV block, type I, with 4:3 conduction ratio.

7–15. Right axis deviation, +115 to +125 degrees.
LPFB.
RBBB.
AWMI, acute (V1–V4).
Sinus tachycardia, 118/minute, high-grade (probably type II) AV block initiated by a premature atrial beat. Junctional escape rhythm, 30/minute in second strip.

7–16. Normal axis, +55 to +65 degrees.
Poor R wave progression.
Late transition (V5–V6).
AWMI, acute (V2–V4).
Sinus rhythm, 83/minute, dissociated from an accelerated junctional rhythm, 75/minute (isorhythmic AV dissociation).

7–17. Normal axis, +85 to +95 degrees.
Low voltage (13.5 mm).
Poor R wave progression.
Late transition (V5–V6).
AWMI, acute (V2–V5).
Sinus tachycardia, 115/minute, brief run (5 beats) of atrial tachycardia, 115/minute.

7–18. Normal axis, +55 to +65 degrees.
Early transition (V2).
Acute pericarditis.

7–19. Normal axis, +55 to +65 degrees.
Early transition (V2).
Sinus rhythm, 75/minute, second-degree AV block, 2:1 conduction ratio.

7–20. Left axis deviation, −40 to −50 degrees.
Poor R wave progression.
IWMI, acute (II, III, aVF).
The QS complexes exhibited by the premature ventricular beats in leads V2 and V3 are evidence of old AWMI. Abnormal Q waves occurred in leads V4–V6 (not shown).

7–21. (ECG of 12/19)
Normal axis, +65 to +75 degrees.

Acute pericarditis.
(ECG of 12/23)
The T wave inversion reflects the postacute phase of pericarditis.
Sinus rhythm, 97/minute, premature atrial beats with aberrant conduction.

7–22. Normal axis, +5 to −5 degrees.
LVH.
Atrial fibrillation.

7–23. Right axis deviation, +115 to +125 degrees.
Early transition (V1).
RVH.
Atrial fibrillation.

7–24. Normal axis, +55 to +65 degrees.
Early transition (V2).
Acute pericarditis.

7–25. (ECG of 4/07)
Normal axis, +45 to +55 degrees.
Low voltage (13.5 mm).
Poor R wave progression.
Late transition (V5).
Left atrial abnormality.
Sinus bradycardia, 50/minute.
(ECG of 4/15)
Left axis deviation, −60 to −70 degrees.
Low voltage (8.0 mm).
Poor R wave progression.
IWMI (II, III, aVF).
AWMI (V2–V5).
Sinus rhythm, 100/minute, premature atrial beats, some aberrantly conducted.

7–26. Normal axis, +5 to −5 degrees.
IWMI, old (III, aVF).
Acute pericarditis (note PR segment depression, lead II).

7–27. Normal axis, +50 to +60 degrees.
Poor R wave progression.
Late transition (V5–V6).
LWMI, old (I, aVL).
AWMI, acute (V2–V5).
Sinus rhythm, 81/minute, premature atrial complex initiating atrial fibrillation.

7–28. Left axis deviation, −55 to −65 degrees.
Poor R wave progression.
Late transition (V5–V6).
Low voltage (11.0 mm).
LAFB.
AWMI, acute (V2–V5).
Sinus rhythm, approximately 83/minute, third-degree AV block with irregular junctional escape rhythm, less than 40/minute.

7–29. (ECG of 6/12)
Left axis deviation, −10 to −20 degrees.
Early transition (V2).
LWMI (I, aVL, V6).
PWMI, old (V1–V3).
(ECG of 6/16)
Left axis deviation, −55 to −65 degrees.
LAFB.
RBBB.
LWMI, old (I, aVL).
Sinus rhythm, 72/minute, premature ventricular beats, normal intraventricular conduction alternating with RBBB in sinus beats.

7–30. Normal axis, +55 to +65 degrees.
Essentially normal ECG.

7–31. Right axis deviation, +120 to +130 degrees.
LPFB.
RBBB.

7–32. Left axis deviation, −10 to −20 degrees.
Low voltage (12.0 mm).
Late transition (V4).
IWMI, recent (III, aVF).
Anterior wall ischemia (V2–V5).

7–33. Normal axis, +5 to −5 degrees.
Early transition (V2).
IWMI (II, III, aVF).
Possible LWMI (V6).
Left atrial abnormality.
LVH.
Anterior wall ischemia (V2).

7–34. Extreme right axis deviation, +220 to +230 degrees.
Low voltage (12.0 mm).
Early transition (V1–V2).

IWMI, old (II, III, aVF).
Possible LWMI (I, V6).
PWMI (V1–V3).

7–35. Left axis deviation, −60 to −70 degrees.
Poor R wave progression.
Late transition (V5).
LAFB.
AWMI (QS in V3).

7–36. Normal axis, +85 to +95 degrees.
RBBB.

7–37. Normal axis, +45 to +55 degrees.
Left atrial abnormality.
LVH.

7–38. (ECG of 12/19)
Left axis deviation, −55 to −65 degrees.
Low voltage (14.0 mm).
Poor R wave progression.
LAFB.
AWMI, acute (V2–V4).
LWMI, acute (I, aVL, V5, V6).
(ECG of 12/21)
Left axis deviation, −65 to −75 degrees.
Low voltage (12.0 mm).
LAFB.
RBBB.
AWMI, acute (V1–V4).
LWMI, acute (V5–V6).
Sinus tachycardia, 130/minute, normal intraventricular conduction alternating with RBBB (strip 1), normal intraventricular conduction alternating with LAFB (strip 2), and normal intraventricular conduction alternating with both RBBB and LAFB (strip 3).

7–39. Left axis deviation, −45 to −55 degrees.
Poor R wave progression.
LAFB.
LBBB.

7–40. Normal axis, +65 to +65 degrees.
Early repolarization pattern.

7–41. Normal axis, +45 to +55 degrees.
LBBB.

7–42. Left axis deviation, −35 to −45 degrees.
NSIVCD.
Left atrial abnormality.
Sinus rhythm, 79/minute, premature atrial complexes with prolonged AV conduction (up to 0.42 second).

7–43. (ECG of 7/12)
Normal axis, +5 to −5 degrees.
IWMI, acute (II, III, aVF).
Possible PWMI (V2–V3).
(ECG of 7/14)
Left axis deviation, −10 to −20 degrees.
Early transition (V2).
IWMI, acute (II, III, aVF).
PWMI, acute (V2–V3).
Atrial flutter with variable AV conduction.

7–44. Normal axis, +25 to +35 degrees.
Early transition (V2).
Possible LWMI (I, aVL, V6).
Possible left atrial abnormality.
LVH.
Acute pericarditis.
Atrial bigeminy followed by short burst of atrial fibrillation.

7–45. Normal axis, +30 to +40 degrees.
Acute pericarditis versus early repolarization pattern.

7–46. Normal axis, +65 to +75 degrees.
Left atrial abnormality.
NSIVCD.
First-degree AV block (PR 0.22 second).

7–47. Right axis deviation, +115 to +125 degrees.
Low voltage (13.0 mm).
Poor R wave progression.
Late transition (V6).
LPFB.
AWMI, recent (V3–V6).
Ventricular tachycardia, average rate 215/minute.

7–48. (ECG of 11/15)
Normal axis, +70 to +80 degrees.
AWMI, hyperacute phase (V2–V5).
(ECG of 11/16)

Extreme right axis deviation, +130 to +140 degrees.
Poor R wave progression.
Late transition (V6).
AWMI, acute (V1–V5).
Possible LWMI (I, aVL, V6).
Sinus rhythm, 83/minute, premature atrial beats with varying degrees of aberrant conduction.

7–49. Left axis deviation, −60 to −70 degrees.
LAFB.
RBBB.
Possible LWMI (I, aVL).

7–50. Normal axis, +5 to −5 degrees.
Probable left atrial abnormality.
LVH.
First-degree AV block (PR 0.22 second).

CHAPTER EIGHT

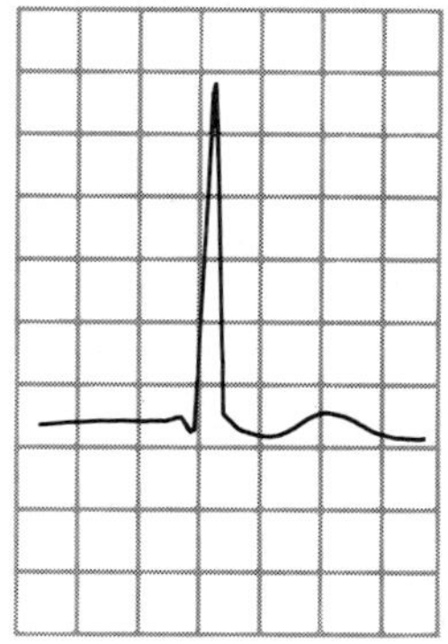

WOLFF-PARKINSON-WHITE SYNDROME

COGNITIVE GOALS

1. Define the term **accessory pathway.**
2. Identify the anatomical substrate of the Wolff-Parkinson-White syndrome.
3. Describe the classic ECG findings of WPW syndrome.
4. Distinguish between type A and type B WPW syndrome.
5. Discuss how WPW syndrome can be distinguished from myocardial infarction.
6. Define the term **preexcitation.**
7. Describe the ECG findings of the Lown-Ganong-Levine syndrome.
8. Describe the circuit typically used during reciprocal tachycardia in the WPW syndrome.
9. Define the terms **orthodromic** and **antidromic tachycardia** and identify how the two forms are differentiated electrocardiographically.
10. Describe how atrial fibrillation can lead to ventricular fibrillation in subjects with WPW syndrome and how ventricular fibrillation is treated.
11. Describe the basis for pharmacological therapy of the WPW syndrome.

Definition

In normal hearts the depolarization wavefront initiated by the sinoatrial node passes in succession through the atria, the atrioventricular node (**1** in Fig. 8–1), the bundle of His **(2),** and the bundle branches **(3** and **4)** before reaching the ventricular myocardium. Early in fetal life the atrial and ventricular myocardia are continuous, but after the first month of gestation a fibrous layer of connective tissue, the annulus fibrosus, begins to separate the atria and ventricles both anatomically and electrically. This process leaves the AV node and bundle of His as the only electrical connection between the upper and lower chambers in the majority of subjects. In a minority, however, this process of atrial and ventricular electrical isolation is incomplete, with the result that additional, congenitally anomalous, accessory pathways persist. These accessory pathways (AP) consist of unobliterated myocardial remnants that make direct electrical connections between the atrial and ventricular myocardia or

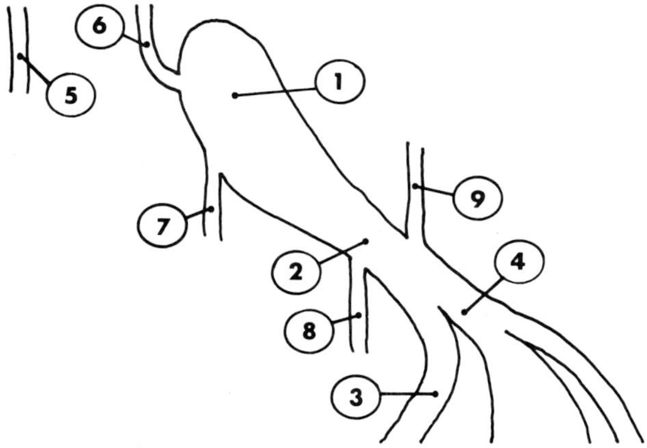

Figure 8–1. Anomalous connections.

ANATOMIC SUBTRATES OF PREEXCITATION
1. **AV Node**
2. **Bundle of His**
3. **Right bundle branch**
4. **Left bundle branch**
5. **Atrioventricular connection (Kent)**
6. **Atrionodal pathway (James)**
7. **Nodoventricular pathway (Mahaim)**
8. **Fasciculoventricular pathway (Mahaim)**
9. **Atrio-His tract (Lev)**

between the atrial myocardium and various segments of the distal conduction pathway. Such anomalous connections permit simultaneous conduction of the sinus impulse over two (or more) anatomically separate pathways, so that ventricular depolarization is then initiated through both the normal and the accessory pathways.

Historical perspective

Anomalous atrioventricular connections were described by the anatomist Kent as early as 1893, although the functional significance of such fibers remained unknown at the time and would not be proved for another 50 years. Today these myocardial fiber bundles are still called **bundles of Kent** (or **atrioventricular connections; 5** in Fig. 8–1) and are known to be the anatomical substrate of the **Wolff-Parkinson-White (WPW) syndrome.** Other types of anomalous connections, more rarely involved in clinically encountered syndromes, were described by Mahaim in 1947 (**7** and **8** in Fig. 8–1) and by James in 1961 (**6** in Fig. 8–1). As early as 1915, Wilson published an electrocardiogram of the yet-to-be-named WPW syndrome and other examples from various authors followed throughout the 1920s. In 1930, L. Wolff, J. Parkinson, and P. D. White published 11 cases thought to represent "function bundle branch block" associated with paroxysms of supraventricular tachycardia (Wolff et al, 1930;

Lazarra, 1979; Rigby and Graboys, 1981). In 1943, Wood and his associates established that the ECG findings in patients with WPW syndrome were related to the presence of accessory conduction pathways of the type previously described by Kent (Wood et al, 1943) and in 1944 Ohnell coined the term **preexcitation** to describe the electrical event responsible for the distinctive ECG features of the syndrome (Ohnell, 1944). Subsequently, ventricular preexcitation was confirmed by epicardial mapping techniques during open heart surgery, and it was established that the destruction of accessory pathways was feasible by both physical and chemical means. It has also been proved that the associated supraventricular arrhythmias, from which the syndrome derives its importance, can be initiated and terminated by programmed ventricular stimulation techniques during cardiac catheterization.

Electrocardiographic manifestations of WPW syndrome

The classic ECG abnormalities of WPW syndrome are (1) a **short PR interval** (less than 0.12 second), (2) a **wide QRS complex** (greater than 0.12 second), and (3) an initial slurring of the QRS complex or **delta wave.** These features are illustrated in Figure 8–2. It should be noted that some cases of WPW syndrome do not strictly conform to the aforementioned criteria, and may present with normal or nearly normal PR intervals or QRS complexes. Such cases may remain undiagnosed unless other factors, such as supraventricular tachycardia or symptoms such as syncope or palpitations, prompt careful scrutiny of the ECG (Krikler, 1975). Because ventricular depolarization is abnormal during episodes of preexcitation, repolarization changes reflected by ST segment and T wave abnormalities may be noted.

In 1945, Rosenbaum and his coworkers (Rosenbaum et al, 1945) classified WPW preexcitation into two major categories, **type A,** in which the major deflection in precordial leads V1 and V2 is **positive** (a dominant R wave), and **type B,** in which the predominant deflection in leads V1 and V2 is **negative** (an S or QS complex). Type A WPW, shown in Figure 8–3, was subsequently shown to represent preexcitation of the left ventricle, producing a V1 pattern reminiscent of right bundle branch block. Type B, illustrated in Figure 8–4, is usually due to preexcitation of the lateral wall of the right ventricle, and produces a V1 pattern similar to left bundle branch block. Atrioventricular accessory connections can also insert into the ventricular septum. Various locations

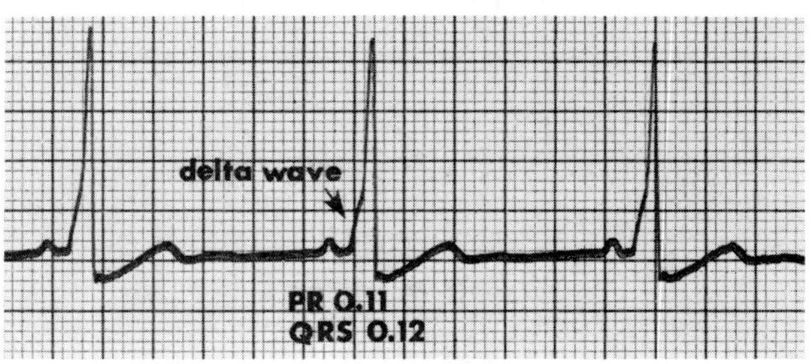

Figure 8–2. ECG characteristics of the WPW syndrome.

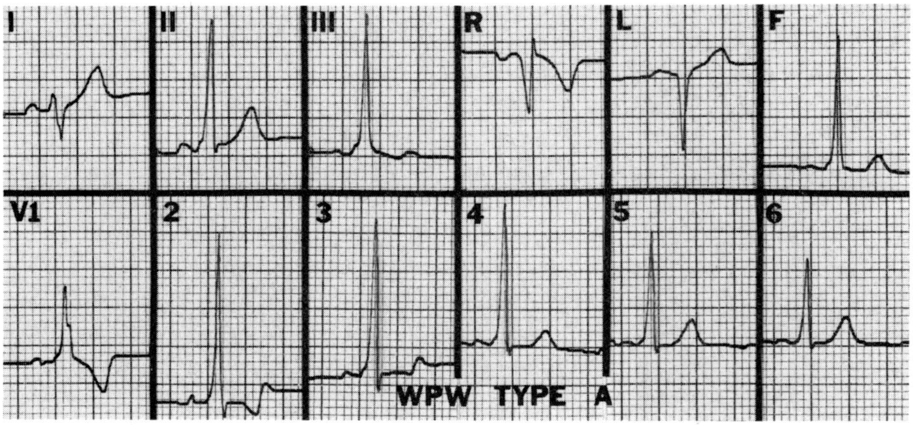

Figure 8–3. WPW syndrome, type A.

of accessory connections at the level of the atrioventricular valves, and the polarity of the resulting delta waves, are shown in Figure 8–5.

It can easily be appreciated from an examination of Figure 8–3 that type A WPW can be misdiagnosed as right ventricular hypertrophy, right bundle branch block, or fully evolved posterior wall infarction (Schamroth, 1980). Negative delta waves in leads II, III, and aVF closely mimic inferior wall infarction, and negative delta waves in leads I and aVL can easily be mistaken for lateral wall infarction. In those cases in which negatively oriented delta waves simulate the Q waves of infarction, the presence of positive delta waves in other leads will usually ensure a correct diagnosis.

Tracings of WPW type B often exhibit negative delta waves in leads V1 to V3 that closely resemble tracings of anterior wall infarction or of left bundle

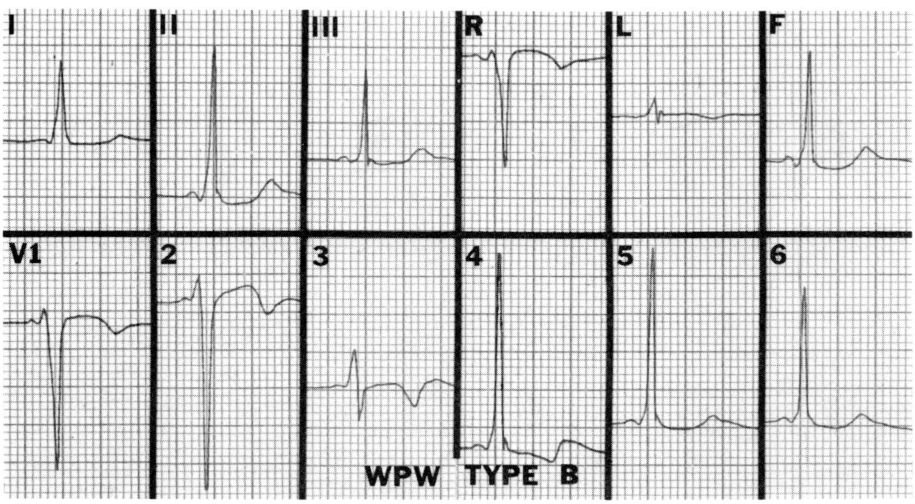

Figure 8–4. WPW syndrome, type B.

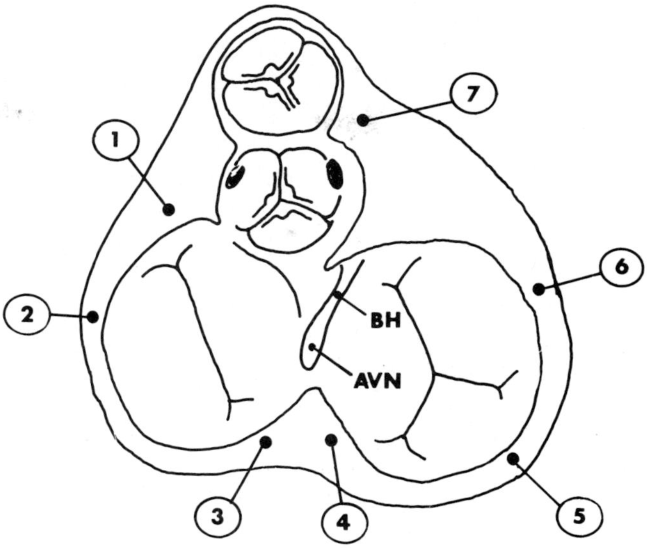

Figure 8–5. Delta wave polarity by site.

DELTA WAVE POLARITY BY ANATOMICAL SITE:

LEAD:	I	III	V1	V6
1.	-	+	+	-
2.	+	±	+	+
3.	+	-	+	+
4.	+	-	±	+
5.	+	-	±	+
6.	+	-	±	+
7.	+	+	±	+

SITE DESIGNATIONS:

1. **Left anterior**
2. **Left lateral**
3. **Left paraseptal**
4. **Right paraseptal**
5. **Acute marginal**
6. **Right anterior**
7. **Pulmonary outflow**

branch block (Goldberger, 1979). When myocardial infarction does occur in patients with WPW syndrome, the preexcitation frequently obscures the diagnostic changes resulting from infarction, rendering the ECG an unreliable assessment tool.

Ventricular preexcitation occurs because the sinus impulse is able to bypass the normal conduction pathway and reach the ventricular muscle by means of an anomalous connection, or Kent bundle, before ventricular depolarization can take place over the normal pathway. Because conduction over the normal path is momentarily slowed at the level of the AV node, the impulse traveling down the Kent bundle reaches the ventricular myocardium first, and initiates ventricular depolarization from the distal point of attachment of the Kent bundle. Hence the term **preexcitation.** As the depolarization wave from the Kent bundle spreads slowly from cell to cell through the ventricular muscle, the depolarization wavefront traveling over the normal path arrives and triggers the remainder of the ventricle in the normal fashion. The result is a fusion beat composed of a **preexcitation component,** or delta wave, and a QRS complex resulting from the ventricular depolarization over the normal path, the unpreexcited component. Because most of the PR interval duration represents slow conduction through the AV node, bypassing the AV node through the rapidly conducting Kent bundle will cause the PR interval to shorten. This sequence of events is illustrated schematically in **panel 1** of Figure 8–6, which shows a typical preexcitation complex. The degree of preexcitation, reflected by both the duration of the PR interval and the width of the delta wave, may vary from time to time or even from beat to beat, or may fluctuate in cyclical fashion, the so-called **concertina effect.** Preexcitation may also be intermittent—present in some beats but not in others, or on some 12 leads but not others.

When anomalous conduction occurs over pathways other than the Kent bundle (compare Fig. 8–1), the ECG features of the **Lown-Ganong-Levine (LGL)**

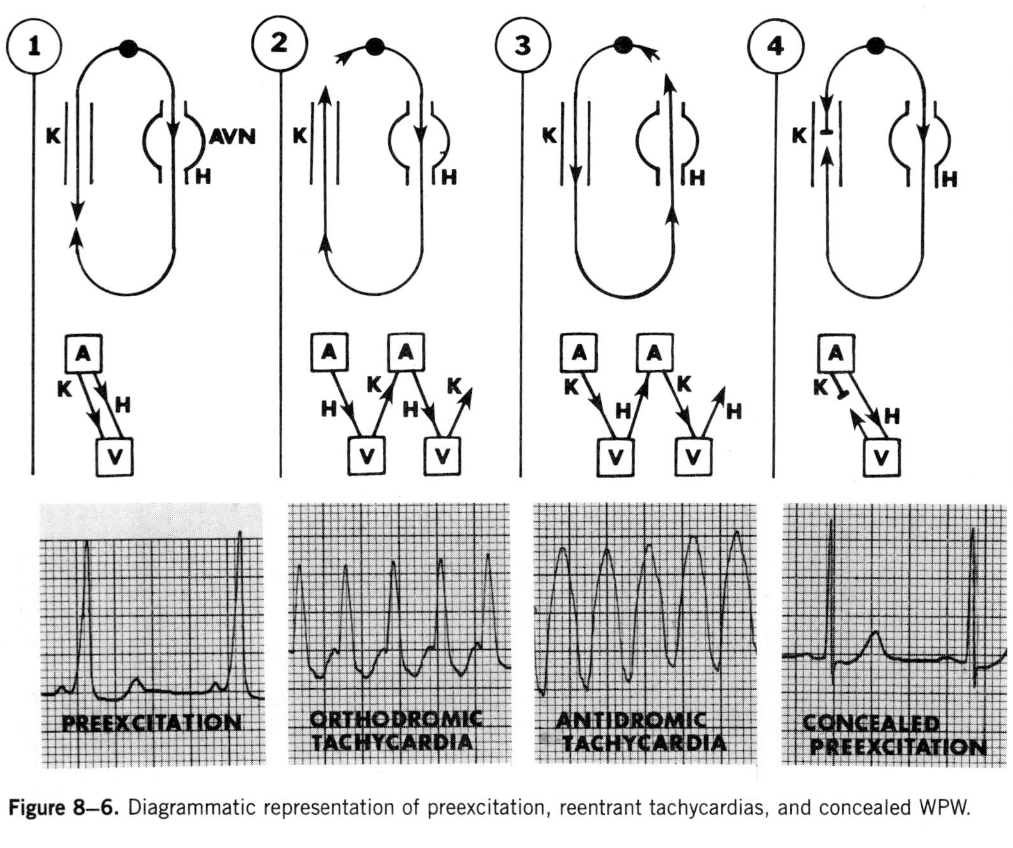

Figure 8–6. Diagrammatic representation of preexcitation, reentrant tachycardias, and concealed WPW.

syndrome may appear. This syndrome is characterized by a short PR interval and a QRS complex of normal width. Rarely, conduction over a Mahaim fiber will manifest itself with a normal PR interval followed by a widened QRS complex with a delta wave. An example of the LGL syndrome, obtained from a 2-year-old male with a history of paroxysms of supraventricular tachycardia, is shown in Figure 8–7. Note the short PR interval, the lack of a delta wave, and the normal QRS complexes. The exact anatomical substrate of the LGL syndrome is unknown, and may vary from case to case (Ward and Camm, 1983). The classification of the varying types of preexcitation is fraught with complexity. The interested reader is referred to the literature for further details (Coumel and Attuel, 1974; Anderson et al, 1975; Lev et al, 1975; Pick and Langendorf, 1979; Wellens et al, 1980; Gallagher et al, 1981).

The WPW syndrome is an associated finding in a signficant number of young patients with congenital heart disease, notably hypertrophic cardiomyopathy, Ebstein's anomaly (in which the WPW is almost exclusively type B), corrected transposition of the great vessels, tricuspid atresia, and endocardial fibroelastosis (Burch and DePasquale, 1967; Marriott, 1983).

The mechanism and incidence of tachyarrhythmias

The incidence of the WPW syndrome is estimated to be in the range of 0.3 per cent of the total population (3 of every 1000 persons). Among those with the syndrome, the incidence of tachycardias is reported in some studies to be as high as 80 per cent.

Most tachycardias associated with WPW syndrome are reentrant or recip-

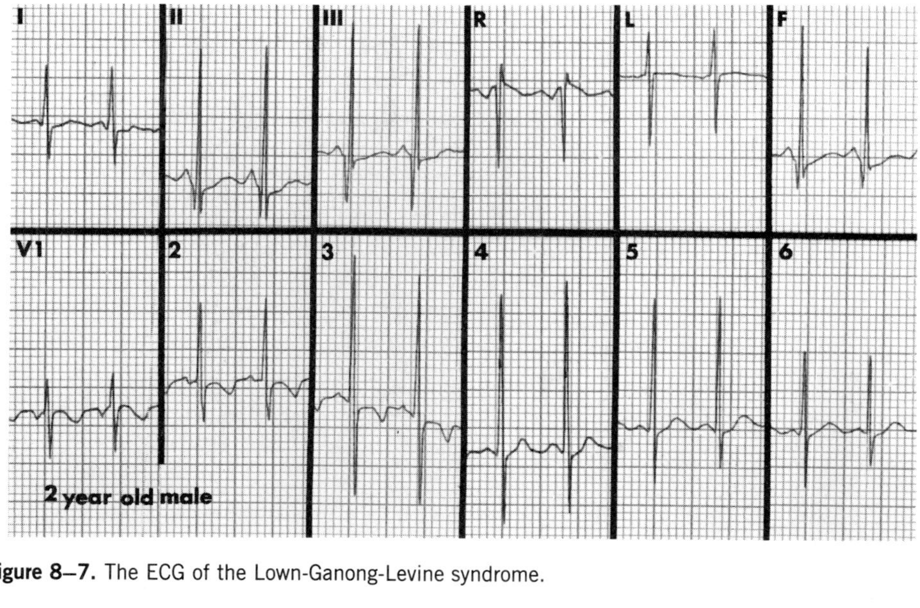

Figure 8–7. The ECG of the Lown-Ganong-Levine syndrome.

rocating arrhythmias. **Reentry** or **reciprocation** occurs when an impulse travels away from its point of origin using one pathway and then reverses its direction, returning to its point of origin using a second path. In order for this mechanism to function, three preconditions are necessary: (1) Two functionally or anatomically separate pathways must exist; (2) conduction in one of the pathways must exhibit unidirectional block; and (3) conduction in the other pathway must be sufficiently prolonged to allow repolarization (recovery) of the first pathway. In cases of WPW syndrome, impulse conduction during tachycardia usually takes place in the antegrade, or atrioventricular, direction through the AV node and His bundle (**H** in **panel 2** of Fig. 8–6) to the ventricles, and then returns to its atrial point of origin using the accessory (Kent bundle) connection (**K** in **panel 2,** Fig. 8–6). The result is a tachycardia with narrow QRS complexes, called **orthodromic** tachycardia because the normal conduction pathway is used for forward conduction of the impulse. Because the Kent bundle is being used exclusively for retrograde, or ventriculoatrial, conduction, the QRS complexes will normalize during the tachycardia and delta waves will disappear. An example of such a narrow-complex, orthodromic tachycardia is shown at the bottom of **panel 2,** Figure 8–6, beneath the schematic drawing of its underlying mechanism.

Another example of orthodromic tachycardia, with its initiating beat, is illustrated in Figure 8–8. Note that after the first two sinus beats, which exhibit the delta wave and widened QRS typical of preexcitation, a premature beat initiates a tachycardia with narrow QRS complexes and retrograde P waves.

Reciprocating supraventricular tachycardias are thought to complicate as many as 40 to 80 per cent of cases of WPW syndrome. Less commonly, the reciprocal tachycardia uses the Kent bundle for antegrade, or atrioventricular, conduction (**K** in **panel 3,** Fig. 8–6), while retrograde conduction takes place through the His bundle and AV node (**H** in **panel 3**). This is the **antidromic** form of reciprocating tachycardia, and because the ventricles are depolarized exclusively through the Kent bundle, the QRS complexes are wide and bizarre. This form of supraventricular tachycardia may be very difficult to distinguish from ventricular tachycardia. An example of such wide-QRS reentrant tachycardia is shown at the bottom of **panel 3,** Figure 8–6.

Between 10 and 20 per cent of patients with WPW syndrome show evidence

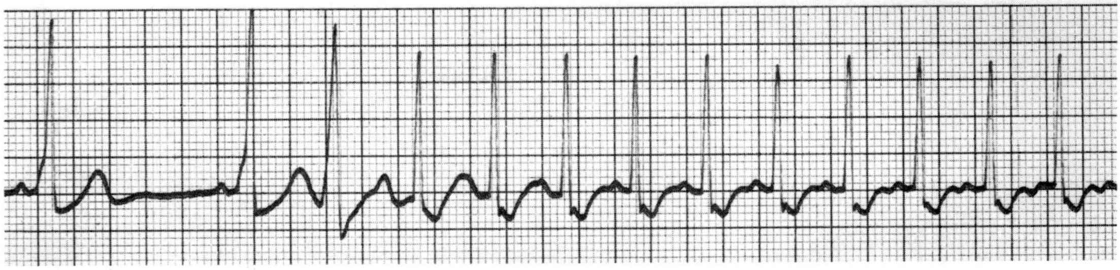

Figure 8–8. Orthodromic supraventricular tachycardia in WPW.

of concealed bypass connections. **Concealed bypass connections** (or **tracts**) refer to Kent bundles that are capable of **retrograde conduction only.** The presence of the bypass tract is therefore not manifest electrocardiographically during sinus rhythm because antegrade, or atrioventricular, conduction does not occur over it, and so overt signs of preexcitation, such as delta waves, are missing (**panel 4,** Fig. 8–6). For this reason, the QRS complex is normal and the WPW syndrome is said to be "concealed." However, during episodes of reentrant tachycardia, the bypass connection functions as the retrograde limb of the reentry circuit. Since only retrograde conduction is possible through the Kent bundle, the patient is protected from extremely rapid rates of ventricular response in the event of atrial fibrillation.

Atrial fibrillation accounts for about 15 per cent of the supraventricular arrhythmias encountered in cases of WPW syndrome. Atrial fibrillation does *not* involve reentrant conduction using the His and Kent bundles to form a circuit. Because the accessory pathway lacks the physiologically slower conduction inherent in AV nodal tissue, atrial impulses are preferentially conducted over the accessory (Kent) pathway. If conduction of fibrillation impulses occurs predominantly or exclusively over the anomalous path, extremely rapid rates of ventricular response can result; cases with ventricular rates of 300 per minute or more have been documented. At such high rates, ventricular electrical activity may become disorganized and ventricular fibrillation may supervene. A case of WPW with atrial fibrillation is shown in Figure 8–9. The widened complexes result from conduction of fibrillation impulses over the accessory pathway; the narrow complexes are conducted over the normal path.

Management of tachyarrhythmias

The location of accessory connections can now be determined in many cases by electrophysiologic studies (EPS), and the conduction properties of the anomalous path(s) can be evaluated in the laboratory. Sometimes arrhythmias can be induced in the EPS lab and the effects of antiarrhythmic therapy evaluated.

The pharmacologic management of WPW employs a number of agents. Beta-adrenergic blockers predominantly affect AV nodal conduction, having little or no effect on the conduction properties of the accessory pathway. Cal-

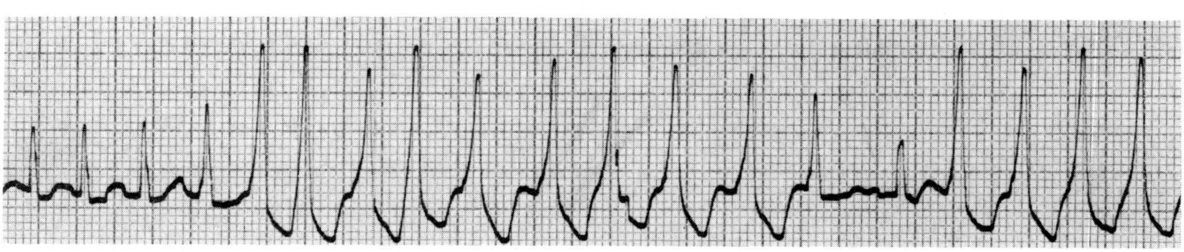

Figure 8–9. Orthodromic and antidromic conduction during atrial fibrillation.

cium channel blockers, such as verapamil, have been shown to be moderately effective therapy. Digitalis, on the other hand, may enhance conduction through the accessory tract and is therefore contraindicated in the treatment of atrial fibrillation and flutter in patients with WPW. Neither digoxin nor verapamil should be used if wide-QRS tachycardia is present. Occasionally intravenous lidocaine is used to break antidromic tachycardia, but in any case in which cardiovascular decompensation is occurring because of rapid heart rate, cardioversion is the treatment of choice.

Drugs that depress conduction in the anomalous pathway by increasing its refractory period are generally considered useful in the treatment of reciprocating tachycardia or recurrent atrial fibrillation, or both. Included is the quinidine family of drugs, notably quinidine and procainamide. More recently approved agents such as encainide and amiodarone affect the refractory period of both the normal and accessory pathways.

Other, nonpharmacologic, therapies include pacemaker insertion and surgical ablation of the accessory tract. In those patients who present in ventricular fibrillation or hemodynamic collapse due to an extremely rapid ventricular response to atrial fibrillation, immediate cardioversion should be done.

Risk stratification

Since the short refractory period of the accessory pathway can sometimes lead to very high rates of ventricular response to atrial fibrillation in patients with WPW, identification of those at risk for this development is obviously highly desirable. This can sometimes be accomplished by using simple, noninvasive maneuvers and observations, including:

1. Identification of intermittent preexcitation
2. Identification of preexcitation that disappears during exercise
3. Identification of complete antegrade block in the accessory pathway (normalization of the QRS complex) following the intravenous injection of ajmaline or procainamide

A positive response to any of these tests or observations implies that the patient may have a Kent bundle with a relatively long refractory period and is therefore probably *not* at great risk for developing dangerously fast ventricular rates in response to atrial fibrillation. Patients in whom preexcitation is a permanent feature, in whom preexcitation does not disappear in response to exercise, or who fail to exhibit normalization of the QRS complex when given intravenous ajmaline are at greater risk for developing high ventricular rates during atrial fibrillation and will probably benefit from more precise risk stratification and study using EPS techniques.

References

Anderson, RH, et al. **Eur J Cardiol** 3:27–36, 1975.

Burch, GE, and DePasquale, NP. **Electrocardiography in the Diagnosis of Congenital Heart Disease.** Lea & Febiger, Philadelphia, 1967, pp 425, 476, 522, 584.

Coumel, P, and Attuel, P. **Eur J Cardiol** 1:423–436, 1974.
Gallagher, JJ, et al. **Circulation** 64:176–189, 1981.
Goldberger, AL. **Myocardial Infarction, Electrocardiographic Differential Diagnosis,** 2nd ed. CV Mosby, St. Louis, 1979, pp 87–90.
Krikler, DM. **In** Krikler, DM, and Goodwin, JF (eds). **Cardiac Arrhythmias, The Modern Electrophysiologic Approach.** WB Saunders, Philadelphia, 1975, pp 144–161.
Lazarra, R. **In** Helfant, RH (ed). **Essentials of Cardiac Arrhythmias.** WB Saunders, Philadelphia, 1979, pp 182–196.
Lev, Maurice, et al. **Am J Cardiol** 36:880–888, 1975.
Marriott, HJL. **Practical Electrocardiography.** 7th ed. Williams & Wilkins, Baltimore, 1983, pp 256–275.
Ohnell, RF. **Acta Med Scand** 152:74ff, 1944.
Pick, A, and Langendorf, R. **Interpretation of Complex Arrhythmias.** Lea & Febiger, Philadelphia, 1979, pp 410–470.
Rigby, WFC, and Graboys, TB. **J Cardiovasc Med** 6:277–293, 1981.
Rosenbaum, F.F., et al. **Am Heart J** 29:281, 1945.
Schamroth, L. **The Disorders of the Cardiac Rhythm.** 2nd ed. Vol. I. Blackwell Scientific Publications, Oxford, 1980, pp 250–271.
Ward, D.E., and Camm, J. **Am Heart J** 105:169–175, 1983.
Wellens, HJJ, et al. **In** Mandel, WJ (ed). **Cardiac Arrhythmias, Their Mechanisms, Diagnosis and Management.** JB Lippincott, Philadelphia, 1980, pp 342–365.
Wolff, L, et al. **Am Heart J** 5:685ff, 1930.
Wood, FC, et al. **Am Heart J** 252:454ff, 1943.

SELF-ASSESSMENT

Multiple Choice

1. Atrioventricular connections that directly connect the atrial myocardium to the ventricular myocardium are called:

   a. Mahaim fibers.
   b. annulus fibrosus.
   c. James fibers.
   d. Kent bundles.

2. The anatomical substrate for the Wolff-Parkinson-White syndrome is:

   a. the Lev tract.
   b. the Kent bundle.
   c. the James fiber.
   d. the Mahaim fiber.

3. The classic ECG features of the WPW syndrome include:

   a. a short PR interval, a delta wave, and a normal QRS complex.
   b. a short PR interval, a delta wave, and a wide QRS complex.
   c. a normal PR interval, no delta wave, and a normal QRS complex.
   d. a short PR interval, no delta wave, and a normal QRS complex.

4. The WPW syndrome is of importance because of the frequent presence of:

   a. ventricular preexcitation.
   b. a high incidence of myocardial infarction and bundle branch block.
   c. a high incidence of tachyarrhythmias.
   d. a very high incidence of sudden cardiac death.

5. The diagnosis of WPW syndrome may be difficult if:

   a. preexcitation is intermittent.
   b. the degree of preexcitation is minimal.
   c. the preexcitation is concealed.
   d. all of the above.

6. Type A WPW syndrome as described by Rosenbaum is characterized by:

   a. predominantly positive QRS deflections in leads V1 and V2.
   b. only positive delta waves in leads V1 and V2.
   c. only negative delta waves in leads V1 and V2.
   d. predominantly negative QRS deflections in leads V1 and V2.

7. The ECG findings of WPW syndrome may closely mimic:

a. myocardial infarction.
b. bundle branch block.
c. right ventricular hypertrophy.
d. all of the above.

8. Reciprocal tachycardia characterized by narrow QRS complexes and retrograde P waves is referred to as:

a. orthodromic tachycardia.
b. paroxysmal supraventricular tachycardia.
c. antidromic tachycardia.
d. the concertina effect.

9. In cases of antidromic tachycardia:

a. the Kent bundle is used for antegrade conduction.
b. the His bundle was used for antegrade conduction.
c. the Kent bundle is used for retrograde conduction.
d. the James fiber is used for retrograde conduction.

10. Concealed bypass connections refer to:

a. Kent bundles capable of antegrade conduction only.
b. His bundles capable of retrograde conduction only.
c. Kent bundles capable of retrograde conduction only.
d. His bundles capable of antegrade conduction only.

11. In cases of antidromic reciprocating tachycardia, the ventricles are depolarized exclusively by means of:

a. the bundle of His.
b. the left bundle branch.
c. the right bundle branch.
d. the Kent bundle.

12. If conduction of atrial fibrillation impulses to the ventricles occurs exclusively or predominantly over an anomalous pathway:

a. a narrow QRS supraventricular tachycardia results.
b. ventricular tachycardia supervenes.
c. rates of ventricular response exceeding 300 beats per minute may be encountered.
d. an orthodromic tachycardia occurs, which must be interrupted by prompt cardioversion.

Practice Strips

Identify the mean QRS axis, abnormalities of transition, voltage and R wave progression, fascicular and bundle branch blocks, infarctions by involved segment, pericarditis, early repolarization, chamber enlargement, and WPW syndrome. When possible the authors have indicated the probable site of the anomalous pathway using the polarity of the delta waves in leads I, III, V1, and V6, as illustrated in Figure 8–5.

8-1.

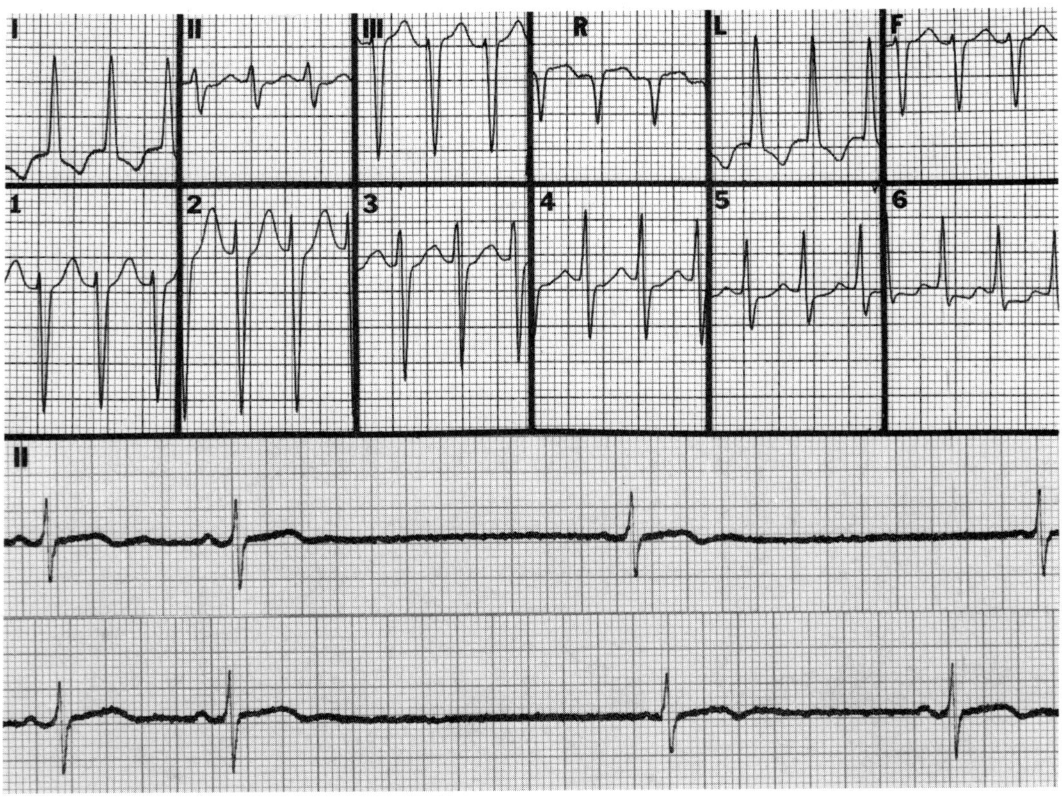

8-2.

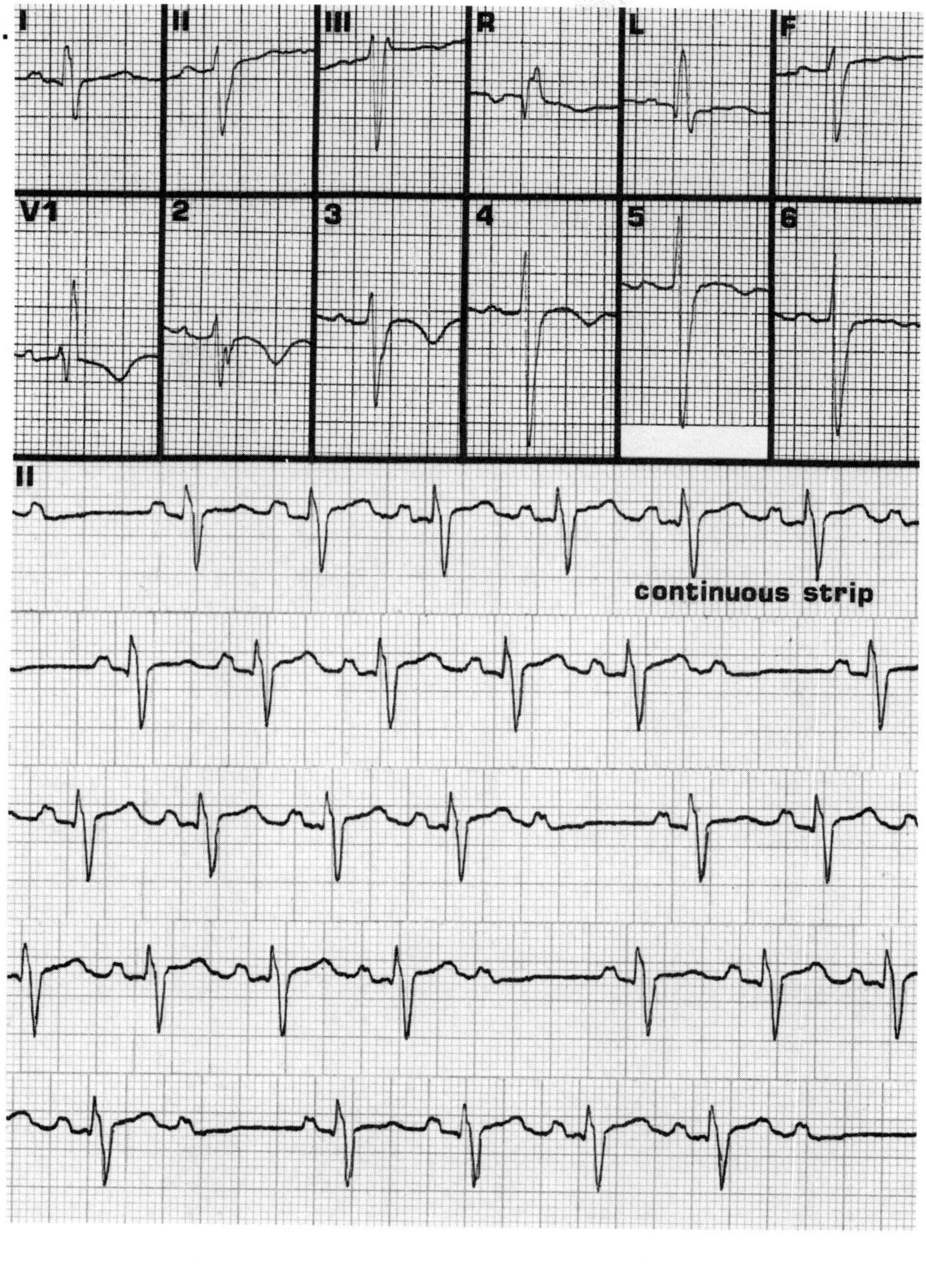

8-3.

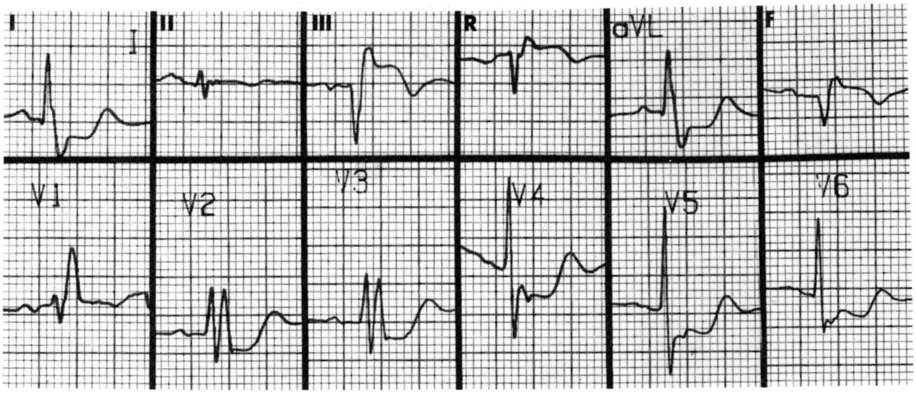

8-4.

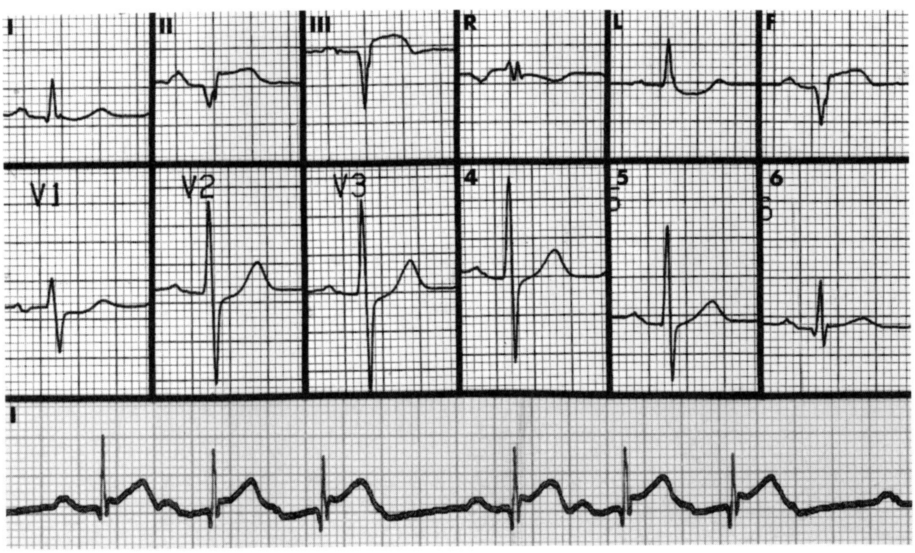

8-5.

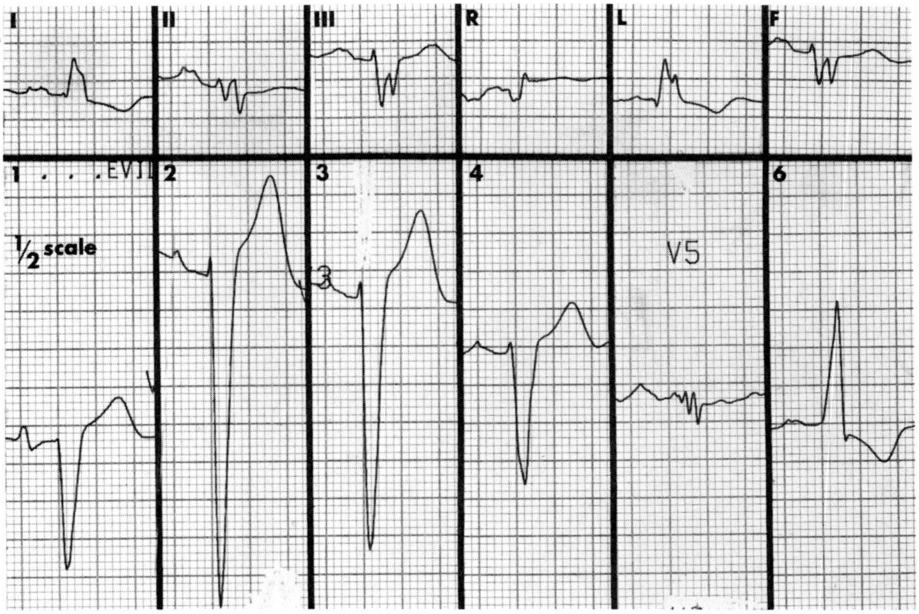
I
II
III
R
L
F
1 . . . .EVJI
2
3
4
6
½ scale
V5

8-6.

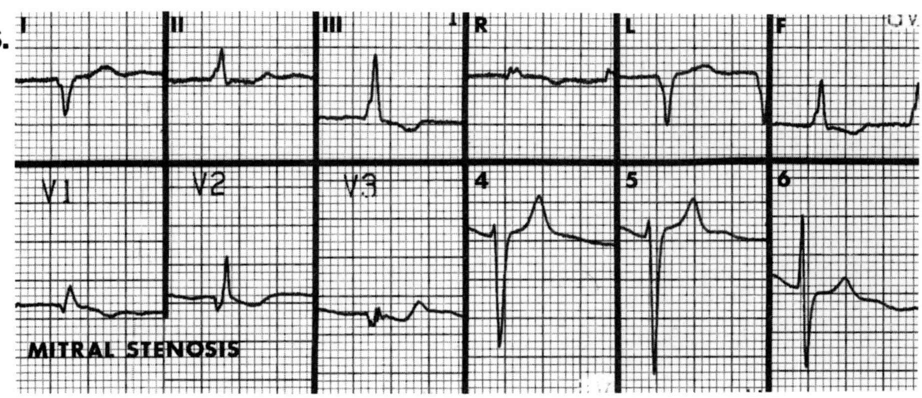
I
II
III
R
L
F
V1
V2
V3
4
5
6
MITRAL STENOSIS

8-7.

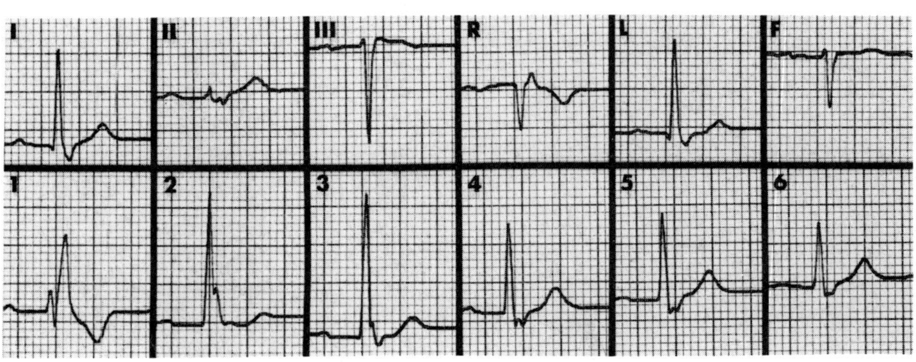
I
II
III
R
L
F
1
2
3
4
5
6

8-8.

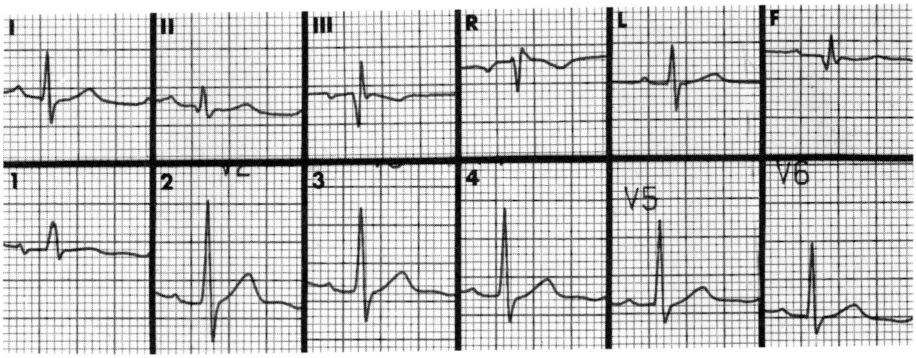
I
II
III
R
L
F
1
2
3
4
V5
V6

8-9.

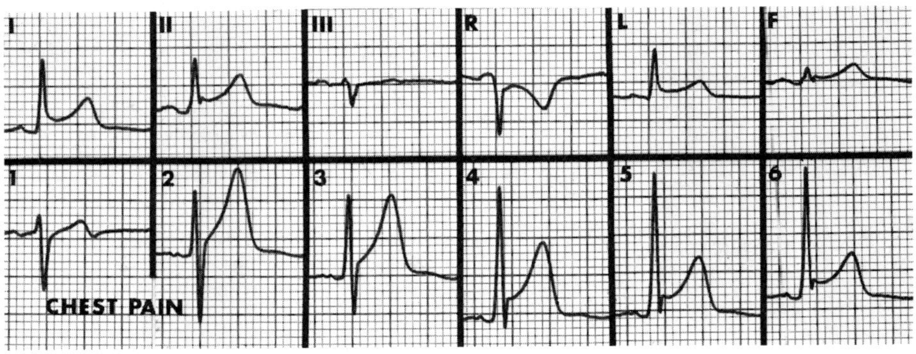
I
II
III
R
L
F
1
2
3
4
5
6
CHEST PAIN

8-10.

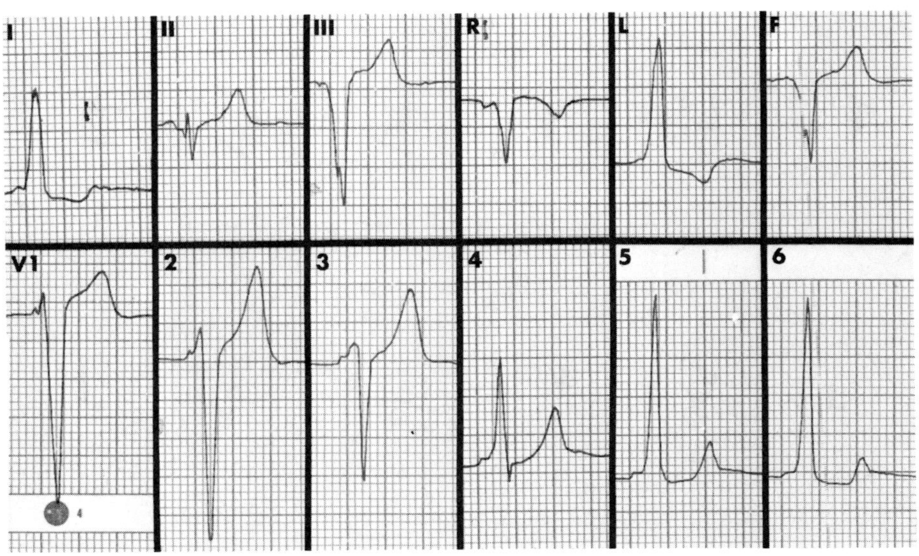
I
II
III
R
L
F
V1
2
3
4
5
6

8·11.

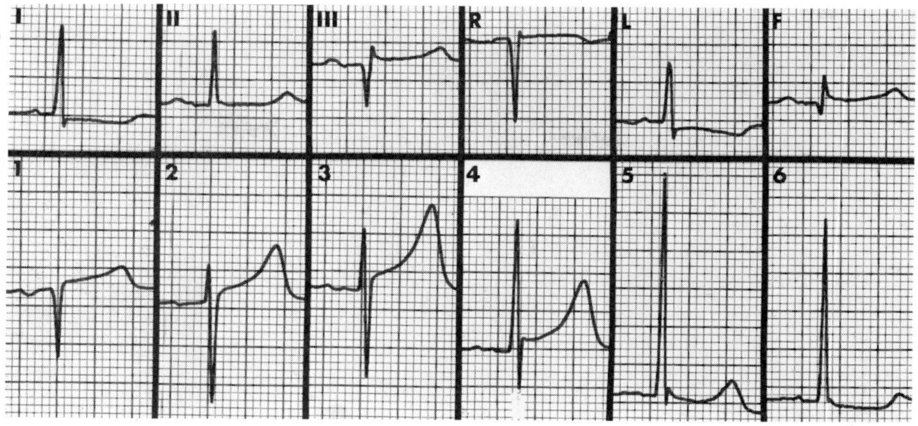
I
II
III
R
L
F
1
2
3
4
5
6

8·12.

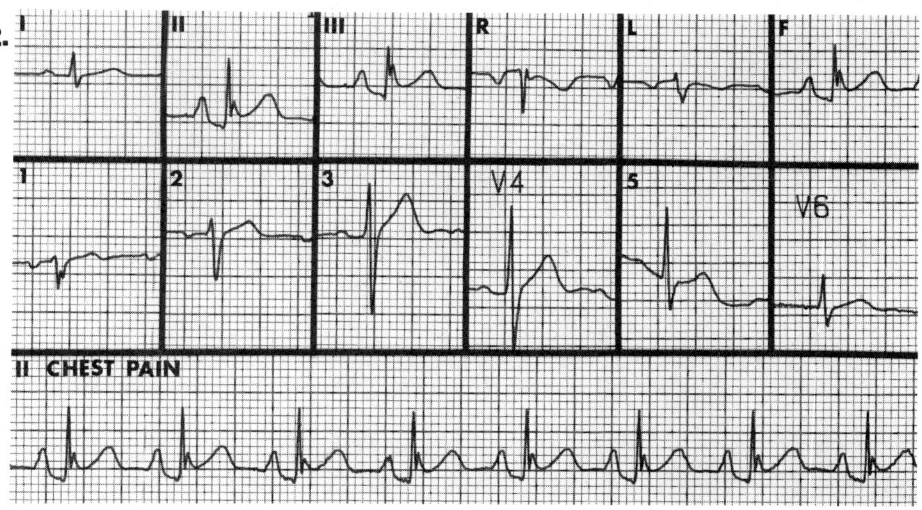
I
II
III
R
L
F
1
2
3
V4
5
V6
II CHEST PAIN

8·13.

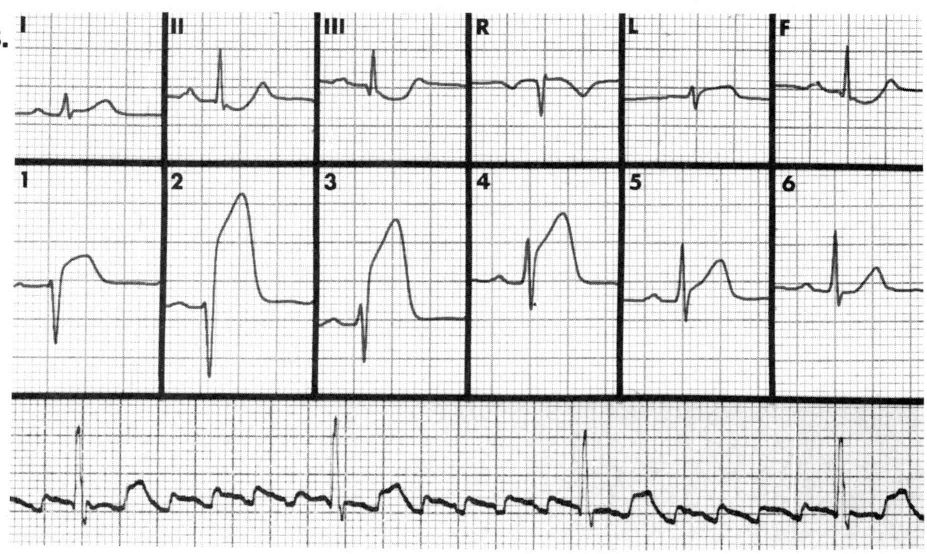
I
II
III
R
L
F
1
2
3
4
5
6

8-14.

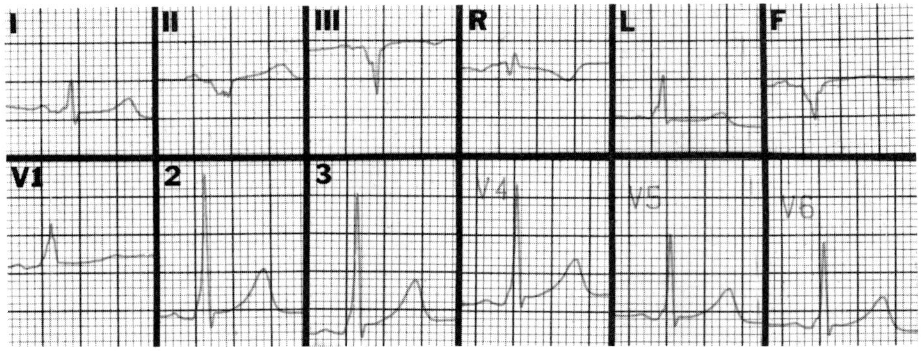
I
II
III
R
L
F
V1
2
3
V4
V5
V6

8-15.

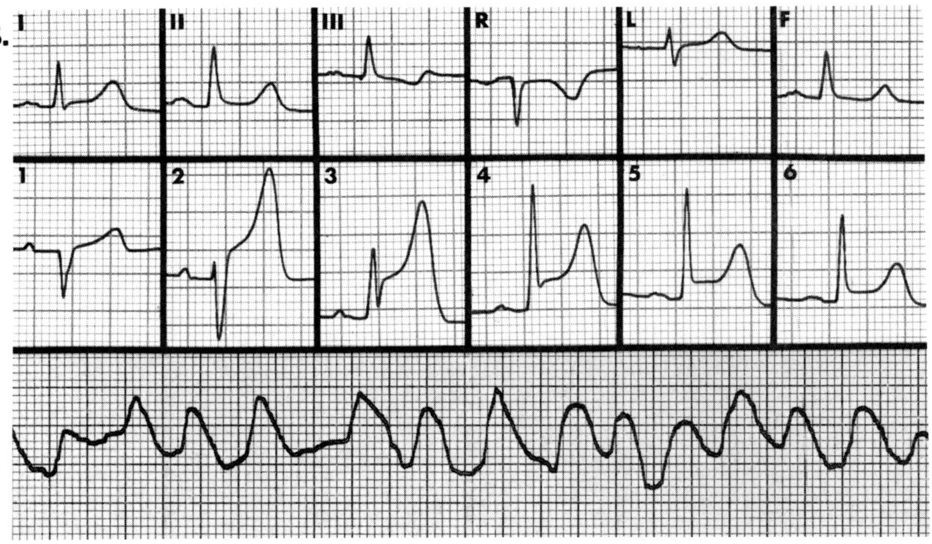
I
II
III
R
L
F
1
2
3
4
5
6

8-16.

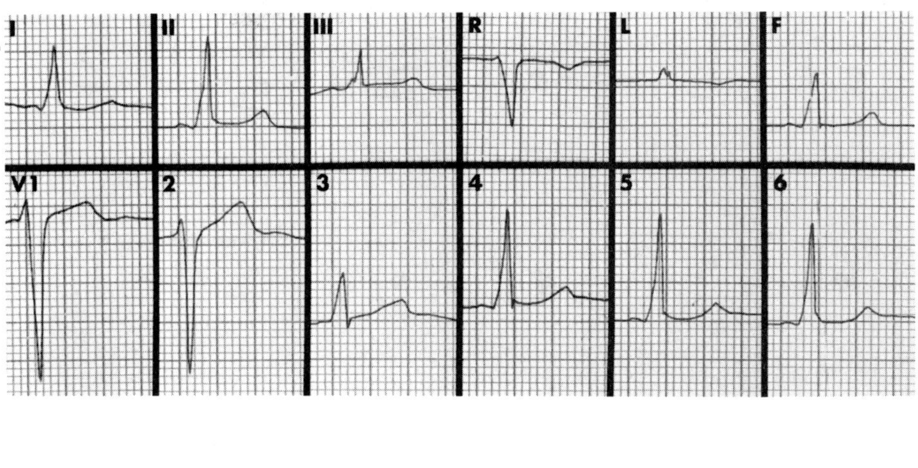
I
II
III
R
L
F
V1
2
3
4
5
6

8-17.

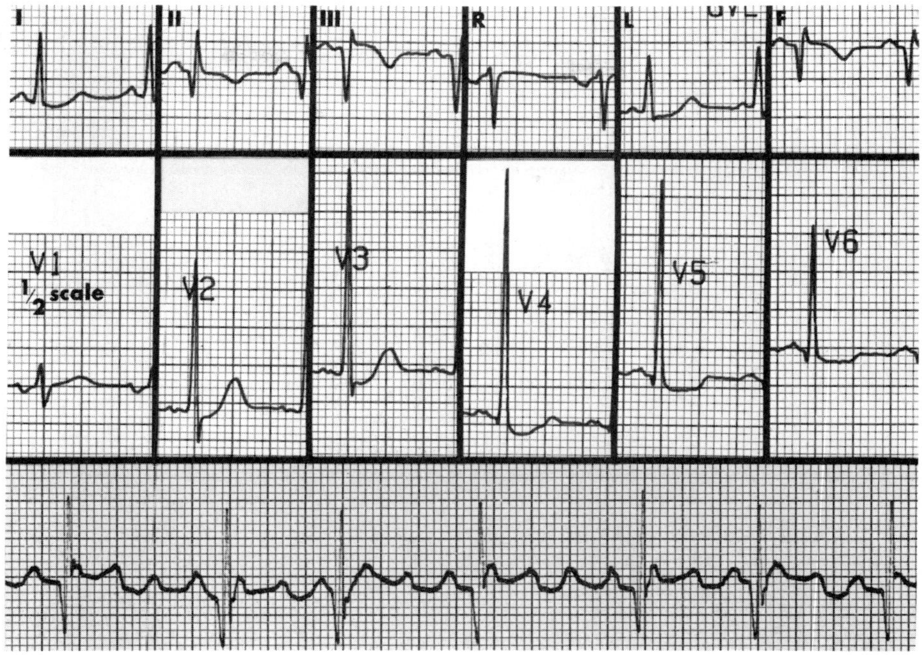

8-18.

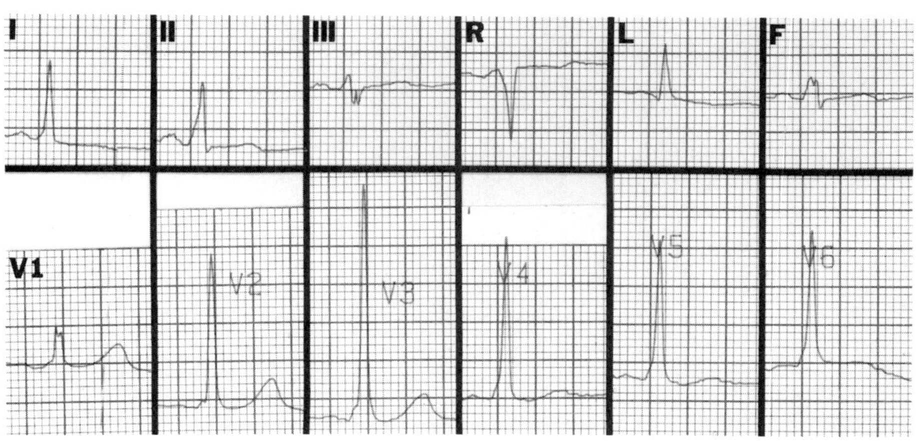

8-19.

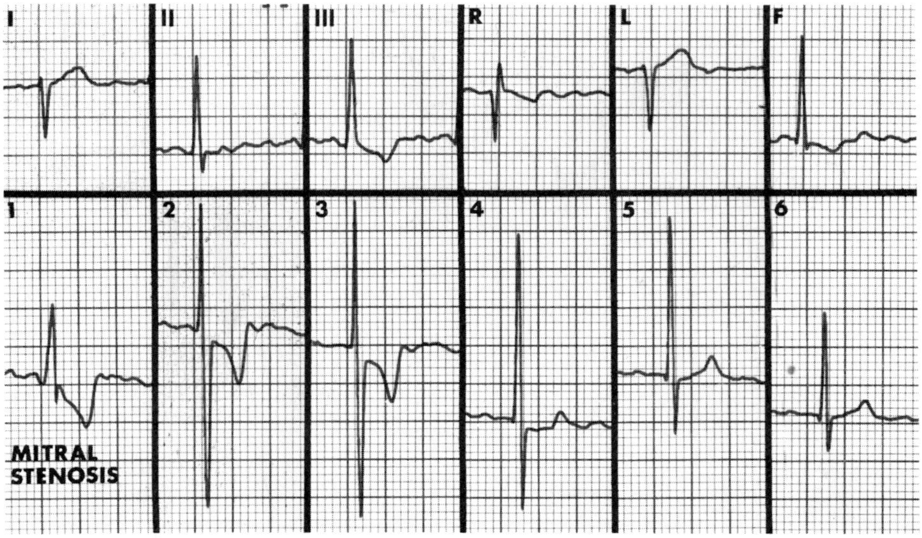

8-20.

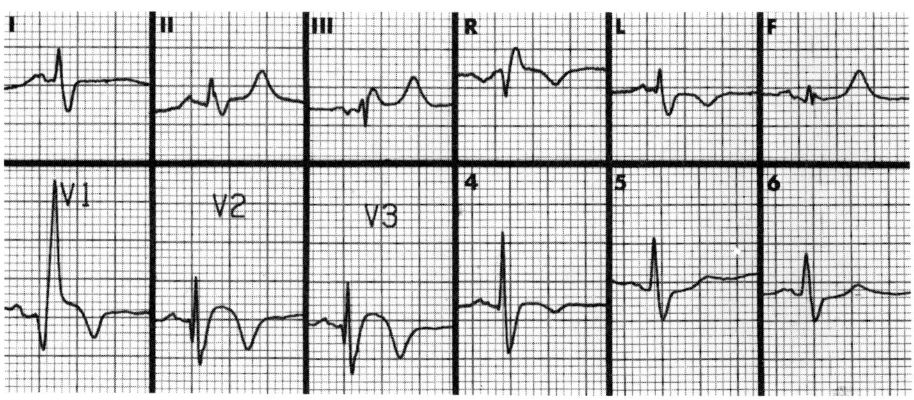

8-21.

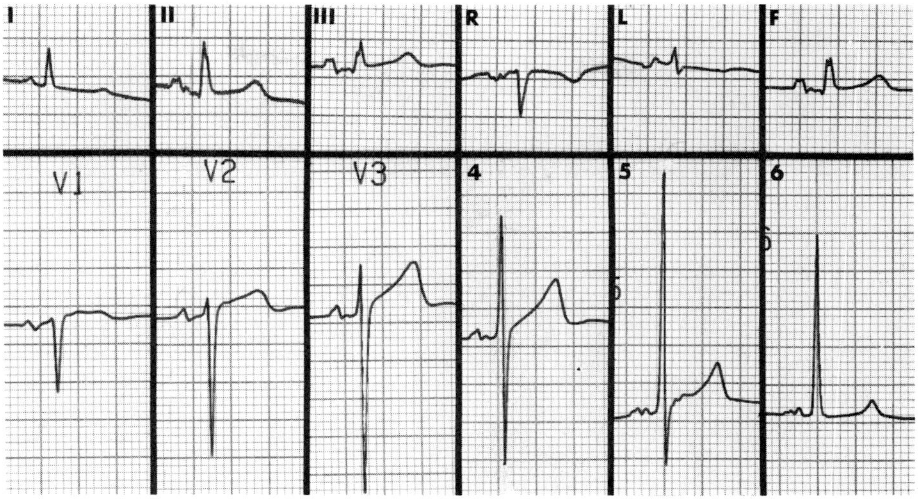

8-22.

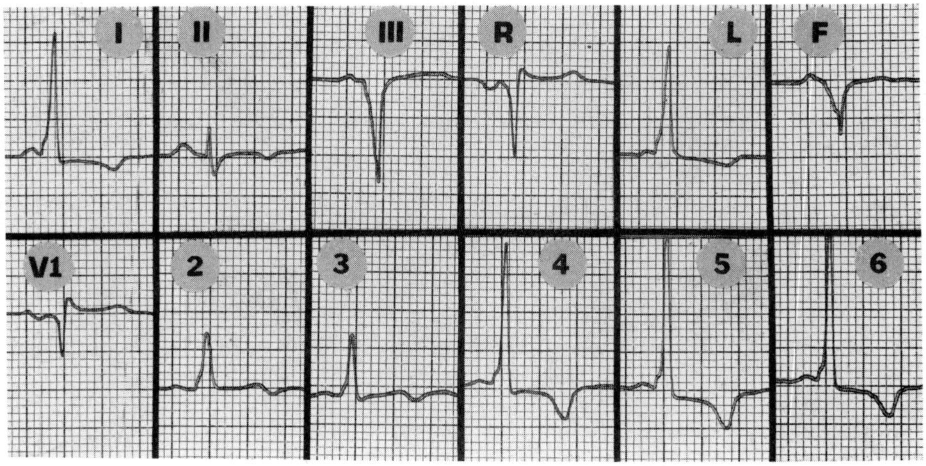

8-23.

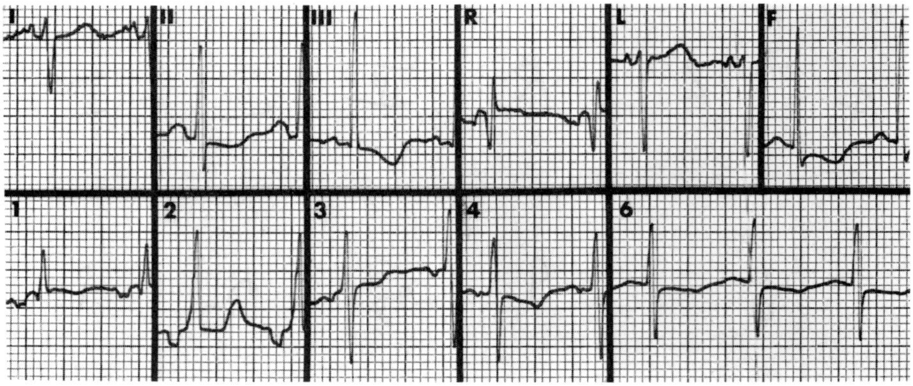

8-24.

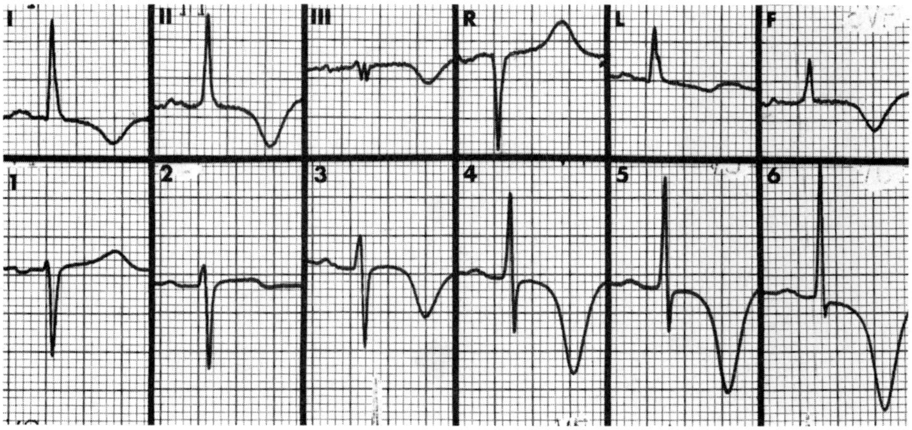

8-25.

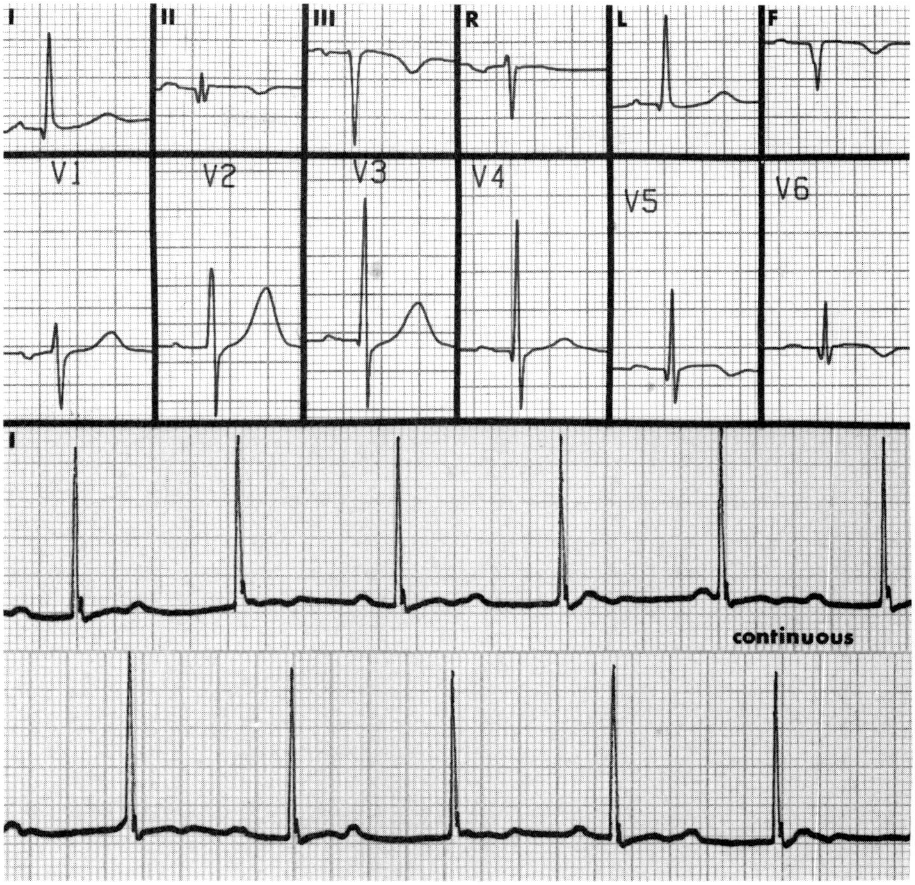

8-26.

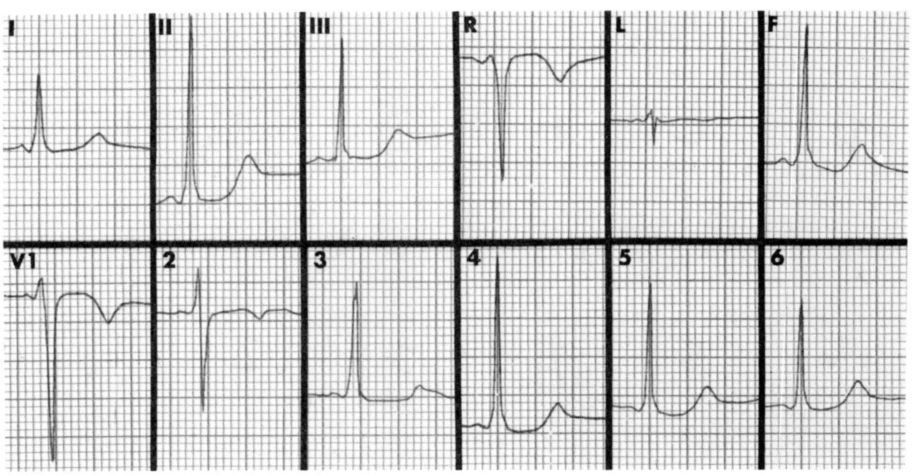

8-27.

8/2 12:47am

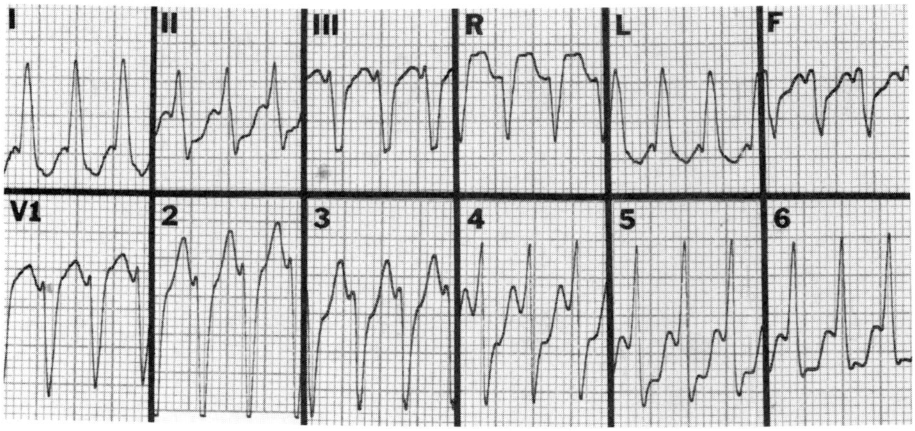

8/2 12:50 pm

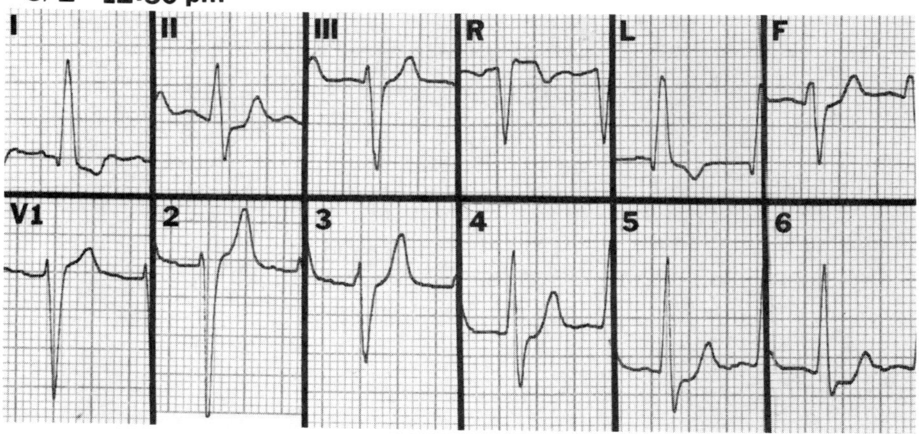

8/3 5:53 am

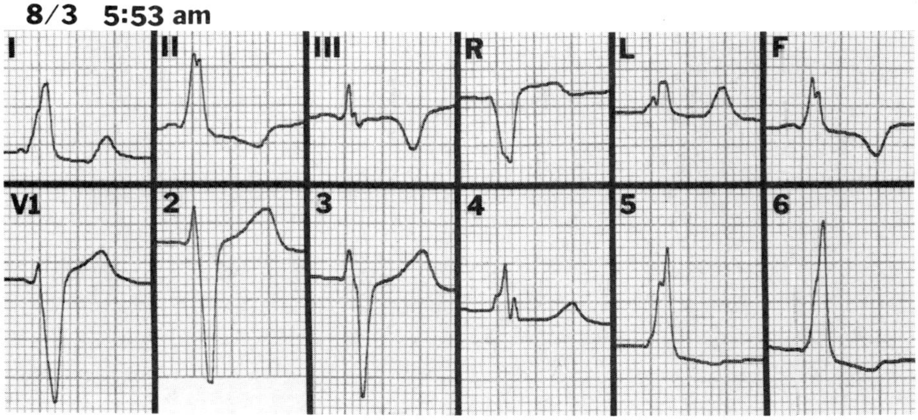

8-28.

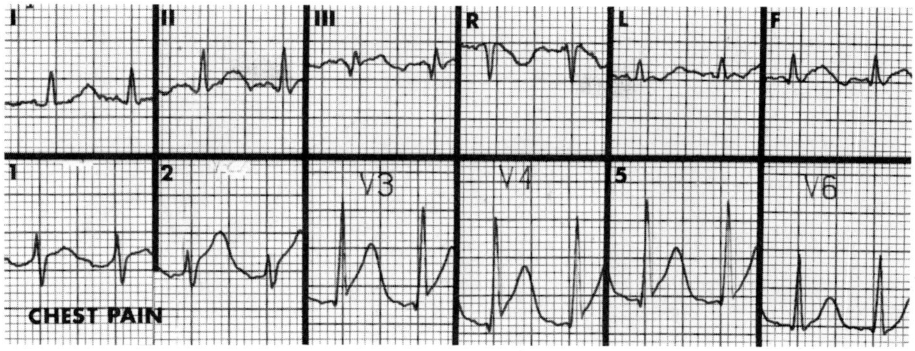
I
II
III
R
L
F
1
2
V3
V4
5
V6
CHEST PAIN

8-29.

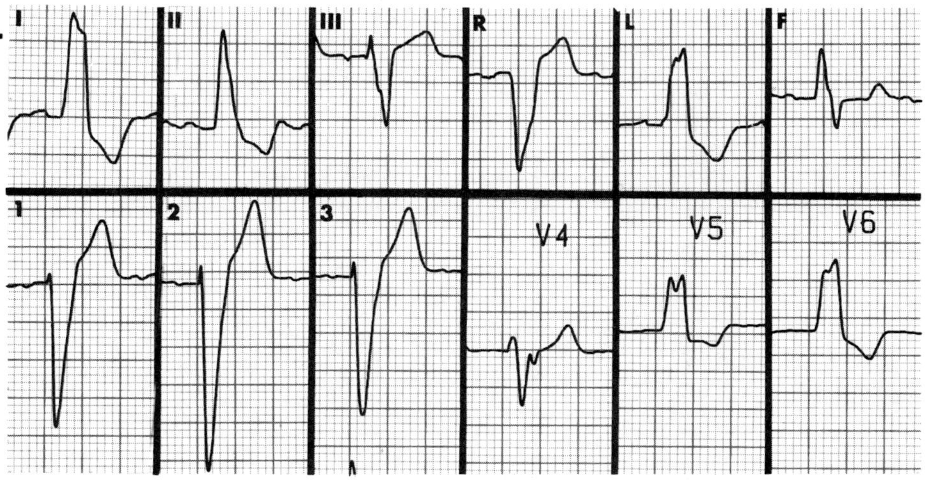
I
II
III
R
L
F
1
2
3
V4
V5
V6

8-30.

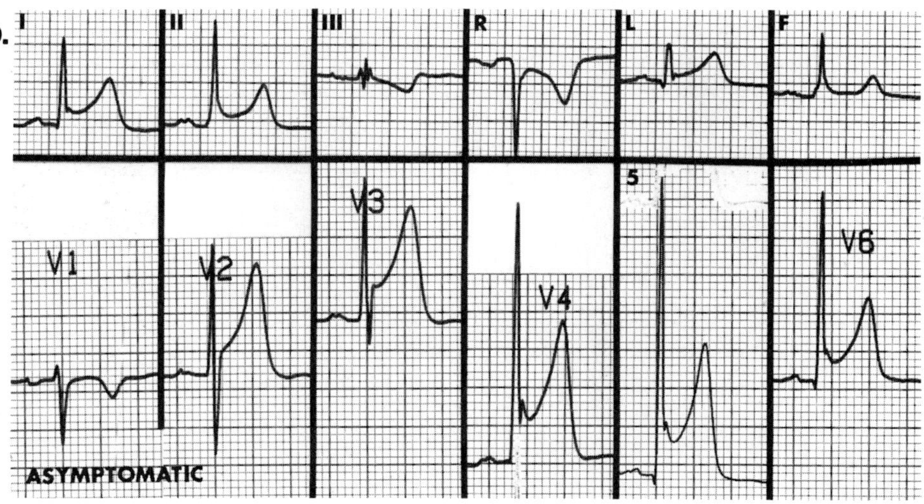
I
II
III
R
L
F
V1
V2
V3
V4
5
V6
ASYMPTOMATIC

8-31.

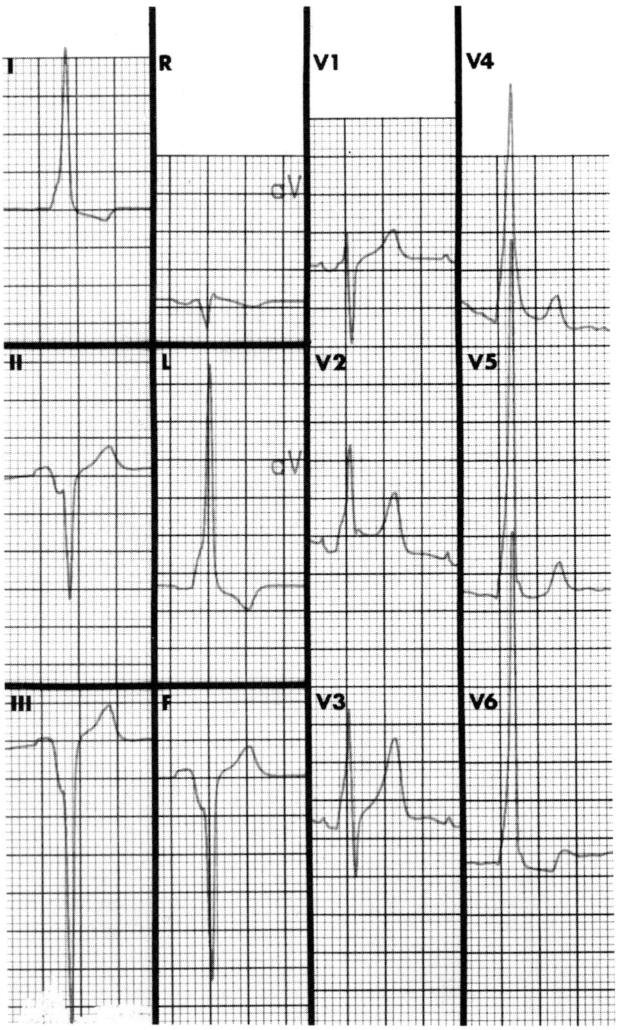

8-32.

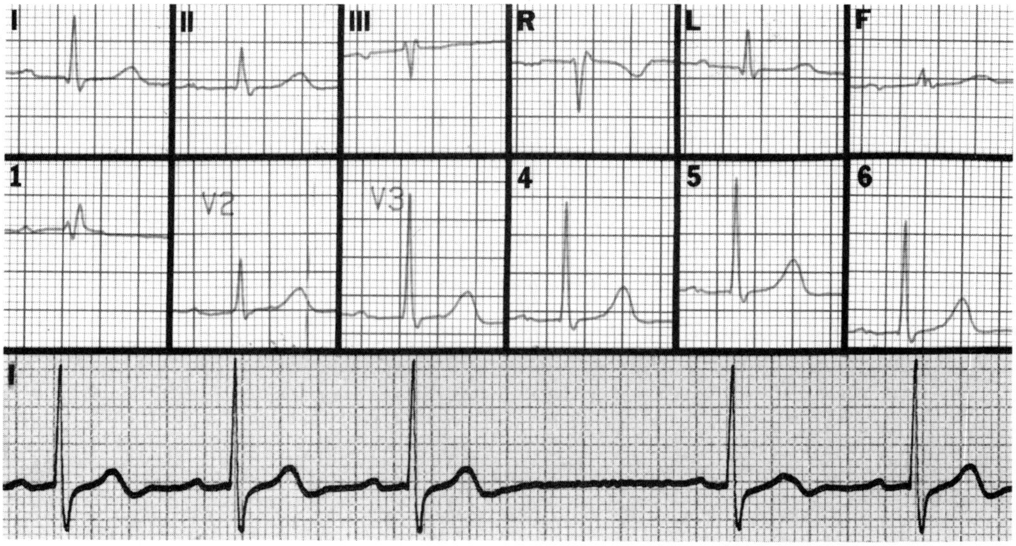

8-33.

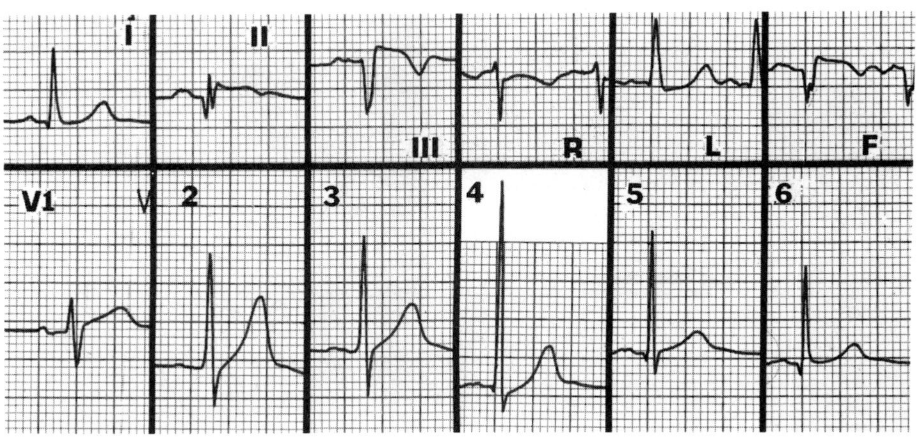

8-34.

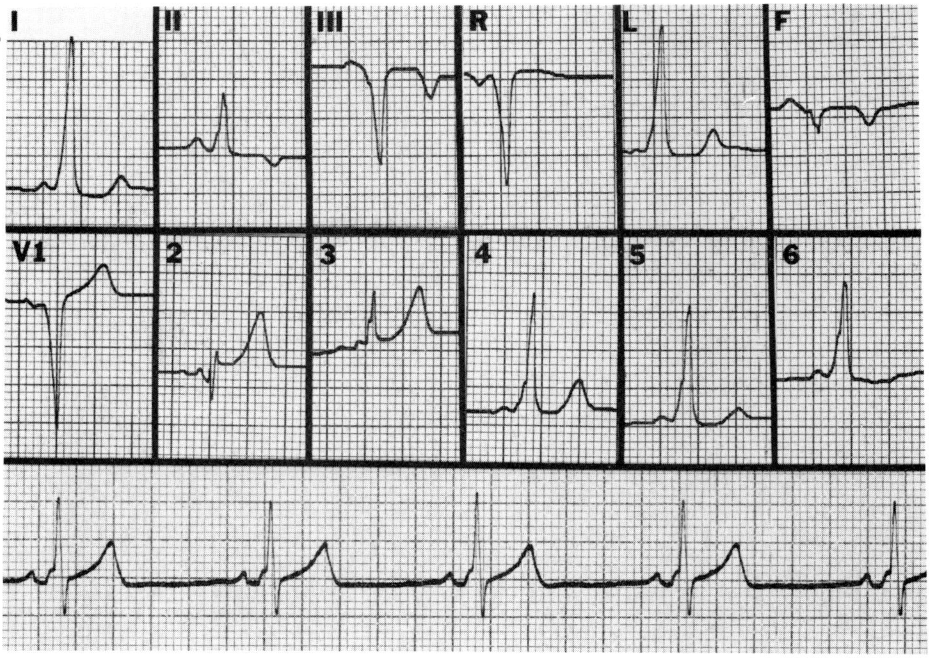

8-35.

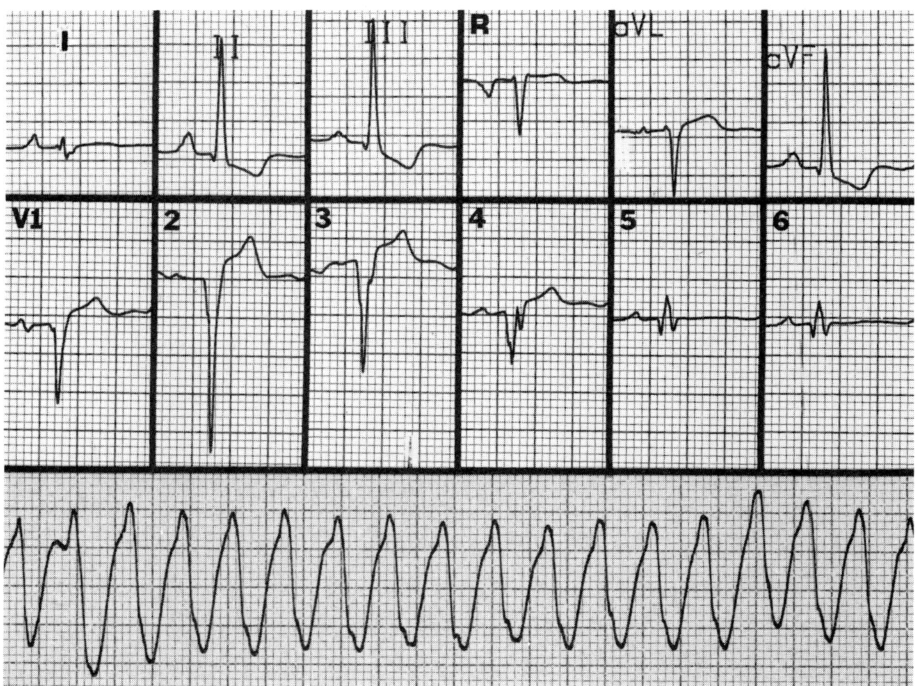

8-36.

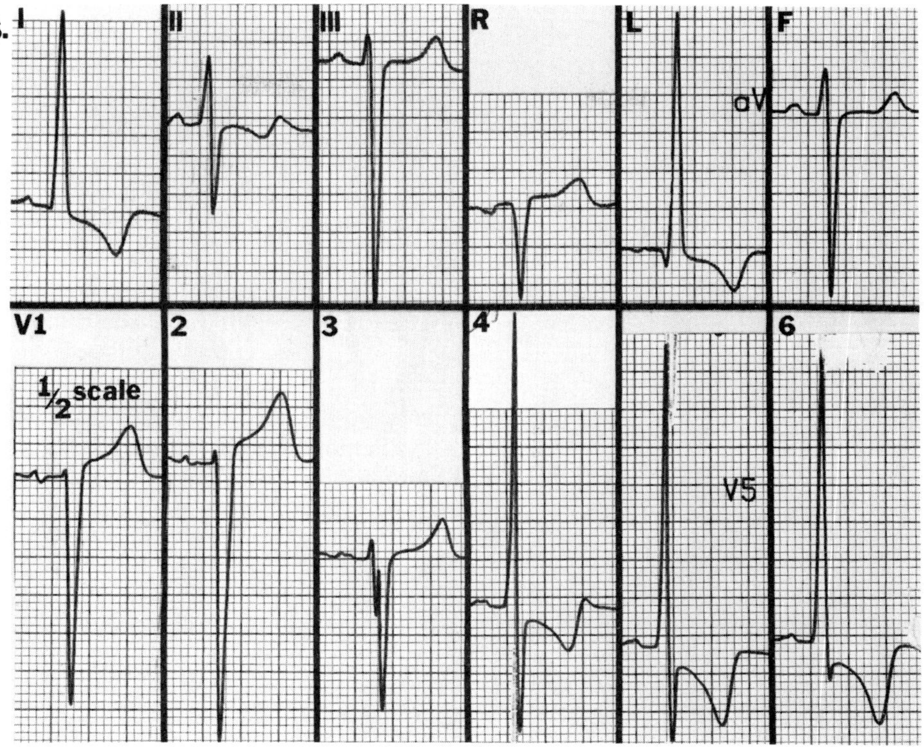

8-37.

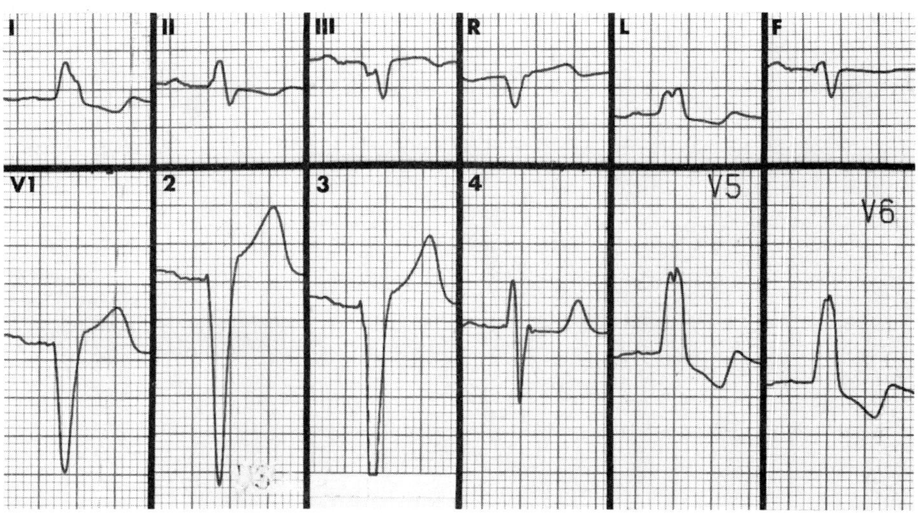

8-38.

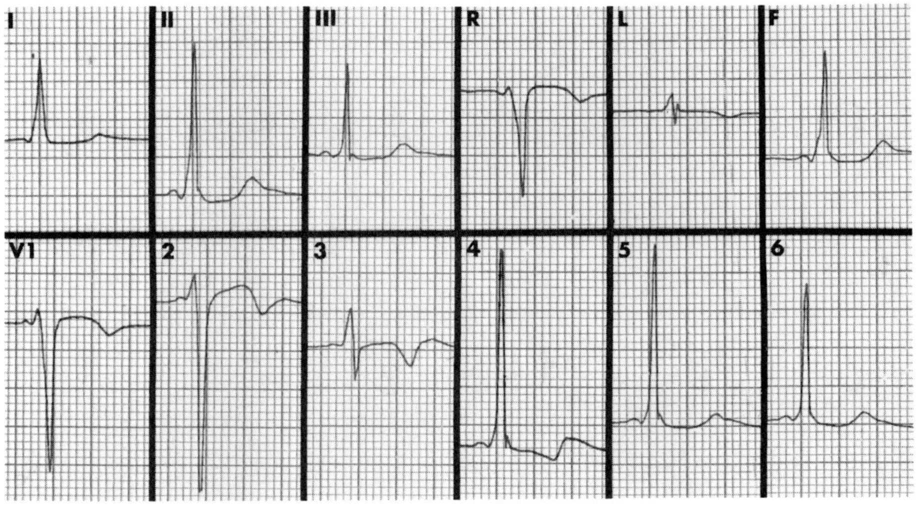

8-39.

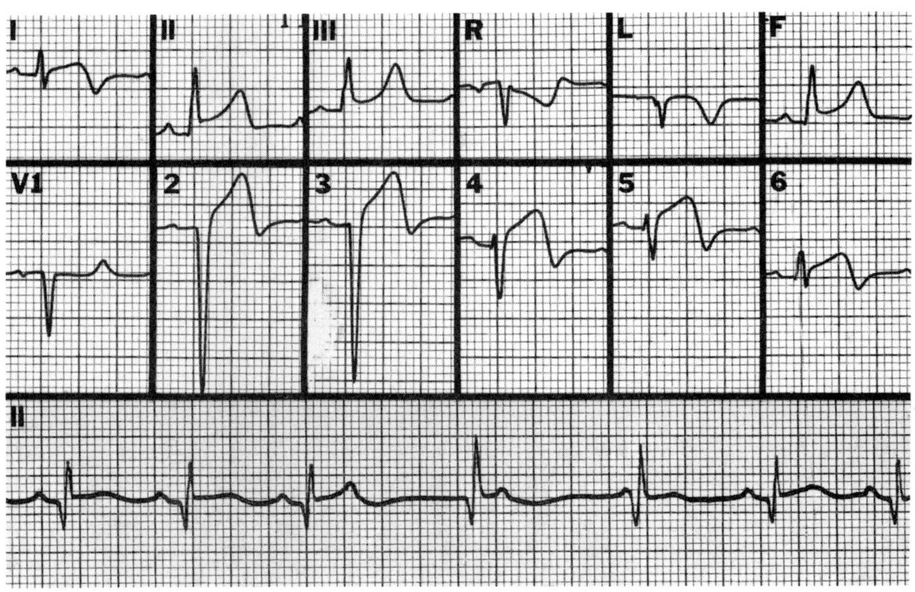

8-40.

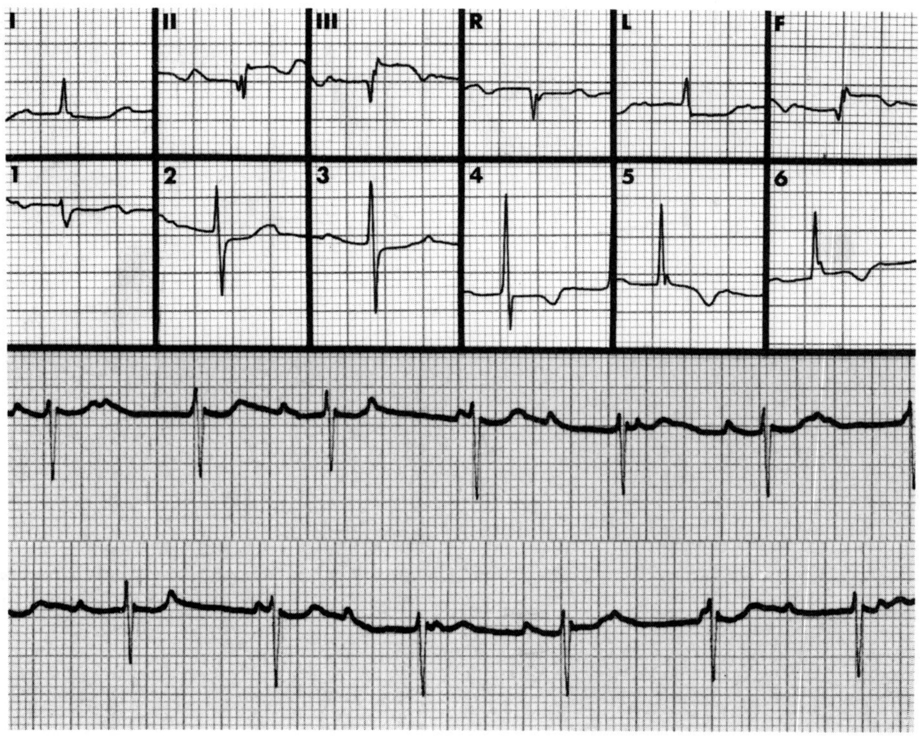

8-41.

3:31 pm

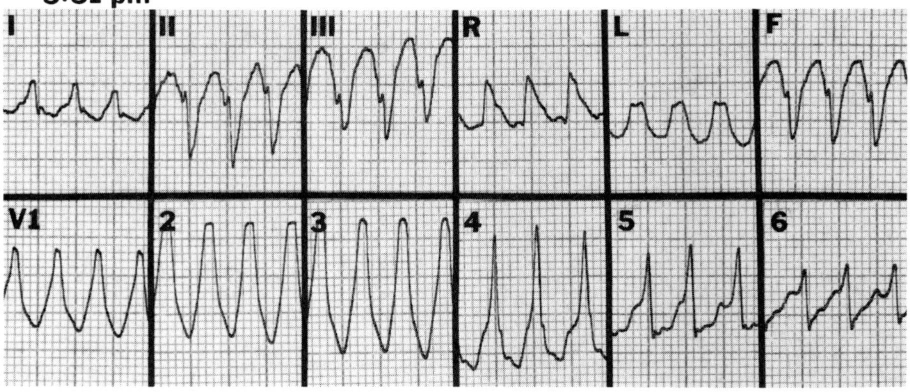

5:18 pm

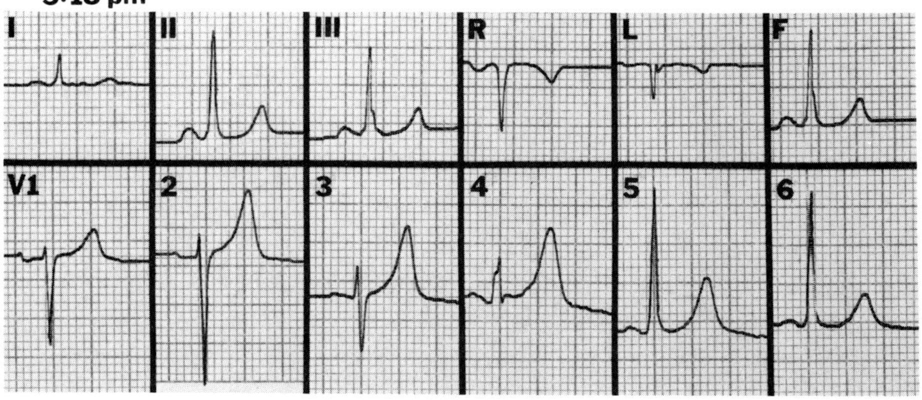

8-42.

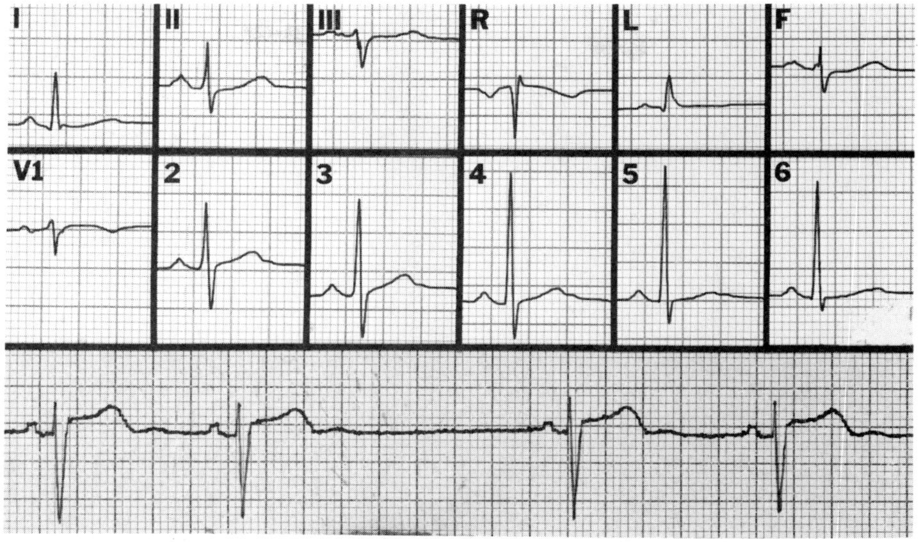

8-43.

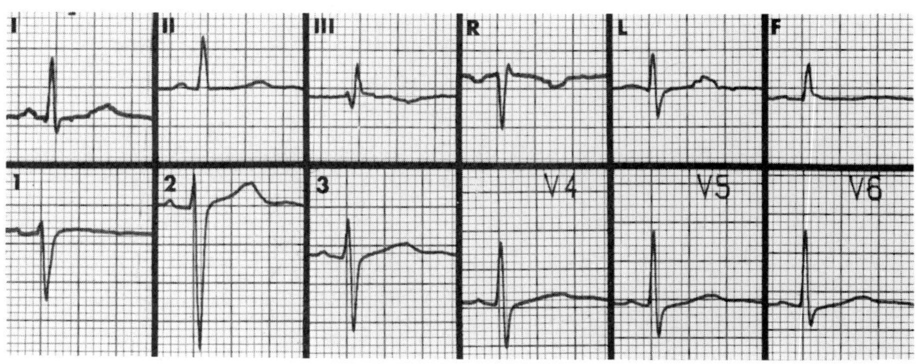

8-44.

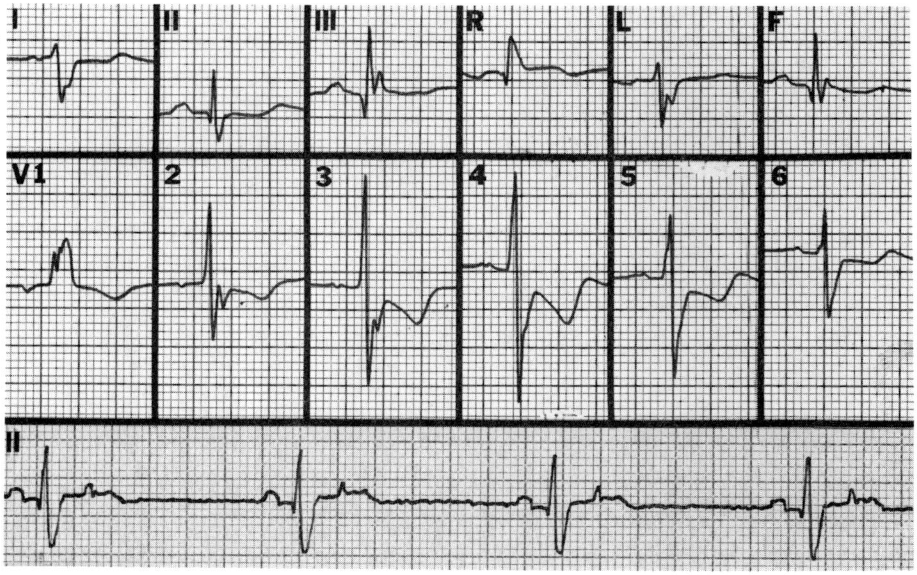
I
II
III
R
L
F
V1
2
3
4
5
6
II

8-45.

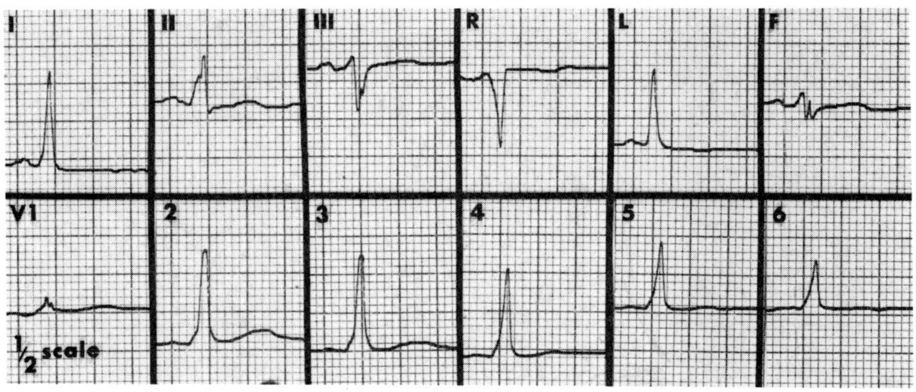
I
II
III
R
L
F
V1
2
3
4
5
6
½ scale

8-46.

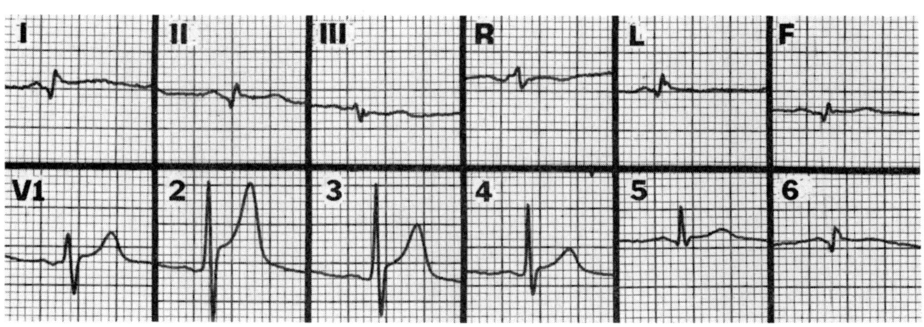
I
II
III
R
L
F
V1
2
3
4
5
6

8-47.

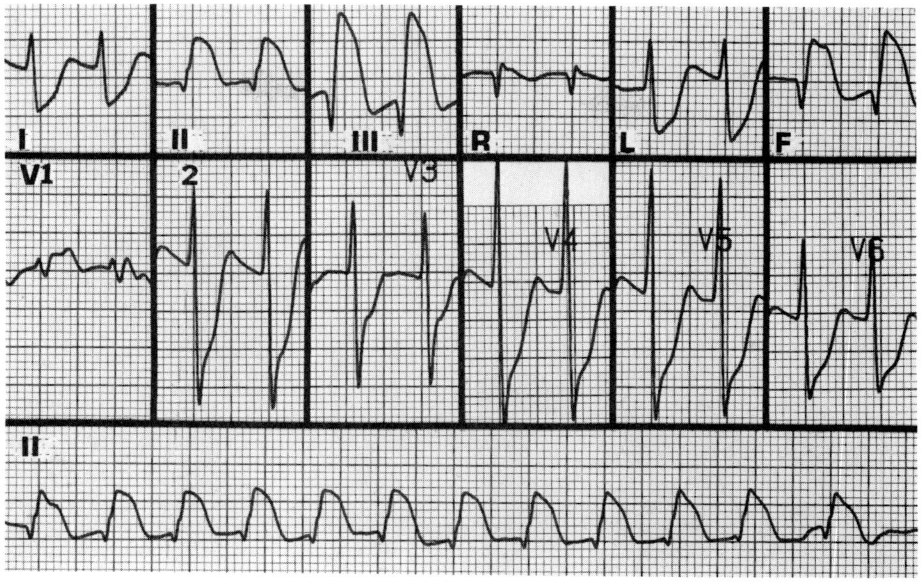

8-48.

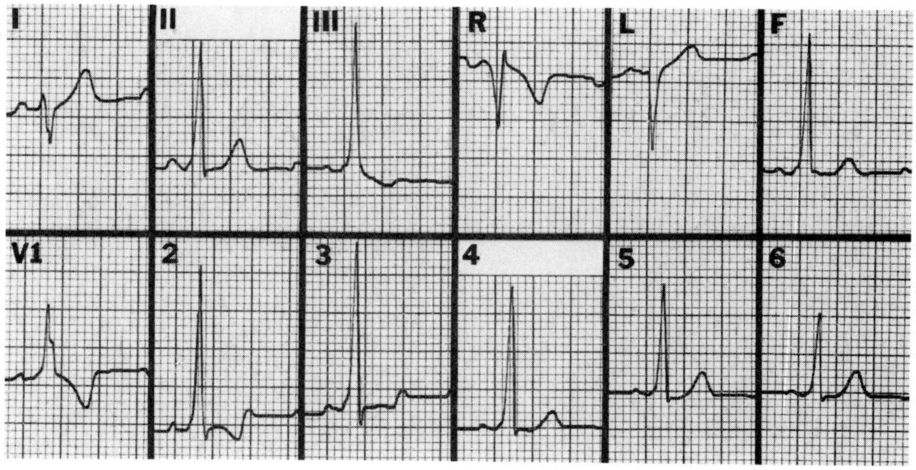

3:14 am

8-49.

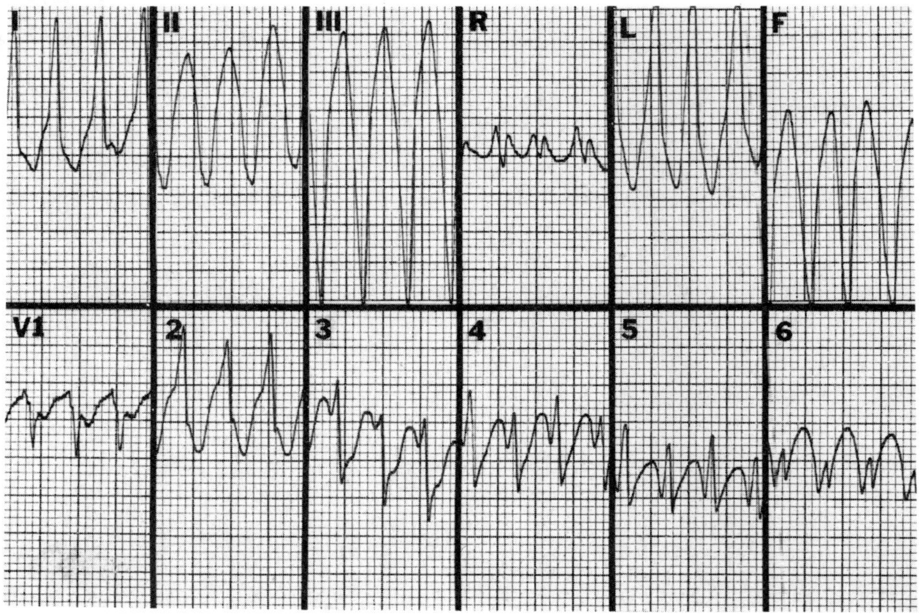

4:34 am

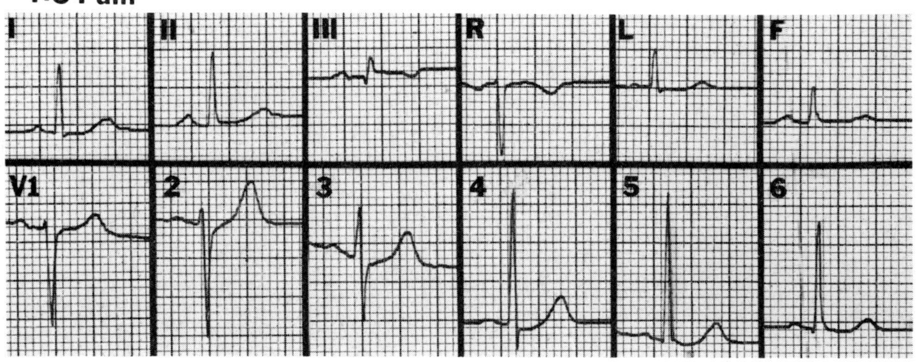

8-50.

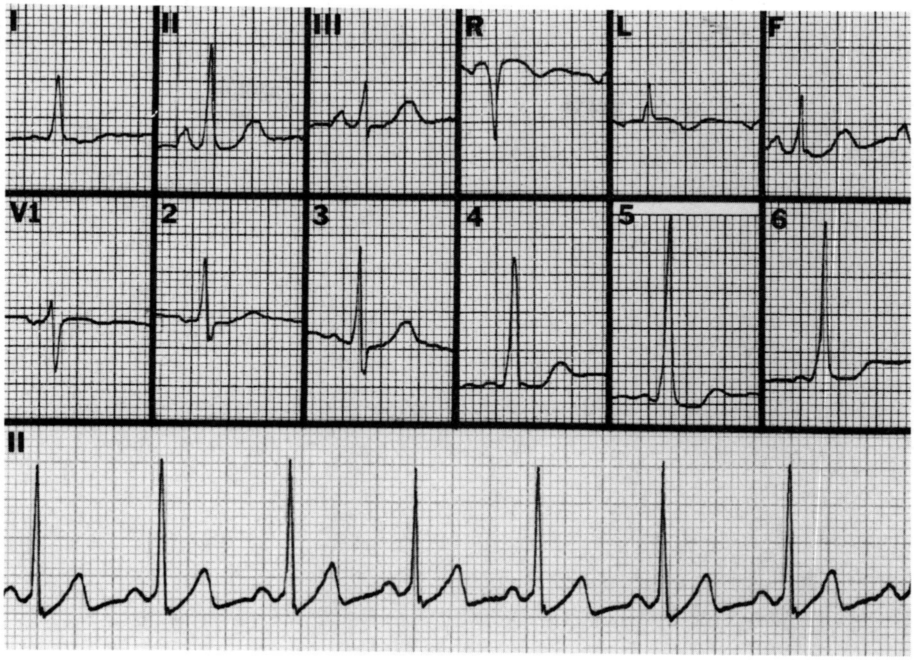

8-51.

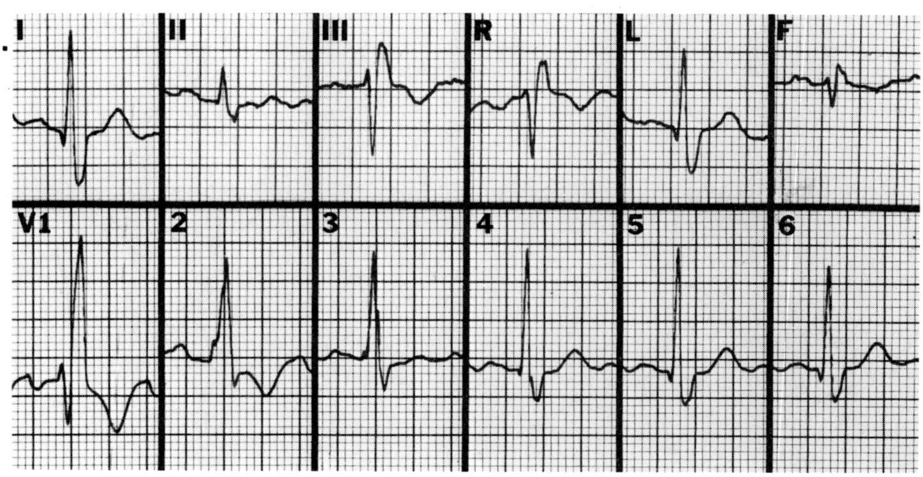

8-52.

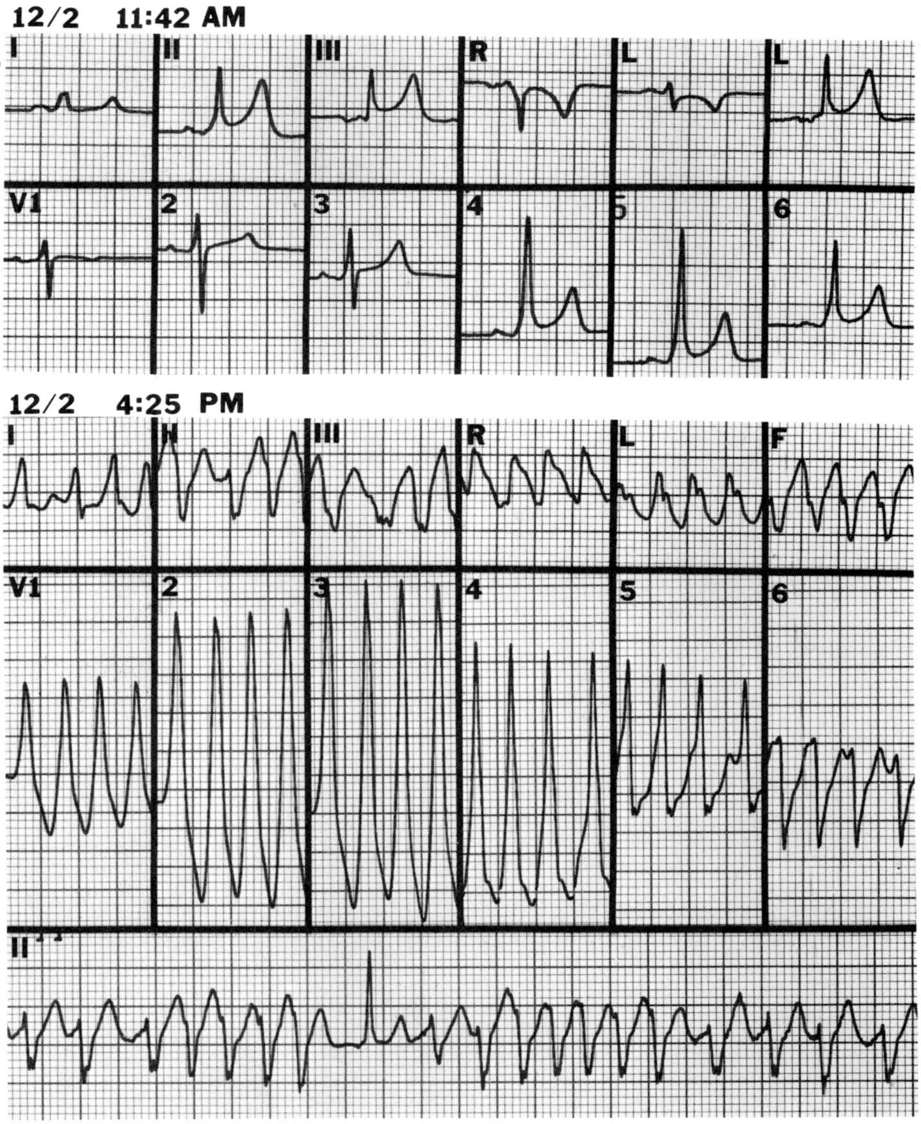
12/2 11:42 AM
I
II
III
R
L
L
V1
2
3
4
5
6
12/2 4:25 PM
I
II
III
R
L
F
V1
2
3
4
5
6
II

8·53.

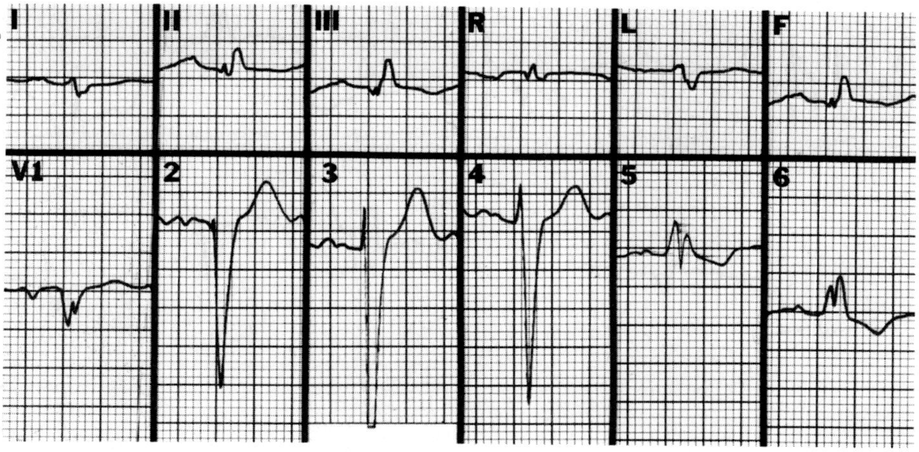

8·54.

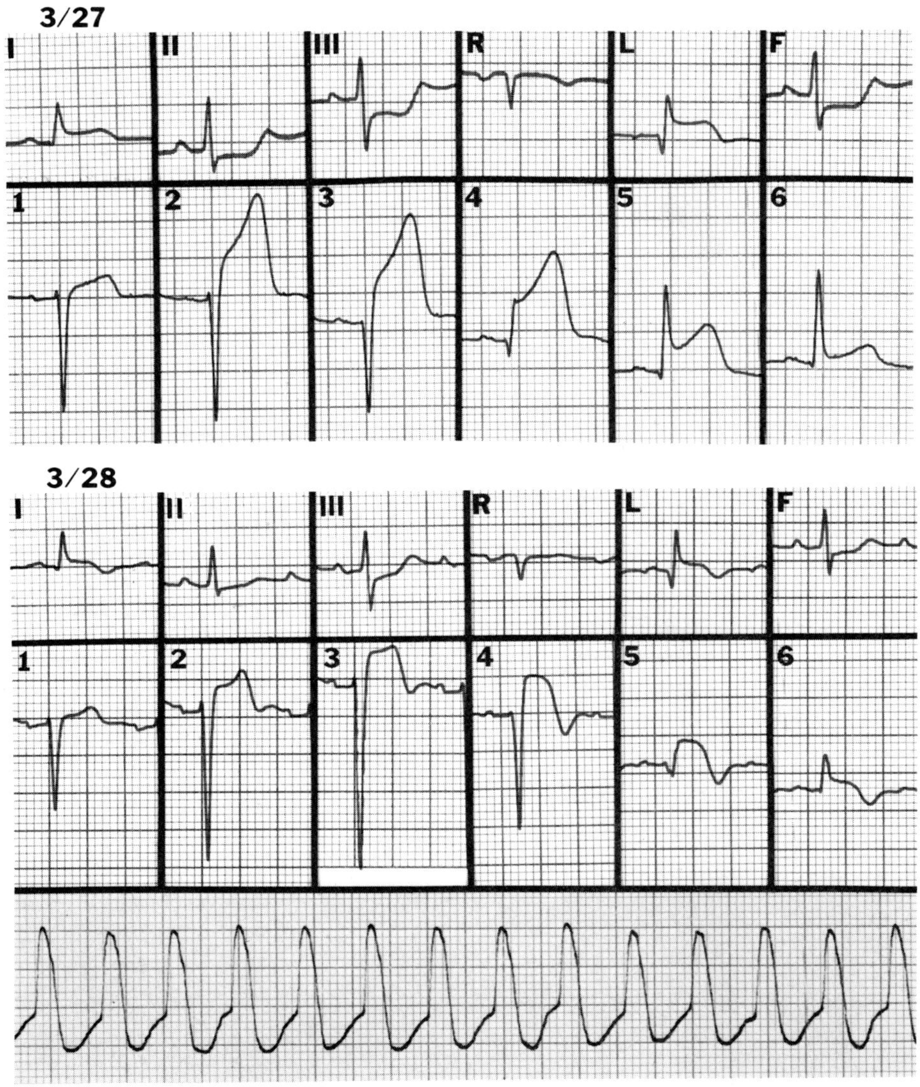

8·55.

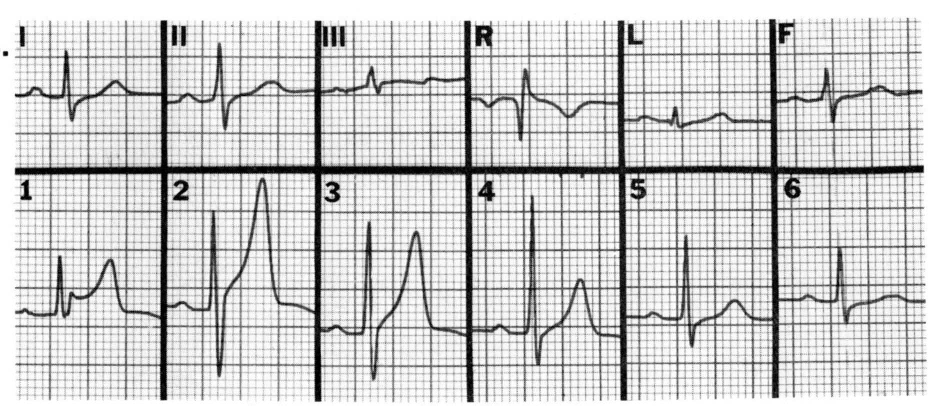

8-56.

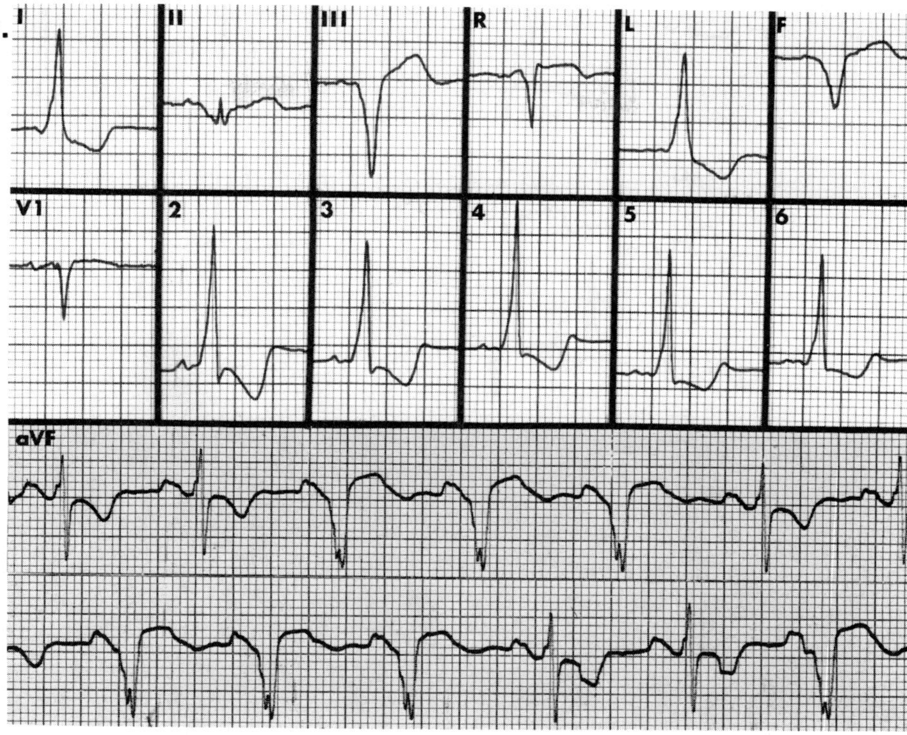

8-57.

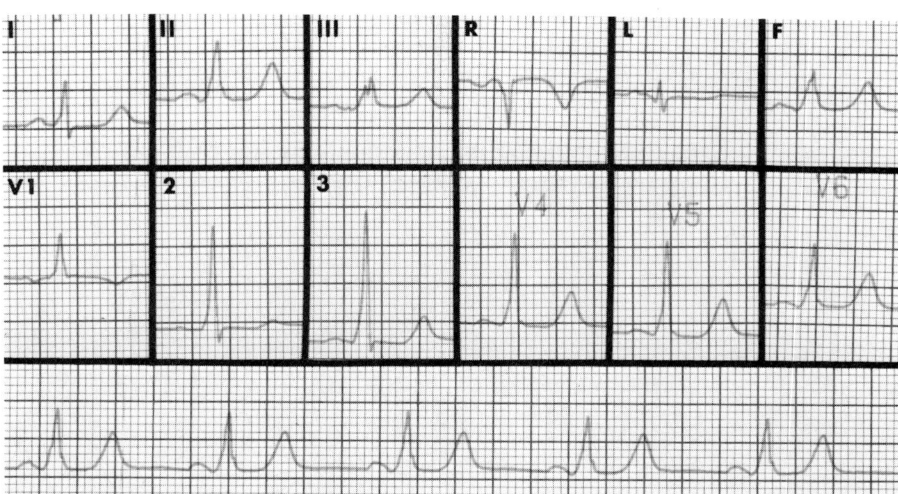

8-58.

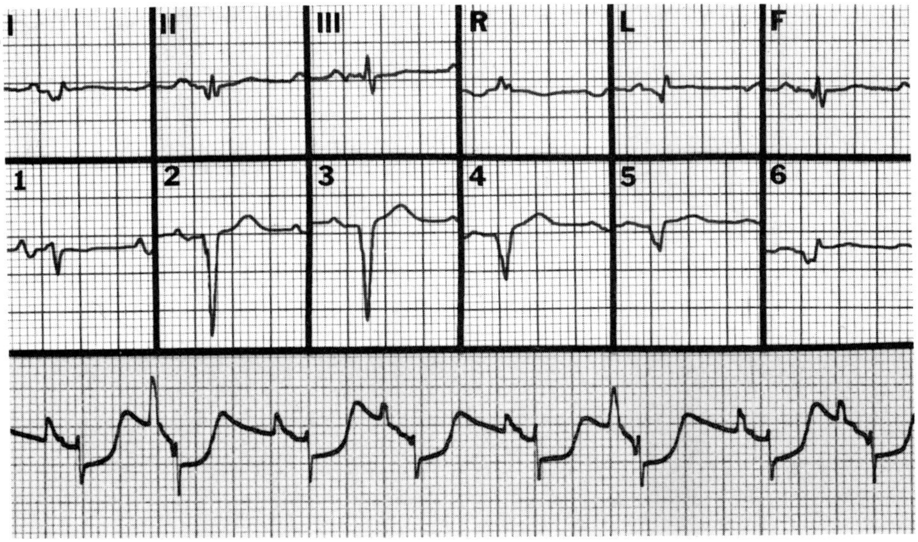

8-59.

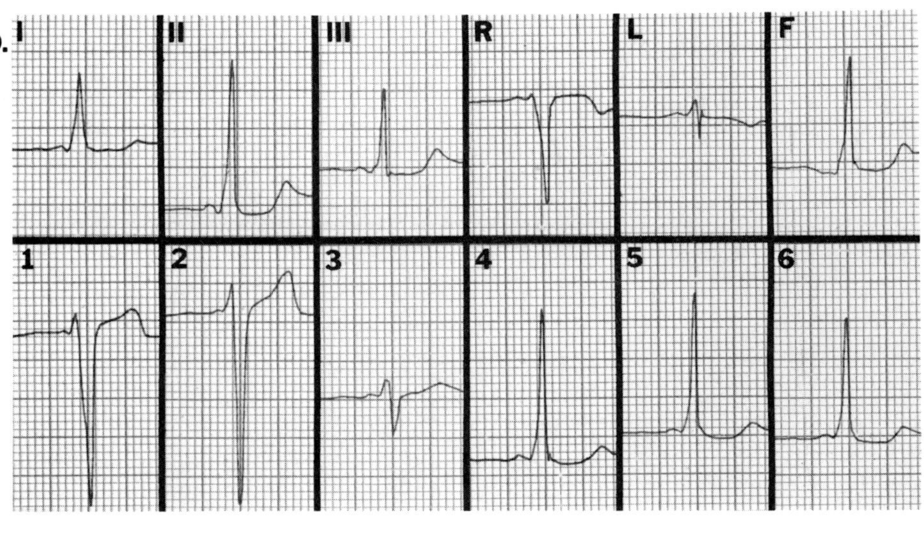

8-60.

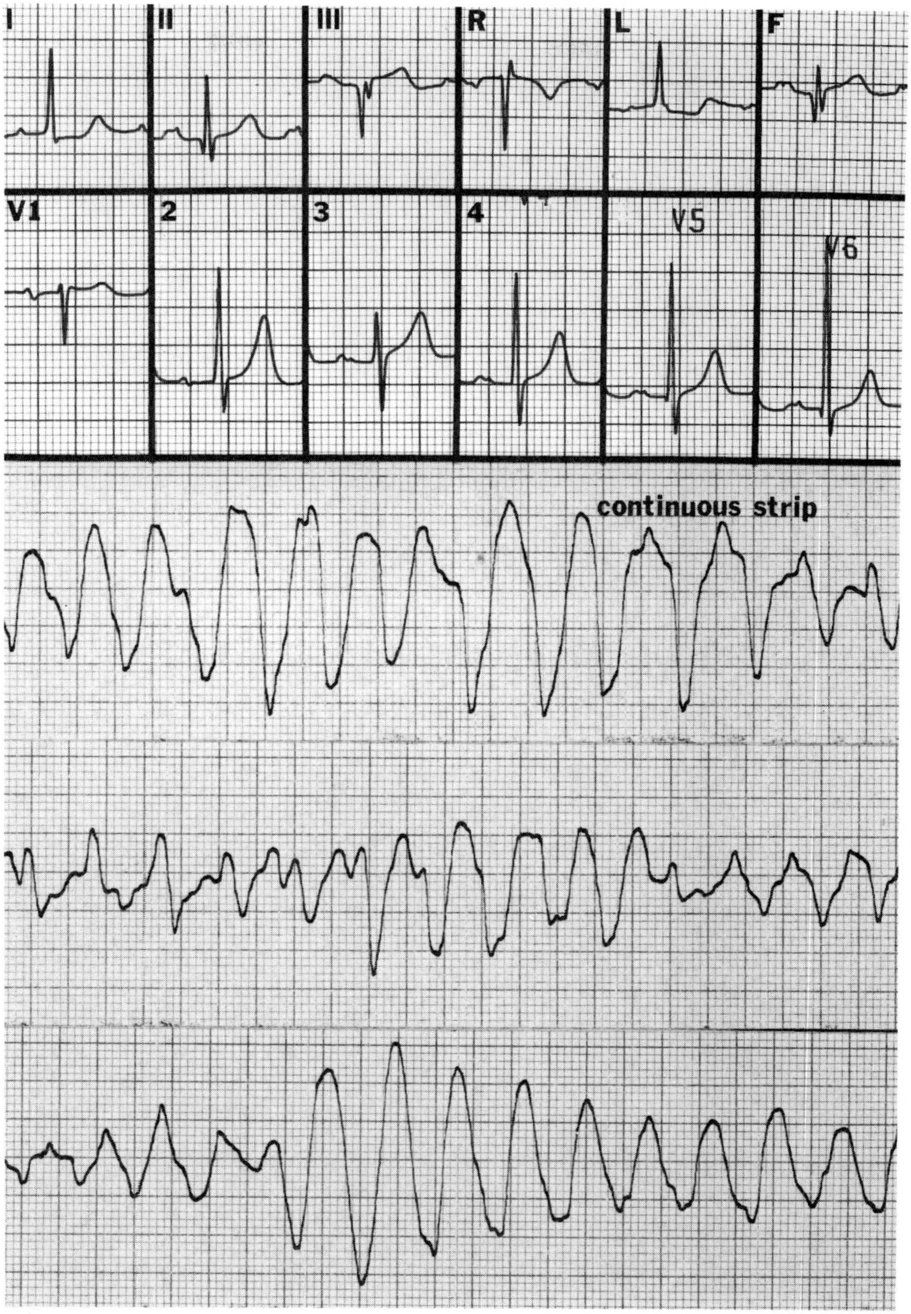

ANSWER KEY

Multiple Choice

1. d
2. b
3. b
4. c
5. d
6. a
7. d
8. a
9. a
10. c
11. d
12. c

Practice Strips

8–1. Left axis deviation, −65 to −75 degrees.
Left anterior fascicular block.
Supraventricular tachycardia in 12-lead, sinoatrial block in rhythm strip (tachy-brady form of sick sinus syndrome).

8–2. Left axis deviation, −55 to −65 degrees.
Left anterior fascicular block.
Right bundle branch block.
Probable Mobitz type II AV block.

8–3. Left axis deviation, −15 to −25 degrees.
Right bundle branch block.
Inferior wall infarction.

8–4. Left axis deviation, −55 to −65 degrees.
Early transition (V2).
Inferior wall infarction.
Posterior wall infarction.
Left atrial enlargement.
Mobitz I (Wenckebach) AV block, 4:3 conduction ratio.

8–5. Left axis deviation, −55 to −65 degrees.
Late transition (V5–V6).
Poor R wave progression.

Left bundle branch block.
Left atrial enlargement.

8–6. Right axis deviation, +115 to +125 degrees.
Early transition (V1).
Right ventricular hypertrophy.

8–7. Left axis deviation, −10 to −20 degrees.
Right bundle branch block.
First-degree AV block (PR 0.22 second).

8–8. Normal axis, +40 to +50 degrees.
Early transition (V1).
Inferior wall infarction.
Posterior wall infarction.

8–9. Normal axis, +5 to −5 degrees.
Acute pericarditis.

8–10. Left axis deviation, −25 to −35 degrees.
Wolff-Parkinson-White syndrome, type B.
Probable right paraseptal pathway (4).
Although the criteria for left ventricular hypertrophy are fulfilled in the precordial leads, WPW frequently mimics LVH so that the diagnosis of LVH cannot be made in the presence of WPW syndrome.

8–11. Normal axis, +5 to −5 degrees.
Inferior wall infarction, remote.
Left atrial enlargement.
Left ventricular hypertrophy.
First-degree AV block (PR 0.22 second).

8–12. Normal axis, +55 to +65 degrees.
Probable right atrial enlargement.
Acute pericarditis (note PR segment depression in lead II).

8–13. Normal axis, +55 to +65 degrees.
Anterior wall infarction, acute.
Atrial flutter, 6:1 conduction ratio.

8–14. Left axis deviation, −50 to −60 degrees.
Wolff-Parkinson-White syndrome, type A.
Probable left paraseptal pathway (3).

8–15. Normal axis, +50 to +60 degrees.
Anterior wall infarction, hyperacute phase.
Ventricular fibrillation.

8–16. Normal axis, +45 to +55 degrees.
Wolff-Parkinson-White syndrome, type B.
Probable pulmonary outflow pathway (7).

8–17. Left axis deviation, −5 to −15 degrees.
Early transition (V1).
Inferior wall infarction.
Posterior wall infarction.
Left ventricular hypertrophy.
Atrial flutter, 3:1 to 4:1 conduction ratios.

8–18. Normal axis, +10 to +20 degrees.
Wolff-Parkinson-White syndrome, type A.
Probable left lateral pathway (2).

8–19. Right axis deviation, +110 to +120 degrees.
Right ventricular hypertrophy.
Atrial fibrillation.

8–20. Right axis deviation, +150 to +160 degrees.
Possible LPFB.
RBBB.

8–21. Normal axis, +55 to +65 degrees.
Probable left atrial enlargement.
Left ventricular hypertrophy.

8–22. Left axis deviation, −15 to −25 degrees.
Wolff-Parkinson-White syndrome, type B.
Probable right paraseptal pathway (4).

8–23. Right axis deviation, +115 to +125 degrees.
Early transition (V1).
Nonspecific atrial abnormality.
Right ventricular hypertrophy.

8–24. Normal axis, +20 to +30 degrees.
Anterior myocardial ischemia.

8–25. Left axis deviation, −5 to −15 degrees.
Early transition (V2).
Inferior wall infarction.
Probable posterior wall infarction.

Atrioventricular dissociation with junctional escape rhythm, probably block-acceleration dissociation.

8–26. Normal axis, +55 to +65 degrees.
Wolff-Parkinson-White syndrome, type B.

8–27. (ECG of 8/02, 12:47 A.M.)
Normal axis, +5 to −5 degrees.
Poor R wave progression.
Orthodromic supraventricular tachycardia, rate 273/minute.
(ECG of 8/02, 12:50 P.M.)
Normal axis, +5 to −5 degrees.
Possible anterolateral ischemia.
(ECG of 8/03, 5:53 A.M.)
Normal axis, +30 to +40 degrees.
Wolff-Parkinson-White syndrome, type B.
Probable pulmonary outflow pathway (7).

8–28. Normal axis, +40 to +50 degrees.
Probable left atrial enlargement.
Anterior myocardial ischemia, probably Prinzmetal's angina.

8–29. Normal axis, +10 to +20 degrees.
Poor R wave progression.
Left bundle branch block.

8–30. Normal axis, +40 to +50 degrees.
Early transition (V2).
Left ventricular hypertrophy by precordial criteria.
Early repolarization syndrome.

8–31. Left axis deviation, −55 to −65 degrees.
Wolff-Parkinson-White syndrome, type B.
Probable right paraseptal pathway (4).
This tracing simulates both inferior wall infarction and left ventricular hypertrophy, neither of which was present in this patient.

8–32. Normal axis, +25 to +35 degrees.
Right bundle branch block.
First-degree AV block (PR 0.24 second).
Sinoatrial block.

8–33. Left axis deviation, 0 to −10 degrees.
Early transition (V1–V2).
Inferior wall infarction.
Probable posterior wall infarction.
Probable left atrial enlargement.

8–34. Normal axis, +5 to −5 degrees.
Wolff-Parkinson-White syndrome, type B.
Probable right anterior pathway (6).
Sinus bradycardia, 55/minute. Note delta waves.

8–35. Right axis deviation, +90 to +100 degrees.
Poor R wave progression.
Anterior wall infarction.
Right atrial enlargement.
Ventricular tachycardia.

8–36. Left axis deviation, −30 to −40 degrees.
Poor R wave progression.
Left anterior fascicular block.
Left ventricular hypertrophy.

8–37. Left axis deviation, −10 to −20 degrees.
Poor R wave progression.
Left bundle branch block.

8–38. Normal axis, +50 to +60 degrees.
Wolff-Parkinson-White syndrome, type B.
Probable pulmonary outflow pathway (7).

8–39. Normal axis, +35 to +45 degrees.
Poor R wave progression.
Anterior wall infarction, acute.
Sinus rhythm, 94/minute, nonconducted premature atrial systole followed by two junctional escape beats.

8–40. Normal axis, +5 to −5 degrees.
Inferior wall infarction, acute.
First-degree AV block (PR 0.26 second) in 12-lead.
Atrioventricular dissociation, probable block-acceleration dissociation (the third QRS complex in the top rhythm strip represents a sinus capture beat).

8–41. (ECG of 3:31 P.M.)
Right axis deviation, +200 to +210 degrees.
Antidromic supraventricular tachycardia versus ventricular tachycardia.
(ECG of 5:18 P.M.)
Normal axis, +55 to +65 degrees.
Wolff-Parkinson-White syndrome with minimal degree of preexcitation (note tiny delta waves in leads II, III, aVF, V5, and V6).

8–42. Normal axis, +15 to +25 degrees.
Early transition (V2).
Possible left atrial enlargement.
Sinoatrial block.

8–43. Normal axis, +40 to +50 degrees.
Normal electrocardiogram.

8–44. Right axis deviation, +130 to +140 degrees.
Left posterior fascicular block.
Right bundle branch block.
Atrial bigeminy (the atrial premature systoles are nonconducted).

8–45. Normal axis, +5 to −5 degrees.
Wolff-Parkinson-White syndrome, type A.
Probable acute marginal pathway (5).

8–46. Normal axis, +20 to +30 degrees.
Early transition (V2).
Low voltage (7.5 mm).
Posterior wall infarction.
Probable lateral wall infarction.

8–47. Left axis deviation, −20 to −30 degrees.
Inferior wall infarction, acute.
Probable posterior wall infarction, acute.
Anterior myocardial ischemia.
Sinus tachycardia, 160/minute.

8–48. Right axis deviation, +90 to +100 degrees.
Wolff-Parkinson-White syndrome, type A.
Probable left anterior pathway (1).

8–49. (ECG of 3:14 A.M.)
Left axis deviation, −60 to −70 degrees.
Antidromic supraventricular tachycardia versus ventricular tachycardia.
(ECG of 4:34 A.M.)
Normal axis, +30 to +40 degrees.
Normal electrocardiogram.
The patient is known have concealed WPW syndrome.

8–50. Normal axis, +25 to +35 degrees.
Wolff-Parkinson-White syndrome, probably type B.
Sinus rhythm, 91/minute, note small delta waves.

8–51. Right axis deviation, +140 to +150 degrees.
Right posterior fascicular block.
Right bundle branch block.

8–52. (ECG of 12/02, 11:42 A.M.)
Normal axis, +55 to +65 degrees.
Wolff-Parkinson-White syndrome.
(ECG of 12/02, 4:25 P.M.)
Antridromic conduction of atrial fibrillation, note single orthodromically conducted complex (narrow QRS) in rhythm strip.

8–53. Right axis deviation, +115 to +125 degrees.
Left posterior fascicular block.
Left bundle branch block.

8–54. (ECG of 3/27)
Normal axis, +5 to −5 degrees.
Lateral wall infarction.
Anterior wall infarction, hyperacute.
(ECG of 3/28)
Normal axis, +10 to +20 degrees.
Poor R wave progression.
Lateral wall infarction.
Anterior wall infarction, acute.
Ventricular tachycardia.

8–55. Normal axis, +55 to +65 degrees.
Posterior wall infarction, acute.

8–56. Left axis deviation, −10 to −20 degrees.
WPW syndrome, type B.
Probable right anterior pathway (6).
Sinus rhythm, 82/minute, intermittent ventricular preexcitation.

8–57. Normal axis, +60 to +70 degrees.
WPW syndrome, type A.
Probable pulmonary outflow pathway.
Sinus rhythm, 67/minute, constant ventricular preexcitation.

8–58. Right axis deviation, +170 to +180 degrees.
Lateral wall infarction, old (I, aVL, V5, V6).
Anterior wall infarction, old (V2–V4).
Left atrial enlargement.
Sinus tachycardia, 115/minute, premature atrial beats.

8–59. Normal axis, +55 to +65 degrees.
WPW syndrome, type B.
Probable left lateral pathway.

8–60. Normal axis, +10 to +20 degrees.
IWMI, old (II, III, aVF).
Possible PWMI, old (tall R wave in V2).
Left atrial enlargement.
Coarse ventricular fibrillation.

Index

Note: Page numbers in *italics* indicate illustrations;
page numbers followed by the letter t indicate tables.